T0327715

Famished

Famished

EATING DISORDERS AND
FAILED CARE IN AMERICA

Rebecca J. Lester

UNIVERSITY OF CALIFORNIA PRESS

University of California Press, one of the most distinguished university presses in the United States, enriches lives around the world by advancing scholarship in the humanities, social sciences, and natural sciences. Its activities are supported by the UC Press Foundation and by philanthropic contributions from individuals and institutions. For more information, visit www.ucpress.edu.

University of California Press
Oakland, California

Library of Congress Cataloging-in-Publication Data

Names: Lester, Rebecca J., 1969– author.
Title: Famished : eating disorders and failed care in America / Rebecca J. Lester.
Description: Oakland, California : University of California Press, [2019] | Includes bibliographical references and index. |
Identifiers: LCCN 2019017205 (print) | LCCN 2019021596 (ebook) | ISBN 9780520972902 (E-book) | ISBN 9780520303935 (cloth : alk. paper)
Subjects: LCSH: Eating disorders—Treatment—Missouri—Cedar Grove. | Eating disorders—Treatment—Moral and ethical aspects. | Eating disorders—Social aspects.
Classification: LCC RC552.E18 (ebook) | LCC RC552.E18 L473 2019 (print) | DDC 362.196/852600977569—dc23
LC record available at https://lccn.loc.gov/2019017205

27   26   25   24   23   22   21   20   19
10   9   8   7   6   5   4   3   2   1

For Daegan, Fiona, and
eleven-year-old me

Bring me your suffering.
The rattle roar of broken bones.
Bring me the riot in your heart.
Angry, wild, and raw.
Bring it all.
I am not afraid of the dark.

— MIA HOLLOW (@miahollow)

Transformation isn't sweet and bright. It's a dark and murky, painful pushing. An unraveling of the untruths you've carried in your body. A practice in facing your own created demons. A complete uprooting before becoming.

—VICTORIA ERICKSON, *Edge of Wonder* (2015)

CONTENTS

PROLOGUE

NOVEMBER 1980

I ease my aching, anorexic eleven-year-old body down into the softest chair in the common area I can find. It smells vaguely of urine and cigarette smoke—I bet Kevin was here before me. I glance up to see him shuffling around the perimeter of the ward, muttering quietly to himself as his slippers make a *swish, swish* noise on the tile floor.

I situate the IV stand next to me. It holds a bag of Sustical, liquid nutrition that supposedly tastes like chocolate. I can't actually taste it, though, because it is being delivered directly to my stomach through the long tube that snakes down from the bag, up through my nose, and down the back of my throat. It is my first "meal" with the tube in, and I sit there watching the brown liquid drop, drop, drop slowly into the tube, petrified. *So many calories! So many calories, oh my god.* What had they said, eight hundred per bag? Eight hundred? That's more than I used to eat in an entire *day,* and now they're pumping it into me for one *meal.* And I cannot do anything about it.

Oh, I fought getting the tube, believe me. I fought with everything I had.

For about a week I had been hiding food under my napkin during meals so I wouldn't have to eat it. I'd also been "water loading" before morning weigh-ins, chugging Shasta can after Shasta can filled with water that I hid under my bed. I knew those things were against the rules. But never in my wildest dreams did I ever think they would shove a tube down my throat to feed me. I'd never even *heard* of such a thing until that morning, when the doctor and five staff members came into my room.

"Why are there so many people here?" my thoughts screamed in my head as they entered, and I felt immediately apprehensive. The doctor walked toward me with a plastic package containing something medical under her arm. She explained to me that my weight was dangerously low and I would die if I didn't bring it up. I had heard all of this before. It scared me, but not nearly as much as calories and gaining weight did. I was prepared to try harder, though, no matter how terrified I was. I felt awful for deceiving the staff—I knew they were just trying to help me, and I definitely didn't want them to feel angry at me. I wasn't trying to lie *to* them—it wasn't about *them* at all. I hated lying. But I was terrified of food and eating the way a person with agoraphobia is terrified of going outside, or a person with claustrophobia is afraid of enclosed spaces. The deception wasn't about anything except pure animal survival.

The doctor opened the package and pulled out a long plastic tube that was bigger than an IV line. She explained that it was a nasogastric (NG) tube and told me what they were about to do with it.

"Wait, you're going to do *what?*" I blurted out, beginning to feel actual fear now. "What if I promise to eat my full meal plan from now on? I can sit near a staff member and show you guys everything on my tray so you know I'm not hiding anything." My words came faster and faster, my voice rising in pitch. "Someone can watch me take every bite! I know it was wrong to hide food. I'm sorry! I'm really sorry! I won't do it again, I promise! I promise!!" But the staff members began arranging themselves around me.

At this point, I freaked out. I completely panicked. I began sobbing, pleading, wailing, promising to do anything that they wanted me to as long as they didn't put that tube in me. "Please!" I begged. "Please, I'll do anything! Please don't! Please *don't!*"

The staff people moved in closer. My panic spiked higher. "Stop! Please STOP!" Two staff members grabbed my arms. Two others took hold of my legs. Someone grabbed my head. I fought like hell, desperately flailing my bony limbs and twisting my sunken body to try to get away. But one anorexic eleven-year-old girl is no match for five grown adults. Still, I thrashed with all my might, begging the whole time for mercy.

Susan, one of the nurses I liked the best, was pinning my right arm to my body and trying to hold my torso still as the doctor approached with the tube. I saw that Susan had tears streaming down her face, even as she held me immobile. The doctor stood before me with the tube. "You will have to cooperate with this next part," she cautioned. "If you don't, there's a chance the tube could go into your lungs instead of your stomach. We *are* going to put it in. You can either cooperate with me here, or we can take you to a seclusion room and put you in restraints and do it there. It's your choice."

I had never felt so utterly broken in my entire life. I had no choice but to let them shove that tube into me, giving them access to my very insides, where they could do as they wished. Finally, all the fight left me, and I became limp and compliant.

Having an NG tube placed is extremely uncomfortable. The tube is flexible, but not *that* flexible. It was inserted up my nose and then curved down the back of my throat, and the doctor had me drink water to help it go into the right spot and not end up in a lung. After it was in, they used a syringe to suction up some liquid; when they saw stomach acid in the tube, they knew it was in the right place.

They fastened the free end of the tube to my right cheek with medical tape. My cheeks were still wet with tears, and the edges of the tape curled up, tickling me uncomfortably as the adhesive pulled away from my skin. No one seemed to notice. "You can rest now," the doctor said. "You'll have your first meal in about an hour."

So here I sit, in the soft chair, with my first meal dripping down into my stomach. I feel the coolness of the liquid as it inches its way down the tube at the back of my throat. I am exhausted and drained from the encounter earlier and sit shell-shocked, feeling vaguely disconnected from the world around me.

"What's that you have there?" asks a patient in her thirties, pointing at the contraption pushing nutrition into my withered body. She is new. I haven't seen her before. "What *is* that?"

"It's a feeding tube," I mumble, really not interested in talking to anyone, let alone having a conversation about the tube.

"Really?" she asks, intrigued. "What do you need that for? What, you don't *eat* or something?" she chuckles, as if that were the most amusing thing in the world.

"Yeah, something like that," I mutter.

"She has anorexia!" Ben, another patient, interjects, like I am some sort of rare zoo animal and he is giving a guided tour.

"Anorexia? What's *that?*" asks the woman. "Oh wait! Is that that thing where you're scared of getting fat? So, you starve yourself? And you get real skinny?" She seems pleased with herself for knowing the answer to her own question. "Hell, I wish *I* could have anorexia for a day!" the woman booms, laughing and grabbing her stomach fat. "Yep, I could really use some anorexia, *that's* for sure!"

Thankfully, the dinner trays arrive, and Ben and the woman head off to the dining room talking about the coming holidays, how much food they will eat, how much weight they will gain.

The smell of the food turns my stomach. I slouch back into the smelly chair, close my eyes, and try not to think of the calories dripping into me.

PREFACE

This book begins with an ending.

On a hot, sticky summer afternoon in 2009, I left the Cedar Grove eating disorders clinic, where I had been conducting research, and drove to the local parish church. As I wound my way through the idyllic Midwestern American suburb, I passed the usual summer scenes: children playing in sprinklers, shoppers at the local farmers' market, families out for a stroll. The sun was shining. It was peaceful and calm, the cheers from the nearby soccer field a joyful soundtrack to an exquisite summer day.

Yet all this small-town charm felt hollow and callous to me, sitting as it did in grisly contrast to where I was headed: a funeral. And not the usual kind of funeral, where mourners bid farewell to Great Uncle Carl or Grandma Nash, who lived full, long lives. This funeral was for a young woman named Allison[1] who had been a patient at Cedar Grove the previous spring. Until three days prior, Allison had been a success story. When she left the clinic, she was healthy, invested in her recovery, thankful to be alive, and eager to get on with her life.

Now, she was dead. She had suffered a heart attack and died on the night of her twenty-seventh birthday.

Allison was not my personal client (I am a psychotherapist as well as an anthropologist), but I had come to know her fairly well during the time she was in treatment at Cedar Grove. She had come to the clinic because one night her father had found her unconscious on the bathroom floor next to a toilet full of vomit. She wasn't breathing. She had no pulse. He performed CPR on her for over twenty minutes, keeping her alive until the paramedics arrived. After that incident, Allison's parents insisted she get help for her eating disorder. Shocked and shaken up by her near-death experience, she willingly signed herself into Cedar Grove the next day.

In treatment, Allison worked hard. She pushed herself to open up in group therapy about her eating disorder, her self-loathing, her family dynamics, and her problematic ways of relating. She received specialized medical, nutritional, and psychiatric support and learned how to nourish her body without capitulating to the overwhelming anxiety and shame that could lead to purging. She worked with an individual therapist on the emotional, psychological, and interpersonal issues underlying her self-destructive behaviors. Over time, she made great strides toward health. By the time she was discharged, four weeks later, Allison was medically and psychologically stable and looking forward to returning to her life.

Four months after that, she was dead.

I don't know what Allison's life had been like since she'd left the clinic. I do know that she had been inconsistent in attending outpatient appointments with Dr. Casey (a psychiatrist and the director of the clinic) and her therapist, Sandra. After her last missed appointment, both had tried to contact her, but she had not returned their calls. One could speculate that perhaps by that point Allison had returned to her eating disorder and was distancing herself from her treatment team during her relapse. This is certainly possible. But because she was an adult, Dr. Casey and Sandra had little option but to wait for Allison to reach out to them if and when she wanted help. She never did.

At the funeral, Carmen and Sheila, two clients who had known Allison at the clinic and were still in treatment there, were sitting in the pew in front of me. They had gotten special passes from the clinic for the day so they could attend. I noticed that Carmen drew uneasy stares from the surrounding mourners. She had a feeding tube conspicuously inserted through her nose, the end of it taped awkwardly to her cheek. In the humid summer heat, the tape curled up at the corners, and her hands fluttered up repeatedly to press it back in place. Sheila, sitting next to Carmen, looked stoic and closed down, staring straight ahead into the distance. Knowing Sheila, I could tell that this face of calm was not what it seemed—she was probably so paralyzed with anxiety that she couldn't bear to make eye contact with anyone. Both young women looked visibly tense, their bodies held tight and rigid in the wooden pew. Carmen cried silently during the service, the tears snaking their way down her cheeks. Sheila sat as still as a stone.

Despite Carmen and Sheila's obvious distress, I was glad to see both of them there. Not only because they had been close to Allison, but also because

I thought it might be a catalyst for them in their own recoveries, perhaps jolting them to awareness that this—death—could happen to them, too.

But later, back at Cedar Grove, Sheila told me that Allison's death had actually made her even *less* hopeful and motivated about recovery than before. "It's just like, why fight it?" she asked me. "Once you have this thing for so long, it's going to kill you one way or another. So, what's the point of trying to get better?"

Sheila's question was more than simply rhetorical. There was something in her tone, the look in her eyes, and the catch in her voice that told me she actually wanted a response. She wanted me to tell her why she should keep trying when she had cycled through treatment on three different occasions, each time having to leave far before she was ready because her insurance ran out, and each time relapsing into a ferocious spiral of bulimia and self-harm. She wanted to know why she should keep trying when her parents had given up on her, her sister had stopped speaking to her, and she had lost three friends, including Allison, in the past year to eating disorders.

"Maybe I just can't do life," Sheila concluded, looking at her hands.

WHAT THIS BOOK IS (AND ISN'T) ABOUT

As wrenching as Allison's death may be, this book is not about the personal tragedy of eating disorders; at least, not exclusively. Nor is it a book decrying the social and cultural factors that persuade girls and women (and, increasingly, boys and men) to abuse their bodies to death through food; at least, not solely. It is not a memoir, although my story matters in what follows. It is not a prolonged analysis of gender dynamics, a sustained critique of neoliberalism, or an impassioned argument against profit-driven healthcare, though these issues are certainly addressed in the text.

Rather, this book is about how and why eating disorders hold such a problematic place in our society and what can be done about it. This involves attending to many sides of the issue. First and foremost, we need to understand with more depth and nuance what these conditions actually are (and are not) and interrogate many of our received assumptions about them and the people who develop them. We also need to pay attention to how clinicians care—and make sense of caring—when facing what appears to be a nearly impossible situation: clients who often don't want to get better, families who are in crisis yet resist change, an illness that kills more people than any other psychiatric condition, and a healthcare system that devalues the very sorts of clinical expertise that seem to help. We need to look at what happens when the dominant logic of care forces eating disorders treatment to operate with an anorexic mentality of scarcity and deprivation that replicates the core dynamics of the very illnesses it purports to treat, catching patients in double binds that keep them unwell. We need to examine how this situation produces contradictory ideologies of recovery and paradoxical renderings of the "healthy subject" that compete for legitimacy in the clinic, producing frictions and roadblocks and vectors of conflict. We need to understand how these processes unfold within an affective atmosphere—a lived, felt experience—of constant precarity, coupled with imperatives for certainty and demands for quantification, prediction, and verification that provide illusions of control. And we need to look at how clients and clinicians alike get caught up in these knots and must struggle to find a way forward, racing against the clock and the specter of disappearing benefits, to access treatment that is complex, contradictory, and—in far too many cases—counterproductive.

This "ambivalent care"[2] has an eerie resonance with the driving issues of eating disorders themselves. Eating disorders, for people in the throes of one, are at heart about feeling unworthy to exist, feeling that they don't have the right to take up space (physical, interpersonal, political, social). Eating disorders are about feeling so fundamentally *wrong* on all levels that the only thing one can do *right* is to disappear, to obliterate oneself, to *non-exist*. Given this, people with eating disorders can never feel "sick enough" to actually deserve *notice,* let alone *care,* despite the fact that care is what they need and crave more than anything. But care is also terrifying. As a person with an eating disorder, if someone cares for you, you are taking something from them, you are a burden. Indebted. You are an actual person in the world with needs, and *that,* for a whole host of reasons we will explore, is completely unacceptable and shame inducing. People with eating disorders therefore often reject care even when they desperately need and even crave it, not because they are "naturally" difficult or resistant to treatment, but because it is almost impossible for them to inhabit a place where accepting care feels morally tolerable.

At its heart, this book is about how both clients and clinicians at Cedar Grove understand practices of care when care and harm are so closely intertwined. And it is about how they make sense of the work of treatment in the face of so much apparent failure, when some clients remain sick or get sicker, and some, like Allison, even die.

In trying to understand how eating disorders, care, and harm are entangled in the contemporary American context, I began research at Cedar Grove in 2002 as an anthropologist interested in cultures of recovery. I soon learned that therapeutic work at Cedar Grove was inseparable from the economics and philosophies of American managed mental healthcare and that economic aims often contradicted therapeutic ones. Again and again, I saw very ill people denied coverage by their insurance companies or given just a handful of days of low-level treatment, barely enough for them to become stabilized (if that), let alone get "better." Insurance companies regularly discharged patients (even those with remaining coverage) or moved them to lower levels of care in blatant violation of accepted best practice guidelines and clinical recommendations. If clients relapsed or worsened after being discharged (a common and unsurprising occurrence), insurance companies routinely concluded that these clients had "failed" treatment and therefore should be denied authorization for further care.

These are deadly diseases. Not everyone survives.

The situation I observed was shocking. How, I wondered, did clinicians and patients make sense of what was happening, particularly against a cultural backdrop that figures people with eating disorders as notoriously "resistant" and "difficult"? What is it about eating disorders that makes them so culturally and therapeutically charged? In part, eating disorders challenge some of our most fundamental beliefs about human nature, human well-being, and human striving. And they also trouble our existing systems of care and the philosophies of the person within which they are grounded. In other words, eating disorders make visible the fractures and paradoxes central to a care system that sells "health" as a commodity.

To understand how eating disorders become potent arenas of contestation, I paid close attention to the ways "care" unfolded at Cedar Grove as clients struggled to get well and clinicians faced decisions about treatment and charted courses of clinical action. I followed how clients became acclimated to clinic life and how they came to talk differently about illness and recovery. I listened as they complained about the contradictory expectations and mixed messages they received from staff, and as staff voiced their frustrations with clients who wouldn't follow protocol. I tracked people's trajectories in, around, and through various levels of care as they struggled to piece together treatment scenarios that would give them the support they needed.

I also took note of the kinds of information clinicians deemed important and how they navigated different sorts of contingencies in deciding what to do in a particular case. I listened closely to how they talked about clients and how they sought support from each other when they were feeling burned out, frustrated, or helpless. And I noticed how clinicians drew on their own personal reactions to clients—what we might variously call countertransference, clinical intuition, expertise, or gut feelings—in sorting through dilemmas of care.

I also came to realize that the sorts of questions I was interested in required a different sort of research approach than standard ethnography. I needed to enter the clinical world in a more direct way, to understand these dilemmas from the inside. I decided to pursue clinical training so that I could practice myself. In 2004, about eighteen months into my anthropological research at Cedar Grove, I entered clinical training through the master of social work (MSW) program at Washington University in St. Louis. I attended classes part-time from fall 2004 through spring 2007 while continuing with my duties as an assistant professor of anthropology. I completed all of my practicum and licensure training at Cedar Grove, which involved running groups, carrying a caseload of individual therapy clients, communicating with insurance companies and families, coordinating client care, planning discharges, and facilitating the process of treatment for clients.

Pursuing my MSW opened up whole new vistas in terms of my ethnographic work at Cedar Grove. Although I had been given quite a bit of latitude as an ethnographer prior to entering clinical training, there were certain limitations to what I could do in that role. For example, as an anthropologist, I could sit in treatment team meetings or weekly supervisions and listen to therapists talk about difficult sessions with clients or struggles they were facing in determining how to best treat someone with limited health benefits, but I had no idea what it actually *felt* like to have to discharge a client knowing she was going to relapse as soon as she walked out the door. I could observe group therapies and talk with clients individually, but I didn't know what it was like to be *responsible* for the health and well-being of someone who was at 73 percent of her ideal body weight but was refusing to eat lunch, or what it felt like to try—and fail—to extend health benefits for someone in desperate need of care.

Once I began my clinical training, I was legally and ethically in a position to do these sorts of things. I not only observed groups at the clinic but also ran them. I began to carry my own client load. I dealt with admissions and discharges, navigated clients' difficult family dynamics, and cared for people who said they didn't want to get better. As I progressed through my training, I took on more and more clinical responsibility. I fielded crisis calls, like the one from a client who slit her wrists and ended up in the ER, another from a client threatening to jump out of her mother's moving vehicle on the highway, and several from exasperated direct care staff asking how to deal with client noncompliance. I talked overwhelmed parents through interventions and supported anxious clients through family therapy sessions. I saw several clients through the entire treatment process—some more than once. I watched some go on to wonderfully productive lives and others descend into cycles of self-destruction.

These kinds of experiences were invaluable in terms of ethnographic insights about the everyday dynamics of clinical work. But there were deeply personal as well as professional reasons for this move. It wasn't just about getting better data. It was about enabling ethical action. I wanted to be able to *do* something when an emaciated teenager curled on up the couch in front of me, ribs and tailbone poking out at painful angles from under her skin, sobbing because she couldn't bear the guilt of having eaten a slice of cheese at lunch; when a young woman disclosed a rape to me that she had never shared with anyone else and then proceeded to disassociate for the next two hours; when a client sliced up her arm with a broken mirror to protest her meal plan increase; when a girl became wracked with sobs so powerful that she broke out in hives every time her parents visited. Writing books and articles is, of course, a form of doing. But I wanted to be more proactive and useful in the moment. And I wanted this "doing" to be guided by more than just my own intuition; I wanted it to be ethical, informed, skilled, and safe.

Certainly, this desire to "do something" was motivated by my own sense of helplessness in the face of such palpable suffering. And I am fully aware that this desire to help risks teetering over the edge of privilege into a savior stance that is as untenable as it is problematic. I had to remain constantly vigilant about my own motivations. But becoming a clinician was about more than just wanting to help in a general sense. It was born of a deep personal commitment—because of my own history with these harrowing illnesses—to alleviate this pain in whatever ways I possibly could, as fraught as that aim may, on some level, be. I can't save the world—alas—but I can at least put my own suffering and capacities into service in some small way. And that's what I tried to do.

My being so intimately engaged in the therapeutic process at Cedar Grove shaped this ethnography in profound ways. Because of my clinical training, and the access and experiences it brought, I am able to provide glimpses into the clinical world that simply would be impossible to obtain through standard ethnographic methods. At the same time, however, it has brought its own challenges. Being in a position of helping vulnerable clients while also conducting research demanded that I continuously think carefully and critically about my own ethical commitments and, at times, make difficult choices. As a rule, when I felt my roles of clinician and ethnographer to be in conflict, I erred on the side of being a clinician first and a researcher second. For example, I did not pursue consent for research with those clients I (or others) thought were either too vulnerable or too overwhelmed to agree to freely or safely. And I considered some issues or encounters off limits in terms of my research—these topics have informed my views, but I have not included them in this book. In other words, my ethical priorities during the research period have placed the needs of the clients first—always and without question.[3]

Outside of the clinic, I became actively involved in the world of eating disorder research and treatment, both locally and nationally. I attended trainings, workshops, and conferences and participated in professional networking events. I helped organize staff fundraising events and educational symposia. I have served on the board of the Missouri Eating Disorders Association (www.moeatingdisorders.org) since 2007 and on the Missouri Eating Disorders Council (www.moedc.org) since 2012. I have facilitated focus groups of therapists, patients in recovery, and family members. Over the course of seven years, I assisted in lobbying for legislative changes to improve access to care for eating disorders in Missouri, testifying in front of state House and Senate committees. I continue these activities today and also see eating disorder clients in my own nonprofit psychotherapy practice. By triangulating these various methods—ethnographic research, clinical training and practice, interviews, and advocacy, along with wide-reaching involvement in broader local and national eating disorders communities—I am able to situate the workings of Cedar Grove within a broader ecological understanding of the world of eating disorders treatment in the contemporary United States. Through this work I have come to understand eating disorders as a special sort of projective domain for articulating and working through of some of our most profound anxieties about what it means to be human and what it means to be in relationships with others.

So, what happened to Allison? Why didn't her progress in recovery "stick?" The standard answer is that eating disorders are intractable and difficult to treat, and that people who have them often resist treatment and don't really want to get better. And that is partially true. But the real reason is much more complex and eludes a simple answer.

It is true that eating disorders are virulent, progressive conditions that do not easily relinquish their hold on sufferers. It is also true that many people with eating disorders are often ambivalent about getting well. But to figure Allison's relapse and death as a product of her *personal* relationship with her illness elides the ways in which care itself becomes complicit in the continuation and exacerbation of suffering. In eating disorders treatment, care and harm become entangled, and the tenor of what anthropologist Lisa Stevenson calls the "psychic life of biopolitics" conditions the terms of recovery.[4] As we will see, in the case of eating disorders, this psychic life is characterized by a structural ethos of withholding, restriction, and deprivation *that moralizes clients' desire for care as itself pathological, even as resistance to care is figured as symptomatic.* This catches eating disorder patients in a dilemma: both wanting and not wanting care are pathologized in treatment and used to legitimate the *withholding* of care as a therapeutic act.

This rendering of clients' *desire for care* itself as problematic reinforces the core dynamics of eating disorders by conditioning clients to understand their own needs for care as illegitimate and even shameful. With eating disorders, where a core part of the illness is believing one doesn't deserve to want or need anything at all, a care system that pathologizes desire and need and withholds care is inherently and profoundly problematic, producing relationships of care that are fraught, ambivalent, and even damaging, although they can also be productive, meaningful, and healing. Understanding these complexities of care will give us insight into the cultural and social conditions of its emergence and can point us toward new modes of intervention.

A BRAIDED TALE

It is true that when people are in a state like Sheila was on the day of Allison's funeral, they can't "do life." I should know. I used to be one of them. Allison's story could have been mine. I could have been the one lying dead in a casket, leaving behind a devastated family and a future life unlived.

I came dangerously close to dying from anorexia twice, once when I was eleven years old and again when I was eighteen. I was hospitalized both times for several months and spent years in outpatient therapy in recovery. Although these are the two episodes where clinicians gave me the official diagnosis of anorexia, in reality they were but two peaks (or valleys) in a much longer and protracted struggle. Between the ages of about eight and twenty-six, I was, at various times, an anorexic, a bulimic, a compulsive exerciser, and a binge eater. I can remember only one brief period during eighth grade when I was not miserably immersed in disordered eating of some form or another. During those bleak years, I learned that there are an infinite number of ways to treat one's body as a detestable, yet constant, encumbrance. I frequently used diet pills, laxatives, stimulants, and anything else I could think of to wrangle, discipline, and punish my body into some sort of semblance of acceptability and to feel, even briefly, that I deserved to exist. It never quite worked.

Having an eating disorder is excruciatingly awful. It is a miserable, grinding, dismal existence. Every second of every day is saturated with fear, anxiety, and self-loathing, with no end in sight. Food and eating (and not eating) become the absolute focus of all your energy and attention. This is not a choice: you literally cannot think of or attend to anything else, at least not without an enormous expenditure of psychological, emotional, and cognitive energy, and even then, any such digression is fleeting and exhausting. Cognitively, you are calculating constantly: how many calories you have allotted for the day, how many you have already consumed, whether or not you counted right—calculating and recalculating and recalculating again, just in case. (To this day, I am a wiz at mental math because of the hours upon hours I spent during my anorexic years adding up, subtracting, substituting, and recalculating calories.) You think about what you just ate. You think about what you are going to eat next, how long you have to wait until then, and how you're going to make it. You think about what you're not eating that you wish you could eat, or you think about how glad you are that you're not eating it because it would clearly turn you into an oozing mass of cellulite. You think about what a horrible person you are because you *want* to eat, even if you know there is absolutely no way you are going to let yourself do it. You think about how to keep yourself from feeling hungry, how to handle it when you inevitably *are* hungry, and how to keep other people from paying too much attention to what you're doing with your food. You wonder what is wrong with you that you can't just eat like everyone else and why you have to live in this misery just to try to look (if not to feel) normal.

Am I well now, all these years later? I think so. My body is healthy. It is strong and fit and active. I have two beautiful children, a wonderful partner, and a supportive community of colleagues and friends around me. But my mind has not forgotten how to torment me, at times sneaking up on me when I least expect it to let me know that it is still there, that capacity for self-loathing and self-destruction. It is critical to understand that eating disorders are not about food—not really. They are about a deep, abiding, toxic shame and self-negation that is so embedded that it may never fully be eradicated. It can be managed and channeled and ameliorated, but once you have had the experience of actively trying to obliterate yourself, something changes. There's a part of you that knows what you're capable of.

As I write this book, I have been free of eating disorder behaviors for over twenty years. I suppose in that sense I am a success story, although I would never in a million years recommend that someone go about recovery the way I did. There are far better ways to do it. And while I no longer engage in eating disorder behaviors, I still struggle daily with the deeper concerns these behaviors expressed: doubts about my worthiness and my right to exist equally with others, a deep sense of shame, and a strong desire to connect coupled with battlement-thick defenses of fear and anxiety. Now, I can name these concerns and address them productively without harming my body. I have no desire to binge, purge, or restrict. I love food and eating and eat pretty much what I want when I want. And I have maintained a healthy body weight through one PhD, two pregnancies, an MSW, therapeutic licensure, tenure, and a number of life crises. I have, I suppose, made it to the other side.

If this were a recovery memoir, I might claim that I answered Sheila's question ("What's the point of trying to get better?") by telling her about the joys of living without an eating disorder and that the whole world is open to her if only she would let go of her illness and seize life. But I didn't. Because I knew how she felt.

And the truth is that there are no guarantees that Sheila or anyone else will actually "get better"—not only because eating disorders are complex and tenacious conditions but also because, as I detail in *Famished*, we live in a society that withholds vital and necessary care that is central to recovery. Sheila was on her third round of treatment at the time of Allison's funeral. She had been an inpatient for three months at a program in another state before coming to Cedar Grove the year prior, only to be kicked out for "non-compliance," and she was now back, provisionally, as the staff assessed her willingness to change. The fact that Sheila, at age twenty-two, had taken out a large personal loan in her own name to pay for treatment, because her parents refused to help with the costs, seemed to indicate a pretty serious willingness to change in my book. But the other clinicians at Cedar Grove remained agnostic.

In any event, I didn't give Sheila my own recovery story. And I didn't give her the typical therapist line about how she's worthy of recovery and owes it to herself to get better; I knew that would fall completely flat. I didn't give her the standard medical spiel about how she would die just like Allison if she didn't turn things around; part of her would have been relieved to die so that the suffering would be over with. I didn't take the researcher angle and ask her what *she* thought the point of recovery was; she would find that (justifiably) obnoxious and dodging. Instead, I told her the truth, as best I knew it, from my own long and harrowing history with these illnesses: the point of trying to get better is that the only alternative is to lie down and die. And she had not fought this hard for this long only to give up now.

But this—survival—is not an obvious motivator for a person with an eating disorder. Not necessarily because she wants to die (though she may), but rather because eating disorders are *themselves* survival strategies. This may seem counterintuitive, given that they can—and frequently do—kill people. What I mean is that they are strategies for *existential* survival that include, but extend far beyond, the physical body. They are about wanting to be seen as a legitimate, dynamic subject, not as a vacuous, static object. They are about wanting one's voice to be heard as a vital contribution, not dismissed as a cry for attention. They are about wanting a *response,* not just an answer. All too often, eating disorders become occasions for the opposite, for silencing and misrecognition, for erasure and denial.

To be absolutely clear: no one chooses to have an eating disorder. *No one.* It is miserable, excruciating, soul-sucking. Every second of every day is torture, and you just want to get through the hours until you can sink into sleep. And then it starts all over again the next morning. *If a person is bingeing, purging, or restricting to the point of putting herself in medical danger, there is something seriously, seriously wrong in that person's life such that destroying herself seems like the only viable option.*

This reality is effectively erased in accounts of eating disorder clients as "resistant" to treatment or as "difficult" and "manipulative." Eating disorders are, in many ways, particularly vexed and vexing conditions, at least as viewed from a mainstream biomedical perspective. When clients don't get better after interventions that clinicians, researchers, and insurance companies think should work, they are identified as "problem patients" and labeled as chronically ill and beyond hope. The possibility that the interventions themselves—and the funding structures that inform them—may be a key source of the problem is rarely considered. As a result, very sick people in need of care frequently go without it and are simultaneously blamed for their "unwillingness" to get well.

The convergence of stigma, misunderstanding, and ignorance that structures the diagnosis and treatment of eating disorders in the American health-care landscape is not an accident or a fluke—it is the result of centuries of gendered, raced, and classed assumptions about who gets sick and why, who is morally responsible for what kinds of suffering, what "health" looks like, and how recovery is to be achieved. Rewriting these scripts will require a full-scale reenvisioning of how we understand eating disorders and their treatment, as well as shining a bright light on the role for-profit healthcare plays in their perpetuation.

In approaching this task, I write this book from three distinct, yet overlapping, perspectives: as a medical and psychological anthropologist trained in analyzing the cultural meanings of health and illness, as a licensed psychotherapist specialized in treating eating disorders, and as a survivor of a long-term eating disorder. This tripartite engagement with eating disorders is unusual, yet, I hope, productive. It is extraordinarily difficult to place such distinct perspectives into productive dialogue with one another, and it raises some challenges.

Specifically, as an academic, writing about my personal history in this kind of detail brings some fairly significant risks. Bringing forth vulnerable personal material to share with the world is not something most academics do. We are supposed to be "impartial" and "objective," at least in terms of our personal emotional lives. But I cannot write a book about eating disorders without including my personal experiences. They are critical to understanding my engagements with the topics in this book. To leave them out would be duplicitous, or at the very least not fully transparent.

At the same time, however, because this is not a memoir, I do not present a cogent and complete account of my history in and through anorexia, bulimia, binge eating, and recovery. Rather, I include snapshots, vignettes, and reflections of different personal events and experiences together with the words of patients and clinicians at Cedar Grove as a way of bringing the reader closer to the experience of living with an eating disorder and to what it is like to inhabit these conditions from the inside. These accounts are woven in and through the text, seeping around the edges in ways that, like an eating disorder itself, are always irrevocably *there*.

WORDS MATTER

Some notes about language: I sometimes talk in generalizations about "people with eating disorders" and occasionally use the first-person plural, *we*, when discussing certain issues (e.g., "We tend to doubt our own material reality . . ."). I wish to be clear that these rhetorical choices do not mean that I presume to speak for all people with eating disorders, nor that I take my personal experience to be somehow emblematic of "the" eating disorder experience. Rather, such choices reflect my knowledge and understandings of these conditions based on my own journey with eating disorders and my over twenty years of ethnographic and clinical work in the field. I am confident in them, and yet no generalizations, no matter how careful, nuanced, or tentative, will ever capture the full extent of people's experiences with eating disorders or anything else, and I remain acutely aware that exceptions, counterexamples, and alternate interpretations may abound. I offer here my perspective on these conditions and their treatment as clearly and as honestly as I can, as one voice in a larger and ongoing conversation.

Also, currently, the majority of people who develop eating disorders are women, and all but one of the clients at Cedar Grove during my research period were female. I therefore refer to clients as "her" and "she" throughout this text. This is not in any way meant to minimize or elide the fact that increasing numbers of boys and men are developing and being diagnosed with these conditions, and I fully recognize that their suffering is just as acute and disastrous as that of girls and women. However, I simply do not have enough firsthand knowledge of boys and men with eating disorders to say anything well informed about their experiences and how they might be similar to or different from those of females. I also do not discuss issues of clients' sexuality or sexual identity much in this text; again, not because it is not critically important, but rather because it did not happen to emerge as central to the questions I was asking.

Regarding race and ethnicity: although the majority of clients who come to Cedar Grove are white, it is by no means a homogenous population, and

African American, Asian American, and Latinx clients are significant parts of the community. To ensure confidentiality, however, I do not identify the race or ethnic background of clients in this book unless it is somehow specifically germane.

Similarly, all names in this text are pseudonyms, and I have significantly disguised clients' stories while still retaining the core elements. All of the quotes, interactions, and vignettes in this text are "true," although I do sometimes use composites or transpose information to protect clients' privacy. Similarly, any treatment dates mentioned in the text have been altered to protect confidentiality.

Numbers (especially weights and calorie amounts) are a highly charged issue in the world of eating disorders and can be acutely triggering for people in recovery. The question of whether to include them in this text is one I had to take seriously. Mindful of these concerns, I largely avoid doing so. On a few occasions, however, providing specific numbers is instructive or illustrative in a particular way that could not be achieved without them. In such cases, I use them.

THE MAGIC ANSWER

I want to be clear at the outset that I do not have a magic solution to the problem of eating disorders. I have very definite ideas about them that have emerged from my own experiences and my decades of research on the topic, but I do not claim to have found "the answer" to healing these illnesses or discovered once and for all what they are "really" about, for the simple reason that eating disorders are not about any one thing. They are extraordinarily complex conditions that entangle (or, better said, reveal and enact the entanglement *of*) biological, psychological, interpersonal, social and cultural struggles about the meaning of existence and the value of persons within our world. While there are some common themes that emerge for people with eating disorders, the actual expressions and meanings that come into play around these themes and the significance they hold for a person's illness and recovery are specific to each and every individual. I cannot promise anyone that they will recover. I know only that it is possible. What I offer here, then, are not answers but rather new ways of asking questions that can help us—all of us—engage those struggling with these conditions with greater compassion, understanding, and awareness.

Provocations

ONE

Introduction

"You *cannot* be serious!" Danya, a dietician, blurts out in the middle of the regular Wednesday morning treatment team meeting at Cedar Grove. Mirroring Danya's incredulity, the rest of us look around at one another, trying to process what we had just heard.

"I'm afraid I am serious," affirms Dr. Casey, the clinic's medical director, speaking up over the mutterings and exclamations of the staff. "I know it sounds crazy—I know! But we have looked at this from every angle. This really is the best option for Hope and for the family."

"Never have I been asked to put an anorexic on a *diet* to make her *lose weight,*" Danya grumbles under her breath. Then, more loudly: "Hope is nowhere near her goal weight. It's going to undo all the progress she's made over the past two weeks. We've just finally gotten her up to where she needs to be calorie-wise with her add-ons! She has worked *so hard*. Now we're going to tell her, 'Guess what? Never mind! Time to start restricting again!'"

"It's an anorexic's dream," quips Joan, the assistant medical director.

"I think she'll view it as punitive," observes Brenda, Hope's therapist. "Like, 'You're bad for gaining weight, and so now we're going to take food away.'"

"That's a real danger," agreed Dr. Casey. "This could totally fuel the anorexia and make everything worse. But really, it's the only chance she's got."

Under what conditions would putting an anorexic client on a diet inside an eating disorders clinic become the "only chance she's got"?

Hope was thirteen years old when she entered treatment at Cedar Grove, one of the youngest clients at the clinic. At the time of the treatment team meeting excerpted above, she had been at the clinic for just under two weeks.

Hope came to Cedar Grove directly from a local children's hospital, where she had spent a week on bed rest under close observation as her vitals stabilized. She had arrived at the hospital not only painfully underweight (at 72 percent of her ideal body weight) but also completely dehydrated—nurses struggled to find a good vein for placing an IV and eventually had to settle for one in her left hand. Utterly panicked by the amount of fluids that were being pumped into her body, Hope found ways to exercise when the nurses weren't looking and to dump fluid from the IV bag so it looked like it had gone into her body when in fact it had gone down the toilet. She refused to eat anything but vegetables in the hospital and would drink only juice (unsweetened), iced tea (unsweetened), and occasionally milk (skim). To stave off hunger pangs, she chewed gum (sugar-free) and sucked on the occasional Jolly Rancher. On threat of an NG tube being placed to force-feed her, Hope began to eat slightly more during meal times. Yet she also increased her exercise to compensate. Her weight continued to go down, and an NG tube was placed.

Hope still had the NG tube in when she arrived at Cedar Grove. Like most who have "the tube," Hope was highly ambivalent toward it. On the one hand, she hated it with a flaming passion. "Oh my god, this thing is awful!" she told me, explaining:

> It hurts, and it moves around, and when I lie down I can feel it down the back of my throat. And the tube gets all crusty in your nose. It's totally disgusting. And then, when they put the liquid in, it's just gross having this stuff running down through your nose and into your stomach. I get stomachaches from the Boost [a liquid nutrition supplement] like a lot of people do. And my body is so slow to digest stuff that I'm still full and it's time for the next "feeding." And I hate how they call it a "feeding," like I'm a horse. Or a baby. I just want it out.

But even as much as she hated the tube, Hope (and others) did find some degree of relief in being able to bypass the actual act of eating. She continued, "I will say, it's nice to not have to deal with meal planning or sitting down to a plate full of food and thinking, 'How will I ever eat that?' It just gets shoved up my nose," she laughed, "and I don't really have to think about it. I think the whole time about all the calories, and that's horrible. But at least I don't have to physically put the food in my mouth and eat it."

Over time at the clinic, Hope began to eat more food by mouth, and by the time of the abovementioned treatment team meeting, she had been off the tube for four days and was doing well.

How, then, did Hope, a dangerously underweight adolescent who was just starting to allow herself to eat, come to be put on a diet *inside* an eating disorders clinic? How was this determined to be the best care the treatment team could provide? Eating disorder clinicians face untenable ethical positions like this on a daily basis. Making sense of apparently nonsensical scenarios like Hope's requires us to radically rethink what eating disorders are and to critically retool our approaches to treatment and recovery. And to do that, we need to understand the fundamentals.

WHAT EATING DISORDERS ARE (AND AREN'T)

Most people today know (or think they know) what eating disorders are. After all, references to eating disorders frequently pepper the covers of magazines ("Angelina Jolie—Anorexic!"), take center stage in movies, or appear in news reports or feature articles. But popular understandings of these illnesses—that they are about wanting to be beautiful, seeking attention, trying to fit in, and/or excelling at control—barely skirt the edges of what eating disorders truly are and what it's actually like to live with one.

Let me start with being clear about what eating disorders are *not*. Eating disorders are not diets that have gone "too far." Nor are they like cocaine or heroin addictions, where an addict can conceivably go cold turkey, detox for thirty days, and essentially be back to baseline as long as they avoid the drug. They are not juvenile temper tantrums, though they can be an expression of anger and rage. They are not "phases" someone goes through. They are not about superficial vanity or self-aggrandizement, though this is how they may look from the outside.

So, what *is* an eating disorder? This seems like a simple enough question, but it is deceptively so. In fact, what an eating disorder is depends on who is asking, and why.

The current *Diagnostic and Statistical Manual of Mental Disorders* (*DSM*)[1] identifies four main categories of eating disorders: anorexia nervosa, bulimia nervosa, binge eating disorder, and other specified feeding and eating disorder.[2]

Anorexia nervosa is characterized by acute self-starvation and the inability or unwillingness to maintain a body weight necessary for normal physiological functioning. Generally, this is accompanied by a deeply held conviction that one is overweight or fat, although instances of non-fat-phobic anorexia nervosa have been documented around the world and even in the United States.[3] The *DSM* identifies a number of subtypes of anorexia nervosa, including restricting subtype (where the person sustains underweight through not eating), purging subtype (where the person restricts intake and also purges through the use of laxatives, vomiting, diuretics, or exercise), and binge-purge subtype (where periods of starvation are punctuated by instances of bingeing on large amounts of food and purging it).

What is not captured in these diagnostic criteria is the lived experience of having anorexia and the way it cripples everyday functioning. People with anorexia are terrified of food and other substances entering their body in the same way a person with claustrophobia is afraid of small spaces. Food and eating send them into utter panic. They starve themselves, even when they are severely underweight, and may also restrict the intake of liquids (including water) and even medications.[4] Their fear and panic is so great that it outweighs any cautions about medical risks—the future possibility of damage or death pales in comparison to the perceived certainty of the immediate danger of eating. Anorexia is extremely harmful, affecting every organ system in the body. The brain starves and can lose mass. The heart can be permanently weakened. The liver and kidneys can shut down. Bones and muscles are depleted as the starving body cannibalizes itself for fuel—I have known nineteen-year-olds with osteoporosis, and one who fell and broke a hip. Some of this damage is reversible if caught early enough. Some of it is not. Anorexia is relatively rare (0.3 percent prevalence),[5] but it is deadly. It kills one out of five sufferers, making it the most lethal of all mental illnesses.[6]

People with bulimia manage their relationships with food differently. Rather than avoiding food completely, they alternate between bingeing and purging, consuming large amounts of food and then ridding themselves of it through vomiting, exercising, fasting, or using laxatives or diuretics. Indeed, the hallmark of bulimia is this alternation between consumption and undoing. Bulimia damages the entire digestive system and places significant burden on the other organs. One woman I knew had so much scar tissue in her throat and esophagus from purging that she could no longer swallow solid food. Bulimia is particularly dangerous for the heart, as it destabilizes the electrolytes in the body, which can cause cardiac arrest. People with bulimia may be of normal weight or even slightly above it, which makes it especially difficult for them to get insurance approval for treatment—to show medical necessity, the person must be at *immediate* risk for cardiac arrest or organ failure before they will be authorized for treatment. The really dangerous thing about bulimia is that someone can have perfectly normal labs and still be one purge away from a heart attack. And labs tell you nothing about a person's actual functionality. I knew a woman who was so consumed by her illness that she quit her job, dropped out of school, and did nothing but binge and purge ten to twelve times *a day,* yet she had normal lab results, so we could not get her authorized for inpatient treatment. Bulimia affects approximately 1 percent of the population, a similar rate as schizophrenia.[7]

People with binge eating disorder binge on food but do not "undo" the binges through purging or other compensatory behaviors, as in bulimia. The distinctive feature of this condition is that the person wants to stop eating but can't. They feel a compulsion to eat, the same as a person with obsessive-compulsive disorder feels a compulsion to wash their hands or check the stove. As much as they may try to not overeat and as much as they may be committed to not bingeing, the compulsion to do so is so overwhelming that they are unable to prevent themselves from doing it. All the while, they feel self-loathing, shame, and disgust, yet they cannot stop. One woman I know described it as "living with a monster. Every day I would swear I wasn't going to do it again, but then it would happen and I couldn't stop it. I wanted to die." Binge eating disorder is the fastest growing eating disorder diagnosis, affecting approximately 3.5 percent of American women and 2 percent of American men.[8]

Other specified feeding or eating disorder (OSFED, previously referred to as eating disorder not otherwise specified, or EDNOS) is a category used to describe conditions that share symptoms across two or more of the other eating disorders or do not meet the duration or frequency requirements of a single disorder. For example, someone may restrict, as in anorexia, but then binge and purge once or twice a week. Or they may oscillate between periods of anorexic restriction, bulimic behavior, and bingeing for weeks or months at a time. People with orthorexia (obsessed with "healthy eating") currently also fit within the OSFED diagnosis, though recognition of orthorexia as a separate disorder is likely on the horizon. Although OSFED is something of an "other" category, this does not diminish its seriousness: more people are diagnosed with OSFED than either anorexia nervosa or bulimia nervosa, and it is just as damaging and deadly. People die from it. Nevertheless, many insurance companies—even those that do actually authorize treatment for eating disorders—often exclude OSFED on the false assumption that people with this condition do not have a "real" eating disorder.

Eating disorder specialists differ on whether they believe the various eating disorders are truly discrete phenomena with their own separate etiologies, trajectories, and patient profiles or whether, instead, eating disorders should be considered as expressions along a spectrum. I endorse the latter view. People often move across different eating disorders during their lifetime, suggesting a continuum rather than fully discrete disease entities. In addition, all of the eating disorders share important core features in terms of sufferers' lived experiences and the issues at stake in their illnesses and recoveries.

Although eating disorders are notable for behaviors surrounding food, body, and weight, the psychological, emotional, and cognitive dimensions of these illnesses run far deeper. On the whole, people with eating disorders tend to view their bodies with abject disgust and experience the weight and shape of their physical existence as intolerable and excruciating. This is generally coupled with a self-loathing that seeps into every crevice of self-knowledge and experience. As one recovering client diagnosed with anorexia described it to me, "I just miss seeing my bones. I miss that so much! Just seeing them through my skin. It made me feel safe to be so near death." People with eating disorders often persist in their behaviors long after they have destroyed relationships, endangered careers, or interrupted schooling. "I saw what it was doing to my life," another client told me. "But the eating disorder just felt so good that I didn't want to give it up. I couldn't. I didn't know who I would be without it." As we will see through the following chapters, eating disorders are what we might call *existential* disorders in that they structure and give meaning to a person's entire life and mode of being.

THE MAP IS NOT THE TERRITORY

The *DSM* definitions of eating disorders describe behaviors and cognitive features that clearly map onto experiences of real people. This is good and important. But do they really capture the phenomenon of what an eating disorder is? Do they capture the sleepless nights spent calculating calories, the depths of self-loathing that lead you to claw at your thighs, the panic that makes you break out in hives when you realize you mismeasured your cottage cheese at lunch? Do they capture the shame that interferes with intimacy for years after recovery, the inability to look at yourself in the mirror without cringing, the almost monumental effort required to allow yourself to take a break, to breathe?

Eating disorders are not simply a collection of behaviors, body weights, lab values, or cognitive distortions. Eating disorders are physically and emotionally devastating conditions where food and eating become the vectors and means by which deep existential concerns are made manifest and struggled out.

With this in mind, I will make a potentially provocative claim: Eating disorders do not exist *within* people; they emerge *between* people. They are not individual psychological (or even physical) illnesses; rather, they are continually conjured as "things" in the contexts of shifting interpersonal, structural, and material relationships within which they do very particular kinds of work. As deeply embodied conditions that entangle existential, phenomenological, and relational concerns, eating disorders manifest as sites where profound issues of intimacy, trust, obligation, and care are struggled out as the illnesses are lived, identified, and treated.

Specifically, one key argument of this book is that eating disorders in the contemporary United States *emerge in and through the circulation of knowledge and practices among treatment providers, research agendas, and insurance companies.* What counts as an eating disorder and what does not is produced through negotiations among powerful interests that, all too often, are motivated primarily by profit or prestige rather than by healing. The result is a clinical "reality" in which patients' "failure" to overcome the double binds within which that reality was created serves to further justify the structures that gave rise to it.

This is *not* to suggest that people are not suffering before, after, or outside of these structures—they most definitely are. But the synergistic aims of these three domains shape what eating disorders are thought to be, how they are diagnosed and treated, how they are experienced, and what happens to people who have them.

How an eating disorder is manifested in a given interaction—what is included as materially important and what is excluded as unrelated (and by whom); how the pieces are thought to interact and hang together; what is thought to cause them; what effects they are believed to have; and how they should be treated—varies not only from person to person but from context to context. One person's eating disorder is never identical to another's, and each is construed differently in different contexts, from the doctor's office to the therapy room, the insurance case manager's docket to everyday life. What delineates the boundaries of an eating disorder and what constitutes its phenomenology are negotiated anew in each and every interaction and in different situational and material circumstances. *Eating disorders, then, emerge and exist between people and in the spaces between people and shifting structures of care.*

In taking this position, I wish to be exceedingly clear. Eating disorders are real. Treatment providers, researchers, and insurance companies do not *create* these illnesses out of nothing. Clearly identifiable patterns of behaviors, beliefs, cognitions, affects, and phenomenological experiences characterize these conditions. Self-destructive behaviors such as self-starvation, bingeing and purging, and compulsive exercise absolutely exist, as do obsessive concerns about weight and shape, distorted perceptions of body image, and fears of getting fat. Symptoms such as osteopenia, low heart rate, and electrolyte imbalance result from these behaviors and have direct physical consequences. Terms such as "social withdrawal," "phobia," "shame," "self-loathing," and "discomfort with intimacy" describe genuine struggles, and these characteristics hang together in recognizable patterns.

But I want to push against this reality in certain ways. When we say a person has an eating disorder, what exactly is it that they have? A pattern of restricting food intake? A distorted body image? A fear of getting fat? Difficulty with affect regulation? Recurrent bingeing and purging behaviors? Problems with intimacy and interpersonal communication? Compulsions to overexercise? Self-loathing? Some combination of these and other features, certainly. But one hundred different people can meet the same diagnostic criteria for anorexia nervosa and yet have profoundly different illness profiles and experiences beyond the narrow set of items outlined in the *DSM*. What, then, is this "thing" we call an eating disorder? What are its boundaries? What aspects of the person are part of it, and what are not? These are not simple or straightforward questions, and how we answer them tells us as much about the larger cultural contexts in which these conditions emerge as about the individuals suffering from them. What constitutes the "thingness" of an eating disorder, then, is a *relational* question, not a psychological or physiological one, although body and mind are deeply involved. Ontologically speaking, the thing termed "eating disorder" unfolds as an interpersonal process.

Contemporary western biomedicine thrives on deriving certainty from uncertainty. By distilling collections of symptoms—pain here, numbness there, dizziness, abnormal lab values, loss of function—into constructs we call "diseases," and designing interventions aimed at restoring "health," biomedicine banks on the correspondence between such disease constructs and actual biological reality. In this way, biomedicine is invested in making claims to truth, where the body becomes the primary bearer of evidence (or lack thereof).

Individuals with what anthropologist Joe Dumit calls "contested illnesses," like chronic fatigue syndrome or fibromyalgia, often experience medical encounters as if they must *prove* their illness and their suffering to others through the mobilization of facts.[9] That is, until and unless these patients can demonstrate through biomedically recognized markers that their diseases are "real," they are treated with skepticism, suspicion, and even scorn. In such situations, biomedical facts come to play a crucial role in how clinicians render judgments about patients, their symptoms, and their claims to care.[10] As Dumit notes, in the biomedical context, "one must have laboratory signs in order to be suffering; one must suffer in code in order to be suffering . . . or one does not suffer at all."[11] Measurement and quantification of the material body's processes come to stand in as proof that something is "really wrong."

Importantly, however, biomedical facts themselves are, as Dumit notes, "susceptible to being framed and reframed by participants" as they attempt to "emplot and counter-emplot each other."[12] In other words, biomedical facts can be used to tell different kinds of stories, depending on the teller, the audience, the evidence, or all three. These facts become critical narrative "flexers" that can leverage different kinds of interpretations of what is otherwise seen as vague or overdetermined information. Often in such cases, there is, Dumit observes, "not enough research and at the same time too many facts," meaning that fights over definitions, diagnosis, response, and prevention come to wield a great deal of power in such situations, despite the fact that they often depend disproportionately on a small amount of underfunded research.[13]

Eating disorders are, in many ways, contested illnesses in Dumit's sense, although with a bit of a twist. They are not contested in terms of their existence—the *DSM* clearly outlines diagnostic criteria, prevalence and incidence data, etiology, and course information, and the American Psychiatric Association (APA) publishes clear treatment guidelines. What is contested about eating disorders is not whether they constitute "real" illnesses but whether and to what extent a given patient is thought to be *suffering appropriately* from an eating disorder and is therefore deemed worthy of care.

This is a key claim of this book, so let me unpack it further. Notably, much of the suffering and debility involved in eating disorders happens *around the edges* of the official diagnostic criteria, in what I call "halo features," such as relentless perfectionism, difficulties with interpersonal boundaries, and challenges in maintaining intimacy.[14] These features effloresce in clinical and anecdotal descriptions of clients and in lived daily experience but are not captured in the official diagnostic coding criteria. Importantly, what does show up in the diagnostic criteria are the elements that appear more choice based (not eating enough, purging, bingeing), skewing the way these conditions are viewed. What is not captured is the constant battering of shame, the paralyzing fear, and the relentless obsessive thoughts. Why do official diagnostic categories leave out such features? Historically, this hasn't always been the case. But as we will see in chapter 4, the shift in the *DSM* in the 1980s to a more descriptive mode of diagnosis (versus an etiological or interpretive one) emerged hand in hand with economic transitions in healthcare funding that focused on increased efficiency and cost savings and were based on outcomes that could be quantified and tracked. Contested illnesses, and indeed all types of psychiatric distress, were reconceptualized beginning with the *DSM-III* as collections of cognitive, behavioral, or biological symptoms that could be objectively measured.

As Dumit notes, in the face of systematic delegitimization, sufferers of contested illness often respond "by emphasizing not the bottom of things, but the surfaces, the micro-tactics of decision making."[15] That is, people learn to express their distress in ways that are locally recognized as legitimate, whether or not these expressions capture the full range of their experiences. With eating disorders, this leads clients, clinicians, researchers, and insurance companies alike to focus on such things as calorie levels, goal weights, and frequency of compliance with clinic programs. Not that these are unimportant things—they are very important. But they are not where the core of the issue lies. In the context of for-profit managed care, however, such biomedical facts come to constitute the reality of what an eating disorder is, shaping the ways care unfolds as a result.

Treatment for eating disorders at Cedar Grove is conditioned by this broader healthcare landscape. Cedar Grove is a private, residential eating disorder facility in the American Midwest that treats anorexia nervosa, bulimia nervosa, binge eating disorder, and other specified feeding and eating disorder. Since its initiation in 2001, Cedar Grove has become one of the premier treatment centers for eating disorders in the United States, particularly known for its top-notch medical care and its use of evidence-based best practices in treatment. Patients come from all over the country for treatment, sometimes waiting weeks or even months on a waiting list to get in (see chapter 5 for more on the clinic's setting and program). The clinic provides three different levels of care: twenty-four-hour residential care, a partial hospital (day treatment) program, and an intensive outpatient program. Patients (as they are called at the clinic[16]) receive comprehensive psychiatric, medical, and psychological assessments prior to admission, and the specifics of a patient's treatment plan depend on these factors as well as on the precipitating events surrounding the development of the eating disorder and a patient's progress while in the program. We will explore this more in section 2.

Cedar Grove and its programs are situated within a broader ecology of mental health services. The American mental health system is composed of a range of levels of psychiatric care for people experiencing different degrees of crisis or difficulty. Inpatient hospitalization serves the most acute cases, when someone is in danger of harming themselves or others or is significantly medically compromised. Generally, this is considered a short-term, targeted intervention to get someone out of the danger zone—then they are discharged. Outpatient care can consist of anything from occasional meetings with a therapist and/or psychiatrist to participation in a day treatment program for several hours a day. Insurance companies often pay for acute hospital care only in cases of marked suicidality or medical instability, and whether and to what degree they cover outpatient care varies. Some cover day treatment (partial hospital treatment) as well as weekly therapy visits, whereas others exclude day treatment and will pay only for once-a-week appointments. It depends entirely on the specific insurance plan a patient has.

Eating disorders treatment requires containment and oversight above and beyond that needed for standard medical or psychiatric care, as well as specialists who know what to look for and how to intervene if needed. This complicates their place within existing services, creating special challenges. As Dr. Casey, Cedar Grove's medical director, told me, "When our patients go to the hospital for medical or even psychiatric issues, they often come back much sicker with their eating disorders. The staff at hospitals are not trained to make sure someone is eating enough, or isn't purging, or isn't exercising when no one is looking. They don't have the staffing power for it. It's just not what they're set up for." The result is that when eating disorder patients are relegated to nonspecialized care, they often get sicker rather than better.

To address these sorts of issues, a third level of intervention occupies a sort of interstitial space between inpatient acute hospital care and outpatient treatment: residential care at clinics like Cedar Grove. Residential care is designed primarily for ongoing, potentially life-threatening conditions that may not currently be medically destabilizing but could become so if not treated, such as drug addiction, alcoholism, trauma, self-harm, and eating disorders. These clinics provide containment along with therapy and oversight in home-like settings that may have medical personnel on staff but are not hospitals.

Some insurance policies cover residential care and others do not. Some insurance plans will cover residential treatment for certain conditions, such as drug addiction, but not for others, like eating disorders. Many insurance companies will pay only for either acute hospital care, which may not be needed, or outpatient treatment, which often does not provide the kind of structure or oversight someone with an acute eating disorder needs. "I'm just not convinced that outpatient therapy works for adolescents," one Cedar Grove therapist told me. "I think they get sicker. It makes them worse. They go to therapy, get all activated, and then go away for a week. To do what? What are they supposed to do with the feelings? The parents don't know what to do and they think their kid is getting treatment, so they don't pay attention. Everyone is in denial: the therapist, the patient, the family, everyone. And the poor person who is sick is left twisting in the wind." In other words, the *very level of care many eating disorder clients need is, more often than not, rendered structurally invisible.*

Places like Cedar Grove exist to provide the critical level of residential care for these clients. But they must do so within a healthcare system that makes the delivery of such care highly problematic. In order to get clients approved for coverage for residential treatment at a non-hospital-based center like Cedar Grove, clinicians often have to justify not only the necessity of care for the individual but the legitimacy of the very existence of these centers as a treatment option.

Why is it so hard to get adequate, comprehensive care for eating disorders? To understand this, we need to take a brief detour into the history of managed healthcare in the United States.

Today's managed healthcare structure originated in early twentieth-century collective health organizations that sought to reduce health costs and increase access to care for workers through the institutionalization of regional prepaid health plans. This approach was formalized by the Health Maintenance Organization Act of 1973, under which HMOs functioned as innovative nonprofit institutions that emphasized provision and integrated services. However, the ground was laid for the incursion of for-profit interests, and by the late 1990s the majority of regional HMOs had been taken over by just a handful of larger managed care organizations, which, following legislative changes, began to run them as for-profit enterprises. With the expansion of managed care in the 1990s, many managed care companies moved from being disinterested gatekeepers to also providing insurance benefits themselves, which gave them a powerful, vested economic interest in minimizing the benefits used, regardless of how necessary or cost effective they were.[17] In other words, what began as a system to protect patients from unscrupulous providers wasting valuable healthcare benefits became a system where the industry regulating the release of benefits is also the industry that profits the most from withholding them.

Today, managed care organizations do what the name implies: they manage care by gatekeeping the release of insurance benefits to patients by (in theory) serving as a kind of middle-person between the physician and the insurance provider (often the managed care organization itself), ensuring that recommended interventions are indeed necessary and not excessive before allowing insurance benefits to be utilized to pay for care. Operating on a philosophy of explicit rationing, the motivating assumption of managed care organizations is that efficiently managed money equates to expertly managed care.

The effect of the transition to managed care on patient outcomes is a hotly debated point. On the one hand, managed care has enabled some types of access to some types of care for some types of patients. At Cedar Grove, for example, a treatment course can easily cost a year's salary or more. Clinicians and clients *need* the managed care system for the clinic to exist, and it is only because of managed care that many clients receive any treatment at all. Insurance enables at least a certain kind of care for a certain kind of client who exhibits a certain kind of suffering. On the other hand, managed care routinely *denies* care to patients, even those who doctors have determined are in dire need of it.

The bottom line is that insurance companies make profits when they pay for the least amount of care possible, and making profits is what keeps their customers—shareholders, not patients—happy. With such priorities, insurance companies have a powerfully motivated interest in the "responsibilization" of the patient as a particular kind of healthcare consumer.[18] In this model, "good patients" are those who are predictable, health seeking, and active in their own recovery. They act to maximize health and minimize harm. They want to get better. They follow recommendations. They can get well. These patients are what we might call the "right" kind of sick in the managed care framework—they are considered good investments of healthcare dollars. "Bad" or "difficult" patients, however, are a different story. They may not want to get better or may not demonstrate this in the expected ways. They may be noncompliant with healthcare providers, and they may even do things to exacerbate their conditions. These patients are the "wrong" kind of sick; they are poor economic investments. The logic of managed care says that healthcare benefits, even if they exist, should not be "wasted" in such situations.[19]

People with psychiatric concerns are, almost by definition, the "wrong" kind of sick in this framework. They frequently act in unpredictable and seemingly irrational ways—they harm themselves, insist they are the messiah, or hoard animals. They may accuse caregivers of trying to harm them or refuse to take their medications. In fact, being flagrantly unpredictable and irrational is often a central part of what distinguishes them as ill.[20]

Within this population, eating disorder patients are renowned to be particularly "difficult" and "resistant," to the point where many clinicians specifically refuse to work with them. It is true that many people in the throes of an eating disorder minimize the risks of their behaviors and insist they do not want treatment. They often actively undermine their own care, appearing to be willfully noncompliant. On top of this, unlike other serious mental illnesses like schizophrenia or depression, eating disorders continue to occupy a space in the popular imagination as a choice—a manifestation of vanity, manipulation, or childish rebellion. Managed care case managers are as susceptible to these erroneous stereotypes as anyone else, and they often have little sympathy for the struggles of clients with "self-inflicted illnesses" (as one case manager characterized anorexia to me when denying a client further benefits).

In the context of for-profit managed care, then, eating disorder patients are not only the wrong kind of sick but also create more work, use more resources, and have worse outcomes than other patients. It is perhaps understandable why insurance companies would treat them with caution. When insurance companies do cover eating disorders, they are especially vigilant about monitoring how healthcare resources are used: they look for clear evidence of progress in a patient's capacity for self-governance and engagement in pro-health behaviors, as indicated by such things as regular and significant weight gain and compliance with program rules. The patient's ability and willingness to act with "right intention"—her *moral agency*[21] as manifested in these outcomes—becomes the barometer of whether she is deemed deserving of care and of the release of additional benefits to pay for treatment.

As we will see in the coming chapters, because of the paradoxes and contradictions built into current care delivery systems, *becoming the "right" kind of patient when one has an eating disorder is almost a logical impossibility until treatment is effective and one is no longer a patient at all.* This poses serious problems when patients' perceived motivations for health have a gatekeeper effect in enabling or restricting their access to care. The consequences are real. In the United States, fewer than one in ten people diagnosed with an eating disorder will access any kind of mental healthcare, and only 35 percent of *those* individuals will receive necessary specialized treatment.[22] This means that for every 100 people diagnosed with an eating disorder, only 3.5 will get care by someone who specializes in these conditions.

Even people who do access treatment for an eating disorder face an uphill battle in terms of getting *enough* or the *right kind* of care. Individuals with eating disorders are regularly discharged when they are still below minimum weight recommendations, and they are often released without access to necessary behavioral stabilization or support, resources, or adequate assistance to help them transition back to the community.[23] One study found that only 3 percent of the ninety-eight health plans it investigated would fully cover the APA-recommended treatment protocol for anorexia.[24] A separate report demonstrated that unlike treatment for other psychiatric conditions like schizophrenia, bipolar disorder, or depression, the average length of treatment for eating disorders is much lower than the APA's recommended standards of care.[25] Many insurance plans provide very circumscribed benefits for eating disorders treatment or exclude eating disorders from coverage all together.

The effects of this situation are devastating. One survey found that one in five eating disorder specialists believe that insurance companies are indirectly responsible for the death of at least one of their patients;[26] 96.7 percent of these specialists believe their patients with anorexia nervosa are put in life-threatening situations because of health insurance companies' refusal to cover treatment.[27] These kinds of problems remain entrenched even after the implementation of the Affordable Care Act (known colloquially as Obamacare): a 2015 study found that while no insurance plan categorically excluded drug and alcohol treatment from coverage and only 5.9 percent of plans excluded treatment for autism, a full 21 percent excluded treatment for eating disorders.[28]

Perhaps, one might speculate, this restricted coverage for care is due simply to the fact that eating disorders are so rare. But they are not rare. Eating disorders constitute an urgent American public health crisis on a grand scale. At least thirty million people of all ages and genders suffer from an eating disorder in the United States.[29] These conditions afflict more than twice as many people as Alzheimer's and five times as many as schizophrenia.[30] An estimated one in five American women struggle with an eating disorder or significantly disordered eating,[31] and eating disorders are the third most common chronic illness among adolescent females, after obesity and asthma.[32] Because of the secretiveness and shame associated with eating disorders, the actual numbers are likely much higher. In addition, many individuals struggle with body dissatisfaction and subclinical disordered eating attitudes and behaviors. A reported 80 percent of American women are dissatisfied with their appearance.[33] According to one study, over half of American females between the ages of eighteen and twenty-five would prefer to be run over by a truck then be fat, and two-thirds of them would rather be mean or stupid than fat.[34] Fifty-one percent of nine- and ten-year-old girls feel better about themselves if they are on a diet.[35] Forty-two percent of first- through third-grade girls want to be thinner.[36] These are girls aged *six* to *eight*. These are dangerous indicators. And eating disorders are the deadliest of all psychiatric conditions—a young woman with anorexia is twelve times more likely to die than a woman her age without anorexia.[37] One in five anorexia deaths is by suicide.[38] Every sixty-two minutes, at least one person dies as a direct result of an eating disorder.[39]

Given the current treatment situation, it is perhaps not surprising that the prognosis for people with eating disorders is grim. Under current policy conditions, only approximately 50 percent of patients with an eating disorder recover; 30 percent improve somewhat, and the other 20 percent remain chronically ill or die.[40] Given the spotty nature of care, those individuals who remain ill often return to treatment multiple times, utilizing additional medical and psychological services and thus reinforcing the perception that these conditions—and the people who develop them—are resistant to treatment.[41]

We might expect that such a deadly and widespread set of conditions might be the focus of a massive research effort. But research on eating disorders, like treatment, is shockingly underfunded compared to other conditions. National Institute of Mental Health research dollars spent on Alzheimer's averaged $247 per affected individual in 2017. For schizophrenia, the amount was $69. For autism, it was $82. For eating disorders, the average number of research dollars spent per affected individual was only $1.07.[42]

Eating disorders are the most lethal of all psychiatric conditions, yet they are among the most excluded from coverage, the least funded in terms of research, and the most rigorously policed in practice. Why might this be the case? In what cultural universe does this make practical, ideological, or ethical sense? And how does care unfurl within such a system? These are the motivating questions of this book. What happens at Cedar Grove is emblematic of this larger set of issues. Indeed, the conditions of care at Cedar Grove extend far beyond this one clinic and represent what is increasingly recognized as a systematic bias against eating disorders in the managed care industry, which has led to legislative action in some states to attempt to protect eating disorder clients and their families from predatory insurance practices (see chapter 12 for a discussion of this).[43] At the heart of the issue is a serious dilemma for eating disorder clients: *How can you become the right kind of patient if you are, by definition, the wrong kind of sick?*

This dilemma has real effects on real people. Shelly, for example, was twenty-seven years old when she came to Cedar Grove for the third time. She was known to be a "highly difficult patient"; the past two times she had been at the clinic, she had stated she wanted to get better but then proceeded to subvert the program at every turn. She hid food so she would not have to eat it at mealtimes, only to binge on it and purge in the middle of the night. She hoarded artificial sweeteners because they can have a laxative effect when taken in large doses, and she snuck in diet pills and laxatives in the lining of her makeup case. She found an area just out of the line of sight of the nurses' station where she could do jumping jacks without being seen. Although

Cedar Grove clinicians recognized these behaviors as indicating that Shelly needed *more* treatment (not less), they were forced to discharge her after two weeks because her insurance company would not release any further benefits due to her noncompliance.

To understand their work with clients like Shelly, clinicians have to devise ways of thinking about patients that enable them to navigate the paradox about mental illness that is inherent in the managed care system. They have to figure out how to care for patients who don't (appear to) want to get well, within healthcare structures that work against them almost every step of the way.

CLINICIANS AS DOUBLE AGENTS

To get care in an eating disorders clinic, clients must learn *how to be sick* in particular ways, but not *too* sick (lest they be deemed difficult or resistant); and *how to be well* in particular ways, but not *too* well (lest they be deemed not sick enough to warrant treatment). Given these conditions, clinicians at Cedar Grove must become what Marcia Angell[44] calls "double agents," constantly negotiating between the requirements outlined by insurance providers and locally derived understandings of what is needed for optimal client care. While this sort of negotiation is common to most areas of medicine in the era of managed care, eating disorder clinicians face particular challenges. They spend much of their time trying to obtain treatment that insurance companies generally do not want to fund, for patients who often do not want it. As Brooke, a Cedar Grove therapist explained it, "Dealing with insurance companies is by far the worst part of my job. You have to fight the insurance companies to get [patients] in, then fight to keep them in long enough for it to do any good. And when you finally get the patient approved for more days, you turn around and they refuse a meal or something and you're like, 'Nooo! There's no way insurance is going to go for that!' Because, honestly, insurance doesn't care."

This grim situation produces daily challenges for clinicians at Cedar Grove, who often find themselves torn between emotionally investing in clients as part of therapeutic interventions—caring for them in all senses of the word—and maintaining enough distance so that failure, relapse, or insurance-mandated discharge does not cause them to burn out—something that, perhaps not surprisingly, is exceptionally prevalent in this specialty.[45] "It's hard,"

Maggie, a therapist, told me. "We heal through [building a] relationship. You can give everything and just have it thrown back in your face, or else someone is doing well but insurance discharges them before they're ready, and they relapse. It can really drain you if you're not careful." Clinicians like Brooke and Maggie are called on to use their affective skills—empathy, concern, attention, emotional containment, de-escalation, mirroring, compassion—with clients as the core of the care they give, but at the same time they must recognize that access to treatment is precarious, eating disorders are tenacious, and clients may not want to—or be able to—get well. Caring may lead nowhere. Clients might get sicker or even die. Or clients may start to get better and then be denied further insurance coverage and have to be discharged. In such a context, understandings of illness that allow for—and even require—the withholding of responsiveness to clients' expressed needs can become especially persuasive as a way of managing the tension between care and detachment. In other words, figuring the client as always already *resistant* to care structures the affective atmosphere of treatment in profound ways, conditioning clinicians and insurance providers to view clients' struggles not as symptoms but as willful noncompliance that delegitimizes clients as subjects of care.

Some clinicians blame the dismal treatment situation on clients themselves, not only for being "resistant" but also for not selecting the correct managed care plan to cover their needs. "Look," said Margot, a Cedar Grove therapist, talking about a client who was upset that her insurance refused to cover residential care, "it's like you went to the store and you bought a blue sweater and wore it for a while. And then you decided you wanted a red sweater. Well, that's too bad—you bought a blue one. That's what you've got. . . . It's a thing with this population," she continued. "They don't do well with limits." Margot sees treatment issues not as a *structural* problem but as an *individual* one that reflects clients' difficulty accepting limits or not getting their way.

Margot's analogy seems to miss the fact that most people have a restricted number of "sweaters" to choose from and that many insurance plans exclude "sweaters" of any color from coverage or forbid red ones specifically. Nevertheless, the rhetorical figuring of clients and their families as rational consumers reflects a cultural narrative of "choice" and "empowerment" that places the burden on them rather than insurance companies for the inability to access care, or on clinicians for not delivering it.

These kinds of machinations speak to the ways in which the precarious nature of eating disorders treatment in the American managed care setting makes clinicians' affective investment in clients feel both critically important and potentially dangerous. To manage this tension, clinicians rely on a variety of strategies that allow them to engage in a *withholding of care* while also construing this withholding to be an ethical and even therapeutic act. In so doing, structures of care, conditioned by economic and political structures beyond the clinic, become folded into ontologies of illness—understandings of what constitutes the very nature of a condition—in ways that reinscribe the very practices of restricting, withholding, and denying basic needs that treatment is supposed to heal. That is, "care" for eating disorders comes to be characterized by practices of deprivation—withholding attention, time, or services—that are framed as therapeutic acts, while clients are induced to be satisfied with less, to deny their needs, and to be grateful for whatever they receive in order to demonstrate their desire to get well.

PARADOXICAL ERASURE: THE DOUBLE BINDS OF AN EATING DISORDER

Such (il)logics regarding recognition, relationship, and care shape every aspect of living with—and recovering from—an eating disorder, and the challenges clients face in treatment resonate deeply with a number of core tensions that animate eating disorders themselves.

People who develop eating disorders often have lived lives of paradoxical erasure. While the specifics are different for everyone, one core common feature I have discerned in people who have developed eating disorders is the experience, often from a young age, of being the focus of heightened attention or scrutiny and also fundamental, devastatingly painful misrecognition. That is, they are surveilled but not seen; monitored but not heard; afforded agency[46] but undermined or delegitimized. These kinds of double binds form what I consider to be the heart of an eating disorder. They happen in families, in social relationships, in treatment, and within society more generally.

Because of this, people with eating disorders often inhabit a space of tension between wanting—needing—to be seen and known, and yet also wanting to disappear from view. Even though they crave to be seen, that experience itself can be overwhelming, especially when that seen-ness has a history of bringing with it other forms of erasure, rejection, intrusion, or physical, emotional, or structural violence. Under such conditions, being seen or looked at can feel fundamentally violating and frightening. Yet being ignored or unseen carries its own legacies of pain. This dynamic of "see me but don't look at me" can be maddening for caregivers and loved ones, who often interpret the simultaneous demand that they *see* and *know* and *acknowledge* the person in front of them, even while she hides and obfuscates and pushes them away, as manipulative and "gamey."

But what most people don't know is that the experience of desperately needing to be seen but simultaneously experiencing that seeing as profoundly invasive and destructive is to be caught in a paradox so painful that it consumes one's entire being. It is like being underwater, with every cell of your body screaming for air to breathe, but the only air available burns and blisters your lungs. What are you going to do? You *need* to breathe it or you will die. You *crave* air, gasp for it. But once you finally let it in, the pain of the burning is so deep and profound that you wonder with each breath how you will possibly survive. And as soon as the worst has passed, there it is again: the growing need for oxygen.

These dynamics of visibility and invisibility in eating disorders are part of broader struggles with interpersonal recognition and connection, which can take many forms. In her compelling book *Abject Relations,* anthropologist Megan Warin argues that eating disorders are, at heart, about regulating interpersonal connectedness, and that people use food and their bodies as a way of constituting and traversing, in carefully controlled ways, the boundaries between themselves and others.[47] Specifically, she focuses on "the abject": those aspects of relatedness that women with anorexia tend to find the most frightening and difficult.

Here, I extend Warin's analysis by considering not only how eating disorders help sufferers manage the abject but also how they are a means for *seeking* connection, for extending an ethical demand to others.[48] That is, they are not just about hiding, rejecting, and pushing away. There is also a very strong tendency in people with an eating disorder to *reach toward,* although this is often hard for others to perceive. Tuning into this is critical for treatment and recovery, because it is where strength and effervescence can be cultivated.

Tuning in requires us to understand that this "push me/pull you" dynamic of "see me!" and "don't look at me!" *is not about the caregivers or loved ones,* or wanting to punish, game, or manipulate them. Rather, we—people with eating disorders—*need* to be seen and *need* our existence to be affirmed because we have no sense of how we appear to others, no understanding of the reality of our own existence. What is reflected back to us is so different from how we experience ourselves that it seems as distorted to us as our own body image seems to others. It just doesn't compute. For example, even today I have to accept that I simply have no concept of what I actually look like or the impact my existence has on others. This can, at times, be highly inconvenient, both for me and the people around me. And this is why people with eating disorders can sometimes appear self-centered or selfish when they don't think about how their actions might affect other people, but this is because *we don't experience ourselves as existing or mattering enough for it to make any difference one way or another.* It takes a significant amount of reeducation and therapy to begin to accept that our existence matters enough to matter. An obsession with looking in mirrors, habitual body checking, the constant need for reassurance and affirmation, and similar eating disorder behaviors reflect the difficulty of trying to make sense of our physical and relational imprint on the world. It is our way of trying to struggle out whether and to what extent we are really *here.*

Specifically, such practices are a venue for articulating and coming to terms with the conditions of becoming *a locally recognized, fully legitimated subject.* By this, I mean being seen, heard, and regarded as someone with legitimate claims to being. This subjectification proceeds along three primary axes.

Visible/Invisible

How is one seen (or not seen) as a full and legitimate subject? Here, I mean "seen" in the abstract sense of being recognized conceptually (i.e., interpersonally. legally, politically, socially, and culturally). But I also mean it in the concrete sense of being literally seen, perceived with the eyes.

In eating disorders, these two senses of being seen are conflated, yet they also sit in tension. People are made both visible and invisible—they become "spectacles" to others even as they try to literally disappear from view and/or hide their afflictions and suffer in secret. They become the focus of attention while also feeling profoundly *un*seen for who they really are. This dynamic persists in the context of treatment, where becoming "visible" means rendering oneself in the local terms of recognition, which are *numbers:* weights, lab values, blood pressures, heart rates. This very process of abstraction that allows clients to be seen simultaneously erases them, as it obscures and submerges the bulk of what an eating disorder is, what it does, and how it is lived. What are the processes of becoming seen—or being erased—in the context of eating disorders treatment, and what conditions them?

Speaking/Silent

How is one's voice heard (or silenced) as that of a full and legitimate subject? How is it cultivated or squelched, and with what effects? Here, too, I mean "heard" both in the abstract sense of one's point of view being recognized and acknowledged, and in the literal sense of having (or not having) a say or of being (un)intelligible to others.

In eating disorders, both these senses of "voice" are at play. Sufferers' behaviors become outward proclamations of pain, grief, rage, and shame, and yet almost no one else can understand what they are trying to say. In frustration, the behaviors may intensify, causing these women to be characterized as so ill that they have no legitimate voice at all. This paradox continues in treatment: in the context of managed mental healthcare, clients are simultaneously induced to develop and use their voices in their quest for (self-responsible) health, and delegitimized as impaired subjects who speak only with and through their illnesses, and who therefore should not be taken seriously. This produces a catch-22 in that, while clients are expected to take charge of their own recoveries, the only time their voices are recognized as legitimate is after the work of treatment is complete. What, then, is the lived experience of speaking and not being heard, understood, or taken seriously in the process of treatment?

Agent/Object

How does one take action as a full and legitimate subject? How does the way one's behavior is interpreted and experienced shift depending on the perceived legitimacy of one's agentic position?

In organizing their lives around and through their eating disorders, sufferers leave themselves vulnerable to cooptation by others, by the healthcare system, and by their illnesses. In the context of managed mental healthcare, the continuation of benefits often hinges on clients' demonstrating that they have developed and deployed "proper" agentic selves. Yet the characterization of eating disorder patients as "controlling" and "manipulative" has a long and deep history (see chapter 2), and this history sheers across these expectations, catching clients in double binds wherein attempts to demonstrate agency—even "proper" agency—become caught up in interpretations about control, resistance, and manipulation that undo the very work clients are being asked to perform. What does it mean to not be an agent in one's own life but rather to perceive oneself as existing solely as an object for others? How does this play out in the context of treatment, where one is simultaneously constituted as an "object" of care and denied the very agentic legitimacy demanded *by* that care?

In answering these questions in the course of this text, we will see that eating disorders—and eating disorders treatments—*articulate and reenact the very kinds of double binds and contradictions that give rise to them.* But eating disorders are more than simple reenactments. They are strategies for *honing* these experiences in very particular ways. This project is complexly engaged—and both strengthened and undermined—in the course of treatment.

LOSING HOPE

Let's return to Hope—Cedar Grove's underweight client with anorexia who was put on a diet *inside* the clinic. This is what happened: Hope's insurance had run out, and the only way she could continue to get treatment was to meet the strict parameters for a randomized controlled trial at a local university that was testing the effectiveness of a particular therapeutic intervention as opposed to meal support through dietician oversight alone. Although it was not assured that Hope would be placed into the group receiving the therapy intervention, as the selection process was randomized, the Cedar Grove clinicians reasoned that if she participated in the research trial, she would at the very least receive free meal support, which was more than what she could get without insurance. By that point, Hope was at 83 percent of her ideal body weight, which was 3 percent higher than what was required to get into the study, despite the fact that the threshold for an anorexia nervosa diagnosis was 85 percent. So the clinic team had to make a decision: discharge her at 83 percent with no support or get her down to 80 percent so she could enroll in the study and get meal support. They chose the latter. What looks like harm becomes a form of care; but what passes as care necessitates harm.

RESPONSIVE CARE

In thinking through these issues in the context of my ethnographic and clinical material, I have found the work of philosophers Dorothée Legrand and

Frédéric Briend to be especially helpful.[49] Writing from a phenomenological perspective, Legrand and Briend argue that eating disorders contain within them what philosopher Emmanuel Levinas characterizes as the "ethical demand of a response" from the other.[50]

Levinas specifically distinguishes "response" from "answer" in his discussion of ethics. An *answer*, according to Levinas, entails the provision of specific information addressed to the question. So, as Legrand and Briend illustrate, the question "What time is it?" might receive the answer "Four o'clock," or even "I don't know." Both are answers to the question about the time. A *response*, on the other hand, is a uniquely interpersonal event, which involves the acknowledgement of one's right to recognition—that is, the right to make a claim on the other, who is ethically obliged to respond. This is not the same as an answer. A clock provides an answer to the question "What time is it?" but does not provide a response, since there is no inter-recognition of subjectivity.

People suffering from eating disorders, Legrand and Briend argue, use their bodies—their starving, malnourished, visibly suffering bodies—to solicit *responsiveness* from their environments; that is, they use their bodies to seek *acknowledgement that they exist as legitimate subjects worthy of recognition as such*. This is different from the "answer" of providing physical nourishment, which can be done without such recognition of one's subjectivity and can, in fact, sometimes become a form of erasure.

ORGANIZATION OF THE BOOK

Famished is organized into four sections. In section 1, I consider the constitution of eating disorders as a certain kind of problem within the epistemological and practical structures of Cedar Grove specifically and contemporary American psychiatry more broadly. Following this introduction, chapter 2, "Rethinking Eating Disorders," offers a cultural analysis of contemporary eating disorder theories, highlighting the contradictory nature of the prototypical "eating-disordered body" and "eating-disordered self" contained within them and considering how this sets clients up for failure in treatment. Chapter 3, "Eating Disorders as Technologies of Presence," presents my understandings of eating disorders and offers a new framework for how to think about them both as lived conditions and as social and cultural phenomena.

Section 2 turns to three key vectors through which the conceptual and theoretical understandings of eating disorders described in section 1 begin to enter into and affect the material world. Chapter 4, "Identifying the Problem," details how eating disorders become objects of concern in the clinic and how particular sets of meanings circulate through research, practice, and managed care priorities, looping around to constitute the reality of eating disorders at Cedar Grove. Chapter 5, "A Hell That Saves You," details Cedar Grove's treatment program as a comprehensive engagement with the physical, behavioral, and emotional lives of clients. Chapter 6, "Fixing Time," considers how competing reckonings of time at Cedar Grove structure understandings of chronicity and recovery and set the framework for the process of treatment at the clinic.

Section 3 takes a deeper ethnographic dive into the treatment process at Cedar Grove and foregrounds clients' experiences of the treatment process. Chapter 7, "Loosening the Ties that Bind," details the first few weeks of treatment, as clients are wrested loose from their lives "outside" and begin to let go of old ways of being and reach toward new ones. Chapter 8, "Me, Myself, and Ed," highlights the core of the recovery process, which involves clients learning to form new sorts of relationships with their eating disorders in which their conditions are part of—but separate from—their true selves. This provokes a profound existential crisis from which clients must return in order to continue their process of recovery; although it is precisely at this point that insurance companies are most likely to determine that a client is "well" and thus mandate discharge. Chapter 9, "'Fat' is Not a Feeling," addresses how clients learn new practices of presencing and get ready to leave the clinic. Detailing how the clinic's program seeks to transform clients' embodied lives, the chapter engages issues of lapse and relapse and identifies what clients find the most helpful in navigating these challenges. It also presents clients' own visions of ideal care.

In section 4, the text considers the implications of the issues discussed in the first three sections for relationships of care in Cedar Grove and beyond. Chapter 10, "Running on Empty," details how the culture of deprivation at the clinic as structured by managed care affects how both therapists and clients come to understand clients' capacities for healthy agency and therefore their deservedness for care. Specifically, I look at attributions of manipulation and noncompliance as sites where these concerns are worked out, albeit usually to the detriment of the client. Chapter 11, "Capitalizing on Care," situates the Cedar Grove therapists and the clinic itself within broader economic changes in the world of behavioral health. I highlight the move toward what I call *therapreneurism,* which sits uneasily with the skills and capacities most necessary for effective therapeutic engagement. In chapter 12, "Conclusions," I offer concluding thoughts about what can be done to ameliorate the significant structural, institutional, and social barriers to effective eating disorder care and point to resources for more information and for getting involved in education and advocacy efforts.

Roller-Skating

I am eight years old. I am roller-skating on the linoleum floor in the sunroom, practicing spins and going backward, enjoying myself. Grandma is visiting from Virginia, and I feel proud showing off for her what I can do. She and Mom sit nearby, smoking cigarettes and watching.

"She has nice legs," my grandmother says to my mother. I am surprised, but pleased at the compliment. Then, after a moment, she adds, "They're a little heavy, but they're nice."

My heart sinks into my stomach. I suddenly feel very vulnerable, exposed. I can tell Mom is taken aback and doesn't know what to say.

"Her shoulders are good, though," says Grandma, and takes another puff of her cigarette.

Rethinking Eating Disorders

Where I come from, it's a very small town in the Bible Belt. Religious. So a lot of people associate anorexia with sin. If I only prayed enough, or if I only went to church enough, if I was only *good* enough, then it would go away. And I think that's one of the biggest things I struggle with—you can feel the judgment when people see you. It's like, "Well, why doesn't she just get over it? Why doesn't she just eat?" or, "She's doing it for attention." That's what I've overheard people say a lot. And that really hurts. "She's obviously got evil somewhere in her or something." I've heard that.

[So] I rebel, I become very bitter. When I was home, I was very bitter towards the town and the community. I kind of just removed myself from religion in general. And I'm very outspoken about my political views and things. Just anything to rebel. I'd be like, "Screw you. You think I'm evil now? Well, gosh, wait 'til something else." It's just very hard.

—KENDALL,
a twenty-year-old woman diagnosed with anorexia

Anorexia nervosa was first identified in the English medical literature in 1874.[1] Since then, scores of academics, clinicians, cultural theorists, journalists, and eating disorder survivors have produced thousands of books and articles about eating disorders for academic and popular audiences alike, with topics as varied as the unconscious psychosexual causes of disordered eating, the neurobiology of starvation, the religious dimensions of anorexia, and family systems approaches to treatment. Clinical texts, therapeutic manuals, autobiographical accounts, and self-help guides abound, offering information, guidance, and hope.

The authors' priorities in these texts are similarly diverse. Psychologically or clinically oriented works tend to focus on the personal psychological and family dynamics thought to give rise to these conditions, as well as on the kinds of treatment interventions that seem to help. Key themes include parent and child attachment styles, developmental processes, gender and sexuality, and emotions such as shame, desire, and fear related to processes of maturation. These texts tend to locate the "problem" of the eating disorder within the psychological life of the sufferer (or, in some cases, the family system), and interventions are aimed at resolving deep-seated conflicts around femininity, sexuality, and separation.

Writing from a very different perspective, cultural theorists and philosophers tend to locate eating disorders within the ideological foundations of Western modernity. Some cite the legacy of Descartes and aspects of the capitalist ethos as primary contributors. Others examine media influences, changes in gender roles following the advent of second-wave feminism, and conservative backlash as the primary cultural conditions that give rise to eating disorders.

In the social sciences and humanities, historians and historically oriented scholars have examined overlaps between eating disorders and medieval religious asceticism, Victorian hysteria, and nineteenth-century fasting girls. Anthropologists and sociologists study such things as the practices that sustain and reinforce eating disorders, including everyday relationships, "fat talk" between girls, and treatments within eating disorders clinics. Cross-cultural research documents the apparent rise in eating disorders around the world in the wake of globalization, leading to the proposition that the West is exporting eating disorders along with our media images, consumer products, models of economic development, and modes of medical diagnosis.

Outside of clinical and academic works, eating disorders have become fixtures of American popular culture. Heart-wrenching autobiographical accounts, guidebooks for parents on how to help a child with an eating disorder, workbooks for people in recovery, inspirational meditation books, therapeutic manuals, informational websites, blogs, and articles in magazines from *Cosmopolitan* to *Good Housekeeping* have flooded bookstore and supermarket shelves over the past thirty years, seeking to educate lay audiences about these illnesses, what causes them, and how to help people who suffer from them. Eating disorders have been featured in award-winning documentaries (*Thin*), blockbuster films (*Black Swan*), HBO features (*To the Bone*), and primetime TV shows (*Rehab*), where visual displays of their self-destructive extremes can be shocking in their intensity. Many college campuses across the United States host annual "fat talk free" events to encourage positive body image among students, and Eating Disorder Awareness Week has become a national phenomenon, complete with T-shirts, ribbons, fundraisers, and posters featuring celebrities promoting healthy eating and self-acceptance.

Given this proliferation of information, why write—or read—yet another book about eating disorders? Because despite—or perhaps because of—more than a century of theorizing and writing about these conditions, pervasive misperceptions and stigma about eating disorders abound, not just in popular media and among the public, but among clinicians and specialists as well.

Eating disorders are often characterized as a form of adolescent rebellion or resistance to authority, and clients are generally constituted as difficult, manipulative, and deceptive. For example, while not an academic source, a 2014 blog post on the *Psychology Today* website entitled "Duplicity, Lies, Manipulation and Eating Disorders: Are you Ready for Treatment?" both expresses and reinforces negative stereotypes of eating disorder sufferers. The author, Judy Scheel (PhD, licensed clinical social worker, and certified eating disorders specialist), prompts suffers to ask themselves the following questions:

1. Do I lie about my symptoms? If so, what purpose does covering up my symptoms serve?
2. Am I the real me with people? Does that matter to me?
3. Does it matter to me that I cover up my symptoms?
4. Do I think others would understand if I told them the truth about my eating disorder?
5. Am I ready to work on being honest about my eating disorder?

While the overall tone of the article is actually rather compassionate, these kinds of portrayals perpetuate perceptions of people with eating disorders as unreliable, scheming, and oppositional to care. These views reflect a profound misunderstanding of these conditions and have very real impacts on sufferers and the kind of care they receive or are denied.

In this chapter, I provide a brief overview of some current approaches to understanding and treating eating disorders, as well as some historical context for their development. I then draw out a number of the assumptions and contradictions that thread through these different models, which, in practice, catch clients in a set of double binds. In this way, we can begin to build an understanding of why and how contemporary approaches to treatment often fail.

WHY EATING DISORDERS ARE "GOOD TO THINK":
FOOD, CULTURE, AND RELATEDNESS

Anthropologists have long observed that food and eating are panhuman modes of social communication and connection.[2] Who procures food; who cooks it; who serves it; how, when, and where it is eaten; what kinds of food are eaten on what occasions; what foods are forbidden and why—within any social group, these kinds of activities and their attendant meanings provide the most basic structures of group cohesion and identity. How food is managed in a group, and how this is understood, enfolds fundamental information about the bonds of connection among members, group boundaries, and group identity.

These social meanings are closely entwined with very real questions of survival. When humans are very young, we are entirely dependent on others to sustain us. Food and nourishment become vectors for the group's investment in an individual person. Food also solidifies relationships and hierarchies, articulates and affirms group identities, and can carry religious and spiritual significances. Food is so symbolically potent because it is the very stuff of life. Without it, we die. With it, we become alive and engaged in social and moral worlds that are negotiated, day in and day out, through practices related to food and eating.

Given this, we can understand how unusual eating behaviors—particularly those that involve rejecting needed nourishment through fasting or some sort of purging—might be very distressing not only to individual people and families but also to social groups as a whole. From an anthropological perspective, rejecting food communicates far more than simply a desire to be thin. It might also communicate a rejection of connection to the social group or to specific others within this group.[3]

In addition to the social meanings attached to food and eating, food is symbolically powerful because of its very materiality. It is a substance that crosses the body boundaries, transitioning from being something in the external world ("not me") to being part of one's physical constitution ("me") and then, through excretion, becoming "not me" again. In this way, food and other forms of nourishment are substances through which we literally incorporate the world, making it part of us as it is transformed into the blood, bones, organs, and tissues we use to live. It also, as we have seen, communicates layers of social embeddedness and relationships. What we eat and how we eat, then, actually *constitutes* the relationship between our "selves" (bodily and otherwise) and the world around us.

Given these particular properties of food and its importance in creating and maintaining self-world relationships, it is not at all surprising that food might become a focus of attention for people who, for whatever reason, are dealing with challenges or questions about themselves and their place in the world. If someone feels lost, confused, anxious, angry, afraid, or conflicted about her purpose in life and her role in the greater social world, developing new behaviors around food and eating is, in fact, a brilliant choice. It kills multiple birds with one stone, so to speak, engaging with social structural arrangements, interpersonal dynamics, and personal psychological concerns all at the same time and also integrating these with the visceral, lived experience of the body.

Eating disorders thus find resonance and purchase across a range of different registers, from the micro level (e.g., psychological, phenomenological, physiological) to the meso level (e.g., affective, behavioral, interpersonal/relational) to the macro level (e.g., social, political, cultural). They crystallize and make manifest concerns at each level in ways that may appear to be contradictory but that in fact "make sense" in the logic of the eating disorder; or, better said, *the eating disorder helps to make sense of life conditions that otherwise would be irreconcilable.* In this way, eating disorders both express and attempt to find resolutions to various psychological, interpersonal, and cultural illogics, even as they endanger the lives of sufferers. Similarly, treatments for disordered eating not only grapple with their specific biological, psychological, and social dimensions but also, more importantly, *postulate how these components are thought to interact with one another.* That is, they enfold and naturalize local cultural understandings of the proper arrangements of micro-, meso-, and macro-level issues. It is here, in the configuration of elements and the conceptual links thought to produce those configurations, that the influence of cultural and historical values and priorities becomes most apparent.

A key argument of this book is that what we now identify as eating disorders are dynamic affective/cognitive/behavioral/phenomenal flows around which we have drawn lines and to which we attribute the status of "fact" but which, in reality, serve as something of a Rorschach test for a given society's prevailing anxieties about relatedness, dependence, vulnerability, and meaning. In understanding how and why these dynamic flows become fixed in time, space, epistemology, and practice, and how this reflects local values regarding self-world dynamics, we can better understand how contemporary frictions and fractures in care occur and how we can better help those who suffer.

THE HAUNTINGS OF HYSTERIA: A BRIEF OVERVIEW OF THEORIES ABOUT EATING DISORDERS

You don't have to be a house to be haunted.

— EMILY DICKINSON

Eating disorders—or collections of behaviors that look a lot like eating disorders—have been part of the human experience for at least as long as recorded history and show up in accounts from Europe, Africa, and Asia. Wherever such phenomena appear, they become sites of contention about bodies, selves, and relatedness and occasions for struggles over meaning, power, and agency. How these phenomena are defined, understood, and treated can reveal much about local investments and priorities regarding human life, human relatedness, and the ethics of care.

What I present here is a curated look at some of the historical antecedents to contemporary understandings of these conditions. It is important to remember that these developments were not linear or mutually exclusive and that multiple understandings can coexist. In fact, this is part of what makes eating disorders and eating disorders treatments so interesting and illustrative from an anthropological perspective—there is no clear consensus about what these phenomena are, why they arise, or how to treat them, and debates about them become ways of struggling out more fundamental questions, such as the nature of human cognition, the relationship between the mind and the body, and the moral dimensions of dependency.

Early Accounts of Disordered Eating

Written accounts of voluntary self-starvation date back to at least the Middle Ages, when extreme fasting and other unusual food and eating behaviors appeared as part of a constellation of practices common to female religious ascetics in Europe. Catherine of Siena, Teresa of Ávila, and dozens of other women across the region reportedly subsisted on nothing but the Eucharist, refusing to eat even when ordered to do so by church superiors, or sometimes vomiting when forced to ingest food. This "holy anorexia"[4] became a site of contention among church leaders, some of whom viewed the behavior as miraculous, evidence of God's grace and a testament to the practitioner's penitential devotion. Others criticized it as a way of making claims to direct divine connection while bypassing the traditional authority (and gender) structures of the church. Still others saw it as the work of the devil luring vulnerable women to crave the attention and notoriety that often came as a result. At issue here was not simply whether a nun ate her evening meal but how the materiality of the temporal body and the immateriality of the immortal soul were linked and with what consequences.[5]

During the Renaissance, self-starvation (again, mostly by young women) accrued different explanatory models as scholars sought to establish a medical foundation for the condition, proposing a variety of different pathogenic pathways. It was during this time that the first description of voluntary self-starvation as what we would now call a mental condition appeared in a 1694 text by Richard Morton, who characterized it as "nervous consumption" and described the association of self-starvation with hyperactivity and excessive studying.[6] A key dimension of debates about these behaviors during this time had to do with whether the disorder was located primarily in the physical body or was instead a disorder of the spirit or the will.

Despite occasional appearances in the medical literature, there doesn't seem to have been another widespread phenomenon of women's self-starvation until the eighteenth and nineteenth centuries, when a number of cases of "miraculous maids" or "fasting girls" became widely known in Britain.[7] Reportedly living on very little food—or none at all—fasting girls captured the public imagination, even as they became sites of contention between medical and religious specialists, both of whom sought claims to authoritative knowledge of the phenomenon. At heart, the question seemed to remain the same as in earlier times: Does this behavior indicate a disruption of the body or a perturbation of the soul? And what is the relationship between the two?

Medical dominion over girls' self-starvation solidified with the first published clinical descriptions of *anorexia hysterique,* by Ernest-Charles Lasègue in 1873, and *anorexia nervosa,* by Sir William Gull in 1874. Both physicians described a series of cases of young girls, and some boys, who refused to eat despite growing increasingly skeletal, and who demonstrated marked fear and panic when forced to eat. A hallmark of this condition was, specifically, the *nervosa* or *hysterique* aspect of it—the fact that no physiological cause could be identified for the lack of appetite and refusal to eat and that food and eating seemed to provoke such pronounced fear and anxiety. The debate during this time again centered on whether this new condition was primarily a bodily illness or an expression of some sort of dysfunction in the will, mind, or moral constitution of the individual.

By the end of the nineteenth century, the question of whether to think of anorexia nervosa as primarily physical or nonphysical in origin was elaborated in the different views of physicians Jean-Martin Charcot (1825–93) and Pierre Janet (1859–1947)—early pioneers of the psychosomatic. Both Charcot and Janet understood anorexia nervosa to be a form of hysteria (that is, an apparently physiological impairment for which no physiological cause could be discerned), and both agreed that anorexia had something to do with the relationship between the psyche and the soma, though they disagreed on the pathogenic pathways and therefore on the interventions to be used for a cure.

Charcot is known as the father of modern neurology and a pioneer in the study of hypnosis and hysteria. While working at the famous Pitié-Salpêtrière Hospital in Paris, Charcot became fascinated with bodily contortions and debilities (e.g., numbness and paralysis)—mostly in young women—that could not be explained physiologically. Drawing on the ancient Greek illness category of hysteria, Charcot first hypothesized that such debilities were due to inherited neurological conditions. As his career progressed, however, he began to suspect that there were psychogenic origins to these symptoms and thus developed strategies of hypnosis to cure his patients by revealing buried sexual conflicts and desires. Charcot found that as these deep, dark sexual urges were unearthed, the hysterical symptoms, like anorexia, seemed to resolve.

Charcot's work on the psychogenic origins of hysteria was continued by his student Pierre Janet. Janet was one of the first to posit a connection between specific past life events and hysterical symptoms, and he was also the first to coin the terms "dissociation" and "subconscious." Putting forward a developmental model of mind, Janet argued that hysteria, as a form of neurosis, resulted from the failure of earlier developmental tendencies to be integrated with higher-level tendencies or from a regression to earlier developmental stages. In the case of hysteria, Janet believed that the body became a vehicle of symbolic communication for distress, whether expressing something about specific events that had happened in the past or manifesting regressed developmental tendencies. By working with patients' bodily symptoms as encoded communications about dissociated memories, affects, and needs, Janet aimed to help patients return to "appropriate" developmental trajectories.

Both Charcot and Janet, then, understood girls' voluntary self-starvation as a form of hysteria linked to submerged sexual conflicts and/or regression to earlier developmental phases. Charcot, however, focused on the neurological pathways by which this hysterical condition became manifest (that is, he took soma as a primary focus), whereas Janet's concern was with processes of dissociation and the psychosomatic expression of past traumatic events (he prioritized psyche).

When Sigmund Freud came onto the scene and began to theorize anorexia in the early twentieth century, the relationship between psyche and soma became the center of a new intellectual and therapeutic movement—psychoanalysis—and anorexia (still considered a form of hysteria) took on a whole new set of meanings. Freud's understanding of hysteria—including anorexia nervosa—brought together Charcot's concern with physiology and Janet's focus on the subconscious in an attempt to provide a synthetic understanding of the relationship between psyche and soma. I will spend some time on Freud's understanding of anorexia and on later post-Freudian developments, as they set the stage for the current landscape of eating disorders treatment.

Eating Daddy's Baby and Throwing Up Mommy

When Freud first tackled the "enigma" of anorexia nervosa in 1918, he proposed a complicated model of oedipal fantasies and forbidden desires that were, he argued, sublimated and articulated in an anorexic girl's unusual food behaviors. He suggested that little girls live a masculine life until the traumatic and earthshaking discovery that they do not have a penis, that they are "mutilated." This discovery leads them to a violent rage against their mother, who "betrayed" them by not giving them a penis and did not prepare them for this devastating revelation. Until this maternal betrayal, Freud tells us, little girls enjoy a phallic sexuality, with their mother as the love object, and they fantasize about having a baby by her. But the discovery that they lack a penis, and the resulting penis envy, propels girls headlong into the oedipal phase, where they seek refuge with their father and direct hatred at their faithless mother.

In this model, food becomes a powerful symbol for the acting out of oedipal conflicts. Food becomes simultaneously a symbol of the mother who is being rejected and the penis the girl does not have but can "enjoy" through sexual intercourse. The anorexic girl, according to Freud, has fantasies of oral impregnation by her father, and food becomes a sexualized symbol of this wish. At the same time, food represents the "poison" transmitted to the girl through the (now hated) mother's breast, leading to an ambivalent relationship to food, and either anorexic or bulimic food behaviors (or both) are the pathological expression of this conflict.

In other words, classic Freudian psychoanalysis considers the anorexic girl to be neurotically fixated on being entered by a penis or, failing this, symbolically enacting her desires through food. She paradoxically desires to be like a man while at the same time wanting to have a child by her father, a child who would then become a substitute for the coveted penis. So great is the girl's envy of the male organ, in fact, that, ironically, even the rejection of food is read as the wish for a penis. Treatment from this perspective, therefore, centers on inducing the girl to give up her phallic aspirations (such as pursuing an advanced education, wanting a career, or becoming involved in politics) and accept her "proper" female roles as wife and mother. As she does so, her need to use food to enact her unconscious psychosexual conflicts will subside.

Bracketing for the moment the various problematic aspects of Freud's model, we can see here that his psychoanalytic take on anorexia seeks to encompass the concerns of both Charcot and Janet with regards to the soma/psyche relationship by transposing these questions into the domains of sexuality and gender. Freud theorized that it is through the shaping of the child's sexual desire, and her sense of herself as a sexual(ized) and gendered being, that psyche and soma can come into conflict, thereby producing hysterical symptoms like anorexia. The resolution of these conflicts, then, would pave the path to healing. In other words, according to Freud, anorexia is first a foremost a problem of improper or incomplete gender and sexual development (the two were inseparable for him), and this theme—albeit in somewhat different configurations--continues to inform eating disorder theories and treatments today.

Post-Freudian Developments

Freud was, from the very beginning, a controversial figure, and even during his lifetime critiques and counternarratives to his understandings of psychosexual development emerged. In terms of anorexia, later psychoanalytic thinkers turned Freud's interpretation a bit, reading food refusal less as a desire for pregnancy and more as an expression of infantilism—a rejection of adult sexuality and a desire to return to the supposedly idyllic time of childhood. In this understanding, the anorexic girl's refusal of food is read as the attempt to achieve a regressive state in which self-induced starvation—leading to a repression of appetite, sexual drive, and signs of physical maturation—enables her to avoid both the maturational issues of sexual development, independence, and autonomy and the frightening prospect of healthy adult female sexuality.

The specifics of this process were conceptualized somewhat differently by different post-Freudian schools of thought,[8] but all maintained the essential commitment to understanding food and eating behaviors both as expressive of existing attachment concerns and enactments of wished-for attachments with caregivers as well as manifesting psychosexual conflicts. Treatment from such perspectives emphasized forcing the patient to relinquish her "regressive" inclinations by refusing to gratify her "infantile" desires, which were read as manipulative strategies to get others to take care of her.

While such understandings of eating disorders may seem antiquated and few eating disorder clinicians today would readily claim psychoanalytic influences, many contemporary models of eating disorders and eating disorders treatment enfold and recast these same principles regarding gender, sexuality, and development, particularly in terms of how they assert that relationships of care should be managed.

Contemporary Psychodynamic Approaches

Psychodynamics is a term used to describe approaches that center on the "inner" workings of the mind and incorporate some notion of a dynamic or changeable unconscious. This is not the same thing as psychoanalysis or psychoanalytic theory, though they are related and share some concepts and terminology. A number of traditional "talk therapy" approaches can be considered psychodynamic, even though they may have absolutely nothing to do with the Oedipus complex and don't involve a couch. In fact, most psychodynamically informed therapists and theorists avidly reject classical Freudian propositions regarding gender, sexuality, and the nature and structure of the therapeutic process and would cringe at being confused with classical Freudian psychoanalysts (or even neo-Freudian analysts) in any way. Nevertheless, because psychodynamic theories do take up questions of how and why people change over time and how therapy can facilitate this process, they engage with many of the same sorts of questions that animated early psychoanalytic thinking—namely, the relationships between psyche and soma.

In terms of eating disorders, despite eschewing many psychoanalytic interpretations, contemporary psychodynamic and psychodynamically informed approaches (e.g., interpersonal therapy, Internal Family Systems Therapy, narrative therapy, and even dialectical behavior therapy) continue to focus on developmental concerns and/or locate the causes of eating disorders within the individual psyche of the patient and intimate relationships within the family system. Although they each take a somewhat different perspective on the process, these models generally figure eating disorders as springing primarily from difficulties with separation and individuation and fears of maturation. Such concerns supposedly manifest in fears of adult sexuality, which the person attempts to avoid by "starving out" secondary sex characteristics and remaining physiologically childlike (as in anorexia) or covering them up with excess flesh to appear less sexual (as in binge eating disorder). A focus on food and eating (or not eating) halts psychosocial and interpersonal development as well, as the eating disorder becomes the individual's primary obsession. Because these perspectives understand eating disorders as stunting the normal developmental and maturational process, interventions center on helping the sufferer become "unstuck" and proceed along the "normal" developmental path. In terms of treatment, this generally means that the clinician, hospital, or treatment center assumes the role of a sort of substitute family whose job is to help restart these stalled developmental processes and guide the client toward individuation. Although Cedar Grove is strongly interdisciplinary in its orientation, this particular strand of psychodynamic thinking deeply informs its program and daily practices.

Taken together, psychoanalytic and psychodynamic understandings of eating disorders as deeply entangled with questions of human development—especially issues of gender, sexuality, individuation, and relatedness—laid the foundation for later theoretical and clinical developments. Despite attempts to create distance from these psychoanalytic roots, current approaches continue to bank on assumptions that linger from these early formulations.

Family-Based and Ecological Approaches

The publication in 1978 of Salvador Minuchin, Bernice L. Rosman, and Lester Baker's *Psychosomatic Families: Anorexia Nervosa in Context* marked a milestone in thinking about eating disorders. In describing the kinds of families most likely to produce a "psychosomatic child" (that is, a child who expresses psychological distress through bodily symptoms), this book made a turn from viewing anorexia as a strictly individual concern to understanding it as the product of a broader family system. It also gave a step-by-step outline of how to treat anorexia, which even then was recognized as one of the most intractable and bewildering of the psychiatric conditions.

Building on the emergent family therapy movement, of which Minuchin was a key proponent, the authors described how stress, individual dispositional vulnerabilities, physiological responses, and family organization and functioning are all mutually affecting and will continue operating as a destructive system until and unless something breaks the cycle—or the child herself breaks. They argued that interventions for anorexia that take an individual approach target only one part of the process and one node in the circuitry—the child may improve, but if the family dynamics remain the same, the child will be recruited back into the system and the symptoms will reoccur. Dysfunctional family dynamics such as enmeshment, overprotectiveness, rigidity, and lack of conflict resolution, and certain relational dynamics such as triangulation, parent-child coalition, and detouring (when parents bury their own conflicts to focus on the "sick" or "bad" child) play a role in the creation of the psychosomatic child—although it is not clear to what extent the authors believed these to be unique features of "anorexogenic" families, psychosomatic families more broadly, or families where psychiatric concerns emerge in general. By offering detailed transcripts of multiple sessions with four "psychosomatic families," Minuchin and his colleagues demonstrate a treatment intervention focused on hospitalization for weight gain and behavior modification for the client in conjunction with therapy for the entire family.

The publication of *Psychosomatic Families* coincided with the heyday of family systems approaches to psychiatric illness and the flourishing of the addictions model[9] and self-help approaches[10] to a variety of conditions, including alcoholism, gambling, and overeating, all of which took an ecological view of human psychic struggles. It was during this time that concepts such as "dysfunctional families," "toxic parents," and "the inner child" came to the fore. Key debates in these movements centered on questions such as: Is the cause of addiction in the body or in the mind? Is suffering caused by dysfunctions in the person or in the environment? How one answers these questions has direct relevance to what one then changes to make things better.

Family therapy has remained a staple of eating disorders treatment, at least for clients who are children, adolescents, or young adults. In recent years, however, family-based interventions have radically transformed. Rather than viewing the family as the proximate cause of the eating disorder, emergent contemporary approaches engage the family as a resource for recovery. Specifically, family-based therapy (FBT) hinges on "empowering" the parents to reclaim their adolescent child's life from the eating disorder by (re) assuming control over all aspects of the his or her eating, as if the adolescent were a much younger child. In FBT, parents do this by deciding what, how much, and when a child will eat, requiring them to eat past their limits, and closely monitoring mealtimes.[11]

FBT specifically does *not* attend to ongoing family dynamics or engage the meanings behind the eating disorder. "Psychodynamic formulations are in your way here," FBT codeveloper James Lock explained in an FBT training I attended in St. Louis, Missouri, on September 26–27, 2016. "This is a strengths-based intervention. We don't look for the etiology." Instead, FBT is intended to be a behavioral intervention for the *parents* to enable them to assume authority and leadership vis-à-vis the adolescent and her eating disorder. "Negotiating with anorexia is like negotiating with a terrorist," said Lock. "First you lose an ear, then a finger, and then you're dead." The idea behind this intervention is that the eating disorder has hijacked the "normal" developmental process by inverting family roles so that the child and the eating disorder assume authority in the family system while the parents feel helpless to act. By, in effect, regressing the adolescent back to an earlier stage of feeding and eating relationships, the parents can regain control and then, ideally, help the child gradually resume self-directed eating in conjunction with undergoing other developmental tasks.

There is much to recommend FBT, and a significant amount of research supports this intervention as successful, at least for certain kinds of individuals in certain kinds of situations (that is, adolescents who live at home with two parents, one of whom can be at home for all meals to supervise the adolescent's eating). But a closer look reveals that the designs of the relevant studies generally purposefully exclude families not likely to be successful in the program, such as those where divorce, trauma, substance abuse, or other mental health issues are present, all of which are very common among this population.[12] Furthermore, measures of "success" that focus on weight gain and compliance with parental instructions do not take full account of clients' experiences or needs. A growing body of literature takes issue with some aspects of the FBT approach, faulting it not only for dismissing and minimizing clients' experiences but also for reinforcing the very family dynamics that can give rise to an eating disorder in the first place.[13]

Cognitive, Behavioral, and Learning Theories

As psychoanalytic and psychodynamic theories began to fall out of favor in the 1970s, a different model of human behavior took center stage: cognitive and learning theories that linked thought to behavior while bypassing the unconscious all together. These theories sought to account for behavior that might not be conscious without resorting to psychoanalytic unconscious explanations.

Cognitive, behavioral, and learning models emphasize the importance of environmental influences on the development of eating disorders, particularly in terms of learned thought patterns and behaviors. Some studies highlight the link between eating and anxiety or depression and point out how individuals can learn to alter these mood states through self-starvation, bingeing, or purging. Others note that as people receive positive reinforcement (either directly, from people in their lives, or indirectly, through images in the media) for losing weight and staying thin, they are more likely to engage in those practices to gain approval and positive regard. Over time, such practices can become habituated to the degree that they are difficult to discard. Social learning theories emphasize the idea that people emulate people they admire, such as peers or celebrity figures, and that this can be a primary motivator for eating disorders. In all cases, faulty cognition and distorted thinking are thought to be the root cause of self-destructive behaviors.

As cognitive, behavioral, and learning theories gained traction in the world of psychiatry, cognitive behavioral therapy (CBT) emerged as a modality of choice for many clinicians, including those in the field of eating disorders. In terms of treatment, this meant an increased emphasis on behavioral interventions focused on here-and-now issues, with less attention given to the underlying or unobservable aspects of these illnesses. While this approach often generated short-term improvements in measurable factors like body weight or frequency of bingeing and purging, many eating disorder specialists continued to insist that psychodynamic factors were, in fact, critical in understanding and treating these conditions and sustaining recovery long-term and were being ignored—a friction in the treatment world that continues to this day. Many of Cedar Grove's daily program activities and homework assignments (therapy assignments clients are to complete outside of session and then share with the group) are based in CBT principles, although clinicians also draw heavily on psychodynamic understandings of the overall process of recovery. The challenges created by this friction are explored more thoroughly in part 2.

Importantly, the shift away from dynamic models focused on the unconscious and toward cognitive-behavioral models concerned with observable and/or quantifiable factors went hand in hand with changes in the economics of healthcare, which were shifting toward a concern with cost-effectiveness, rationing, and "evidence." The rise of managed care, then, reinforced the ascendance of CBT and vice versa, a circuit that is explored in detail in chapter 3.

Biology-Centered Models

As noted above, understandings of biology and biological processes have long been central to understandings of disordered eating. But beginning in the 1990s, biologically centered models of eating disorders entered a new era. In concert with the broader disciplinary shift within psychiatry toward a focus on the biological correlates of psychiatric illness, and in conjunction with new technologies such as gene sequencing and fMRIs, the framing of eating disorders as first and foremost *biological* illnesses began to take hold.

Some research in this vein has focused on the genetics of eating disorders, suggesting that genetic factors may account for up over 50 percent of the risk of developing an eating disorder at some point during the life span.[14] Other work has focused on the body's reactions to severe malnutrition, positing that common features of anorexia like hyperactivity, obsessive thinking about food and eating, and a desire to eat alone may in fact be responses to acute starvation.[15] Studies of topics like neurotransmitters, endocrine function, metabolic processes, and genetic factors have come to dominate eating disorder research all over the world in the past twenty years.

So central has the biological narrative become in the field of eating disorder research that a statement issued by NIMH president Tom Insel (himself a father of a daughter in recovery for an eating disorder), and later circulated widely in news and social media and among eating disorder clinicians and advocates, officially identified anorexia as a "brain disorder" and specified future research pathways regarding the pathophysiology of eating disorders that should be expanded.[16] Eating disorder practitioners and advocates heralded this declaration as an unmitigated success and huge step forward for eating disorder awareness because it was seen to legitimize eating disorders as "real" illnesses in ways that they had not been before. It also supported efforts to get eating disorders classified as "serious mental illnesses" under current mental health parity laws. I take up this issue—including the risks of such a position—in chapter 12.

Treatment approaches based on biological models generally focus on weight restoration and the stabilization of medical indicators like blood pressure, heart rate, and lab values. Such an orientation is an important part of Cedar Grove's overall treatment program, although it exists alongside other modalities and approaches.

Focusing on the biological dimensions of eating disorders is essential, and locating their causes in biology may go some distance in reducing stigma and, perhaps, increasing access to some forms of care. But I want to raise some important questions here that we will return to throughout this book: Why must a condition be labeled "biological" or "biologically based" for it to be legitimized? Why is biology the arbiter of reality? And what happens to our collective moral responsibility in terms of social, institutional, and cultural change if we relegate eating disorders to the realm of biology? By insisting that eating disorders are primarily biological, we risk doing an end run around the pervasive and destructive structures, relationships, and practices that enable eating disorders to emerge and fluoresce. This figuring of biology as a proxy for legitimacy is an issue I will return to throughout this ethnography, as it has a great deal to do with the double binds inherent in eating disorders treatment.

Feminist/Cultural Models

Feminist/cultural models of eating disorders locate the pathology of the conditions not in the individual psyches of sufferers but in the cultural values and proscriptions within which women (primarily) try to make sense of their existence. They contend that a legacy of Cartesianism that devalues "the body" coupled with ideologies of self-improvement, autonomy, and austerity amid plenty as a moral virtue produces anorexia, in particular, as a "crystallization" of Western culture.[17] In such views, a woman with an eating disorder is not pathological or sick (as she is considered to be in the other perspectives). She has simply taken cultural lessons about the value of women to their logical extreme by embodying the injunction to take up as little (physical, social, political) space as possible while also denying herself pleasure in the pursuit of "higher" aspirations (resulting in anorexia nervosa) or by embodying the consumption patterns of a capitalist culture (resulting in bulimia nervosa). Because feminist approaches understand eating disorders as manifesting values that minimize, degrade, and silence women, interventions built on such perspectives (e.g., narrative therapy) favor helping women claim space for themselves in all realms of their personal and social lives as well as actively challenging the prevailing images and narratives that perpetuate the devaluation of women.

Interpersonal and Phenomenological Models

Interpersonal or phenomenological models of eating disorders build on psychodynamic, biological, behaviorist, and feminist/cultural models by focusing on the subjective, embodied experiences of eating disorder practices and the ways people use them to negotiate interpersonal dynamics situated within structures of power. From these perspectives, the causes of an eating disorder have less to do with individual pathology (as in psychodynamic or behavioral approaches), biological adaptation (as in biological approaches), and cultural messaging (as in feminist/cultural approaches) and more to do with how eating disorders function to shape interpersonal connectedness and the experience of living in relationship with others. Treatment from such an orientation (e.g., interpersonal therapy and to some degree dialectical behavior therapy) is focused on helping the person with an eating disorder develop new modes of interpersonal relating as well as new ways of living within their own embodied emotional worlds.

ENTANGLING PSYCHE AND SOMA: EATING DISORDER THEORIES AS PHILOSOPHIES OF EMBODIMENT

Theories are cultural artifacts. They are ideas generated by cultural beings in particular cultural and historical contexts for particular reasons. They are addressed to perceived questions or problems that are deemed important enough to puzzle over, and they offer hypotheses about those issues in ways that make sense of them according to prevailing cultural logics. As such, theories reveal a great deal about what people are concerned about, how they understand the world to work, and how they reason about that world.

While they each have different emphases, these various approaches to understanding eating disorders are not mutually exclusive, and most eating disorders clinics and eating disorder clinicians use some combination of them. For example, a CBT therapist might draw on psychodynamic or inter-personal understandings when working with family members, or work within a feminist-informed framework. A psychodynamically oriented therapist might also use CBT interventions or attend to biological factors. Cedar Grove draws on all of these approaches in crafting its program.

What stitches all of these approaches together, despite their differences, is a set of core cultural concerns about the relationships between "the body" and "the self" in eating disorders, which become a practical and pragmatic reality in clinical care. That is, these different understandings of eating disorders not only grapple with the specific biological, psychological, and social dimensions of these illnesses but also, and more importantly, *postulate how these components are thought to interact with one another.* While they may have quite different ways of thinking about this process, each model articulates a vision of how the psyche and soma interact.

For example, take three commonly accepted "facts" about anorexia: (1) women diagnosed with anorexia are usually emaciated; (2) women diagnosed with anorexia tend to be perfectionists; and (3) women diagnosed with anorexia are often high academic achievers.[18] One might interpret the coexistence of these factors very differently depending on the theoretical or practice orientation adopted. A more psychodynamic perspective might link these elements through a narrative about pre-oedipal and/or oedipal conflicts that lead a woman to reject her femininity and strive for characteristically "masculine" traits (e.g., a body with no curves, a focus on achievement). Or, taking a more interpersonal view, the narrative might be about a deep need to be accepted and approved of, or the need to feel some control over one's environment in a chaotic family situation. A feminist/cultural narrative might focus on messages that tell women they should take up the smallest space possible (socially, politically, physically) and that they must be "perfect" in all ways in order to be valued in a patriarchal society.

Each of these explanations, in addition to offering a conceptual model of eating disorders, engages fundamental questions about the *nature of being human*—how the biological, psychological, and social dimensions of human experience interact. Does the biological index the social, or the other way around? Does "pathology" emerge because of a woman's resistance to cultural norms or because of her submission to them? To what extent does culture get "inside" us? And, most critically, *how* do these things happen? Each model implicitly entails a series of propositions about the *metaphysical* (What constitutes the nature of being?) and the *existential* (What constitutes the meaningfulness of being?) dimensions of human existence that situate them in dialogue with broader social and cultural trends while at the same time lodging them firmly in the physicality of the human body. What animates these theories are propositions that seek to explain how energy, investment, and meaning move across these various domains. In other words, *theories about eating disorders telescope shifting cultural concerns and anxieties about meaningful human experience.* They enfold assertions about how the material (soma) and nonmaterial (psyche) aspects of being relate to one another, why it matters, and whether and how people can change.

Why is this important? In producing knowledge about disordered eating, contemporary Western psychiatric understandings of eating disorders constitute a collection of paradoxical subjectivities that, in practice, censure certain kinds of ethical demands from certain kinds of subjects. As such, recovery from these conditions according to such models is often highly problematic.

PARADOXICAL PATIENTS: PSYCHIATRY'S CORE CONTRADICTIONS ABOUT EATING DISORDERS

What, then, do current theories tell us about contemporary American beliefs, concerns, and anxieties about embodied subjects? Despite their differences, a set of core concerns or ambivalences about bodies, selves, embodiment, and dynamics emerge. Three issues in particular predominate: (1) boundaries and flow, (2) patterning and regulation, and (3) intensity and amplitude. These concerns manifest in three central constructions of people with eating disorders in American psychiatry: they are perceived as (1) both dysregulated and hyper-regulated, (2) both depleted and depleting, and (3) both fragile and resistant. These ambivalences create a number of double binds for people diagnosed with eating disorders that become exacerbated under the conditions of managed mental healthcare

Dysregulated/Hyper-Regulated

Eating disorders, historically and across theories, are generally construed as pathologies of control. The narrative usually goes something like this: someone feels out of control regarding things in her life, so she turns her focus to something she *can* control—food. While this formulation is not necessarily untrue, it is only one part of the story. Yet questions of control—over patients' bodies, over food and eating, over exercise, over how time is spent, over emotions—and attendant questions of power often eclipse other issues, especially in the context of treatment. Here, I want to tweak this conception a bit, to trouble the notion of "control" as a heuristic, and to tease out how it functions as a social artifact.

Across models of eating disorders, the eating-disordered body is constituted as, paradoxically, both hyper-regulated and dysregulated; that is, it is both rigidly controlled and wildly out of control at the same time. Like the theme of hunger (taken up later in this chapter), "regulation" bridges multiple domains and levels of analysis, from the molecular to the philosophical, and this has profound implications on how these conditions are understood and treated.

Physiologically speaking, eating-disordered bodies are generally viewed as desperately trying to regulate themselves under extreme conditions, and many of the physical symptoms associated with eating disorders can be understood as regulatory processes that have been thrown into overdrive. For example, because they have lost the body fat needed to keep the body at a stable internal temperature, people with anorexia often shiver uncontrollably or grow soft downy hair on their skin. Menstruation ceases because the state of the body signals to the hormonal system that conditions are not optimal for reproduction and scarce resources should be otherwise allocated. Bulimic bodies that have been purged of nutrients crave them with intensity, leading some people to binge not only on chips and ice cream but also on things like carrots and bananas as their bodies try desperately to attain equilibrium.

Experientially, too, people with eating disorders often *feel* extremely dysregulated and out of control, even though their lives may appear to be rigidly structured around imposing and maintaining control and self-regulation. These positions are not at odds; in fact, they go hand in hand. For people with eating disorders, self-imposed mechanisms of regulation and control often feel like the only things standing between them and complete and utter chaos—physically, psychologically, emotionally, and interpersonally. For those with anorexia, maintaining control over food intake (amount, type, location, etc.), affective relationships, physical contact, and sensory pleasures can help contain a body whose needs are experienced as terrifyingly big and strong. A similar thing often occurs for people with bulimia, though they tend to vacillate between tight control and the experience of "breaking points," where the control no longer holds and those needs break forth, thereby confirming their belief in the power and magnitude of their appetites. For people suffering from anorexia, bulimia, or binge eating disorder, then, a driving fear is generally that if left to her own devices, the person and her appetites (for food, but not only for food) would be completely uncontrolled and uncontrollable. For a person with one of these conditions, the line between hyper-regulation and dysregulation is a very fine one indeed, and one that she must walk with careful and conscious deliberation every second of every day. I explore these practices of tinkering and fine-tuning in more detail in chapter 3.

These dynamics of regulation play out interpersonally as well, and an eating-disordered person's relationships with others often parallel their relationship with food. People diagnosed with anorexia, for example, generally tend to be restrained and constricted in relating with other people, in the sense of how much of their own needs or opinions they express and to what extent they allow themselves to depend on others. Often highly solicitous of others, eager to meet others' expectations of them, and driven by a desire for total self-sufficiency, many women diagnosed with anorexia choose or enact relationships where they are constantly giving of themselves to other people and rarely asking for things in return. The contrast between this mode of relating and the fact that severe anorexia actually demands that others step in and *take care* of the ill person is part of what can make others in the person's life feel that she is manipulative, resistant, and difficult: If she needs help, why doesn't she just ask for it? Why does she insist she is fine when she's clearly not? Why does she resist getting better? There are many complicated answers to these questions, but one reason is that needing or asking for *anything* is anathema to the majority of people with anorexia. So, in effect, their illness does it for them, behind their own backs, as it were. The interpersonal experience both for the person with anorexia and for the people around her, then, is often one of hyper-regulation *and* dysregulation—rigidly maintained boundaries, avoidance, and rejection of overtures of care coupled with physical indicators that the individual is in serious trouble and could die from her behaviors.

Questions of interpersonal regulation and dysregulation often arise for friends and family of people diagnosed with bulimia as well. Unlike those with an "anorexic" mode of interpersonal relating, people diagnosed with bulimia tend to be overtly intense in their connections to others and also more vehement in their rejections of others. They often enact their struggles with food and vice versa in their interpersonal relationships, with issues of neediness, shame, and desire coming to the fore. At Cedar Grove, for example, clinicians observed how some clients diagnosed with bulimia would "binge" on their therapists. That is, they seemed desperate for constant contact with their therapists; never appeared to get enough attention, feedback, care, or one-on-one time from them; constantly sought their therapists out in between groups or during breaks; routinely ran over time in session; devised ways of finding extra interaction time; and so forth. Or they might "binge" on other clients, forming intensely close friendship bonds and becoming inseparable with someone (or a series of someones). Other times, clinicians described clients as enacting a form of "purging" in therapy and other interpersonal relationships. Certainly, therapy is meant to be a place for verbalizing and processing emotional material, and most people experience the therapy hour as, to some degree, an emptying out of internal distress. But for some people, therapy and other close relationships become arenas for "vomiting out" their emotional insides in more disorganized or less adaptive ways.

For example, Mallory, a twenty-year-old woman diagnosed with bulimia, would talk nonstop from the very beginning of her therapy session to the last second of it, not letting her therapist get a word in. "It doesn't feel like a relationship," her therapist Brenda told me. "She talks *at* me, just spewing out everything without any kind of filter. When clients do that they're not receptive to what you might have to offer." It was not a two-way street. When this dynamic is at play, the client is often so overwhelmed with anxiety or self-loathing that she feels she *has* to get it all out, as quickly and as completely as possible, to reduce her distress. Frequently, however, the person on the receiving end of this kind of emotional purging feels "dumped on." Their subjectivity or input does not seem to matter; they are simply a receptacle for the purged feelings. Although we have probably all been both the "dumper" and the "dumpee" at different times in different relationships, what marks this form of relating as distinct is that it can be the predominant mode through which an individual attempts to connect with others in their immediate environment. While the "dumper" may feel a good deal of relief after such an encounter, the "dumpee" often feels resentful, hurt, and confused. In both cases, this is not an optimized form of healthy connection.

Given these dynamics, many people diagnosed with bulimia often either experience extremely intense and challenging relationships with others or have learned to avoid interpersonal connections because they have been told that they are "too intense" or "too needy" and have suffered painful interpersonal rejections. They then often develop interpersonal styles that aim at regulating dysregulated forms of relating.

While different models of eating disorders interpret issues of regulation in different ways, all point to issues of "control" as central concerns in eating disorders. In CBT, for example, clients utilize various tools and strategies to learn how to control their unruly or distressing thoughts and behaviors while also supposedly relinquishing controlling attitudes. In psychodynamic therapies, clients take control of their lives by releasing their desire to control others. Therapies based on feminist models, by contrast, encourage women to assume *more* control of their lives and the terms of their own self-definitions as a pathway to healing. In terms of treatment and relationships of care, the focus on control sets up an oppositional relationship between clients and caregivers where control becomes a central defining logic of relating in the clinic. Clients are encouraged to control their eating disorder urges while at the same time letting go of the urges to control. As we will see in chapter 7, much of Cedar Grove's program hinges on such practices of constraint and regulation even as, in therapy, clients are encouraged to embrace expansion and abundance.

In addition to all of this—and perhaps most importantly—I want to highlight the gendered dimensions of this focus on control. Why, after all, is a desire for control bad? Who among us does not want to have bodily integrity, to feel a sense of mastery over our lives and our environments, over what we do, with whom we are intimate? A desire for control is only considered pathological when it is viewed as an *illegitimate* desire, a claim for more space or authority than is deemed "reasonable" for a given person. *This is a gendered and gendering construct.*

Now, I do not want to suggest that control is a nonissue when it comes to eating disorders. It can absolutely overrun a person's life such that experiences of joy and feelings of freedom are squelched. But we could just as easily engage this from the view of wondering why the person feels unworthy or unable to embrace these other feelings. That is, instead of pathologizing *control,* we could instead focus on encouraging clients to allow themselves to experience *freedom* and *growth.* This may sound like the same thing, and the difference is subtle, but it is critical. Control is not the problem. The problem is not feeling or being authorized to fully exist. When we focus on control as the issue, *we pathologize the individual for what is a cultural, social, and structural problem, and we reinscribe the message that she is not deserving of the basic structures of subjecthood in our culture.* An individual person cannot, of course, overturn those structures. But she can be equipped with methods that can help her navigate them in ways that enable her to exist more fully.

Depleted/Depleting

If the constitution of clients with eating disorders as dysregulated/hyper-regulated focuses on issues of control, the next theme has to do with the dynamics of *intentionality* and *flow*.

Perhaps the hallmark of an eating-disordered body—especially for people with anorexia—is that it is literally starving to death. Eating-disordered bodies are understood, from a medical perspective, to be chronically "hungry"; they exist in a perpetual state of craving resources for survival, resources that are not forthcoming. Deprived of essential nutrients and calories, the eating-disordered body begins to consume itself, progressively breaking down muscle, bone, and organ tissue to stay alive. Even in the binge-purge cycle of bulimia, where massive amounts of calories may be consumed in a given episode, the body can become critically malnourished, with dangerously low levels of essential nutrients (like protein) and electrolytes (like potassium and sodium). A person who binges on ice cream and cookies, purges, and then repeats the cycle (or restricts her food intake the rest of the day out of fear of another binge) will produce a body that is just as "hungry" for the components it needs to survive as an anorexic body. The eating-disordered body, then, craves what it lacks, and it is only through extreme intervention by the individual that it does not receive that sustenance.

Experientially, people diagnosed with eating disorders *feel* their bodies as hungry bodies, though what this means and how they relate to it differs depending on the particular constellations of symptoms they are dealing with as well as the specifics of their own life histories. Although people diagnosed with anorexia often insist they simply never get hungry, in my experience with clients and in my own experience with anorexia (and further supported by other autobiographical accounts), this is not exactly true, or at least not for most people. While it is certainly the case that hunger and fullness cues can become extremely dysregulated in people with eating disorders so that it is difficult for them to confidently identify what it is that they are feeling, most people diagnosed with anorexia do frequently feel hungry. *Extremely* hungry. That hunger may pass if one waits long enough, or a person may be able to convince herself that one Triscuit and a stick of gum is really enough to make the hunger go away. But once they are out of the deepest depths of the illness, every single person in recovery that I have spoken to has told me that hunger was a chronic and abiding experience during their anorexia. Yet rather than propelling them to eat, that hunger was experienced by most of them as confirmation that they were doing something "good" by denying their bodies what it so clearly craved.

People diagnosed with bulimia and binge eating disorder tend to situate hunger somewhat differently. While every person's experience is unique, one common theme for many women struggling with bulimia is that the only way they have found to make the sense of hunger or craving go away is to binge and purge (though some use other methods, such as self-harm, as well). For many of these women, feeling hunger is not a comfort or a confirmation of self-sacrifice, as it often is in anorexia. Rather, it generates intense experiences of panic—so intense, in fact, that they will do just about anything to avoid it, or get rid of it once it appears. Often, these women speak of feeling their hunger to be a bottomless pit, as if there were no end to it and that if left to their own devices they would eat and eat and eat until they simply died from ingesting too much food. For many of these women, the lines between wanting, craving, and physical hunger are often so blurred that it is extremely difficult for them to figure out what they are actually feeling, and the anxiety of sitting with whatever that feeling may be is so great that it seems intolerable.

Interpersonally, people with eating disorders are often seen by others as "hungry" for attention, as if they are trying to draw emotional resources from the environment and people around them, grasping and depleting the energies of others as if they need that attention as a form of sustenance.

I will take this theme up in more detail throughout the course of the book, but here I want to separate out some issues. Most women with eating disorders are ambivalently situated in their interpersonal relationships. Often, they want and need empathy and care, but they do not think they deserve it or that they *should* want it; and they believe they certainly shouldn't *ask* for it. *Ever.* So they may try to get that empathy and care in indirect ways while simultaneously pushing others away or rejecting offers for help. This can be exceedingly frustrating for others, and it is one example of why people with eating disorders are often experienced as manipulative or difficult. But it need not play out this way if we simply pivot our orientation just slightly. What feels like manipulation or attention-seeking begs the broader question of *why* someone would feel she has to go to such complex and elaborate lengths to get what we might consider to be a basic human *right* in a relationship: to be *recognized*. And it flags to us that, rather than feeling she deserves to be the center of attention, a person diagnosed with an eating disorder might feel unworthy of even the barest existence. Yet the idea that people with eating disorders are "starving for attention" has characterized much of the clinical and popular thinking about motives and treatments over the past hundred years, leading to unhelpful or even harmful interventions.

Elaborating on another dimension of the eating-disordered body/self as "hungry," cultural theorists have examined eating-disordered bodies as a materialization of consumer practices in postindustrial modern society. In this formulation, material excess, coupled with moral injunctions that favor self-denial and accumulation (consistent with the Protestant ethic), generate contrasting forces that promote conspicuous consumption while also casting such consumption as vulgar and morally weak. In this dynamic, overindulgence is a gendered, raced, and classed practice, with sensuality, excess, and disinhibition generally marked as female, nonwhite, and lower class and self-control generally coded as male, white, and upper class.

This situation produces a number of internal contradictions. On the one hand, the desire for more—more goods, more services, more quality, more land, more workers, more success—is the driving engine of the capitalist machine and is associated with various sorts of privilege. On the other hand, when this desire for "more" is expressed by beings who are nonwhite, non–upper class, and/or gendered female—and when the desires are for things like more rights, more equality, more space, more voice, more sexual expression, more freedom—they are often dismissed as overreaching, overstepping their place, or even being pathological. Eating disorders, in this view, represent an enactment of these logics in one of their most extreme and visible forms—that is, they involve shrinking the self (material and immaterial) so dramatically that one literally becomes the constricted, docile subject that prevailing structures of privilege and power require. Treatment for eating disorders, in this view, might be read as normalizing practices aimed at rehabituating clients to "acceptable" cultural expectations rather than critiquing those expectations as themselves flawed.

Regardless of theoretical approach, we can see that eating disorders are generally conceptualized as deriving from some sort of challenge in self-realization stemming from a truncated or misdirected flow of energy, attention, or investment that results in a dynamic of depletion that renders the body, self, and subject perpetually "hungry." What emerges in these different approaches to eating disorders is a view of clients as both physically and psychologically malnourished, craving, and grasping, and as existing in a state of raw deprivation. They are viewed as being both physically and psychologically depleted, which is thought to drain and deplete those around them.

How might this view of people with eating disorders affect relationships of care? As I explore more in chapter 10, when clients are perceived as perpetually ravenous and needy, clinicians feel the need to be constantly on guard, to vigilantly focus on boundaries and limits, and to be cautious with what they give lest they be "consumed" by the clients' needs. Like the focus on control, this leads to an oppositional relationship between client and caregiver, and it is exacerbated by an insurance system that prioritizes conserving resources and is suspicious of greed and waste. At the same time, clients are deemed "resistant" if they do not recognize their illness and willingly accept care. Clients, then, find themselves in a double bind: if they resist care they are deemed noncompliant, but if they accept care they are found needy and depleting.

Fragile/Resistant

If the theme of dysregulated/hyper-regulated speaks to issues of control, and that of depleted/depleting deals with interpersonal boundaries and flow, the third theme—fragile/resistant—has to do with issues of amplitude and saturation. By this I mean the intensity (or lack thereof) of energy, attention, and investment across multiple domains.

A body ravaged by an eating disorder is materially brittle. Its bones become weak and prone to fracture. Its skin is thin and papery. Its hair breaks off or falls out. Its teeth may be corroded, its esophagus burned raw by stomach acid, its muscles atrophied, and its capacity to endure cold radically compromised. It is a body whose vitality and strength have been sapped and whose very structure—bones, organs, life systems—teeters on the edge of collapse.

Given these characteristics of eating-disordered bodies, medical treatments often include the institution of a calorically and nutritionally sufficient diet and the administration of nutritional supplements (calcium, magnesium, iron, and potassium supplements are commonly used) to replenish and strengthen the body from within. Without such interventions, the eating-disordered body is seen to be at risk of eroding from the inside out.

Yet changes to the body during treatment can come in fits and starts, bringing additional concerns to the fore. If an underweight person gains weight too quickly, she can develop "refeeding syndrome" (potentially fatal shifts in fluids and electrolytes that can occur when nutrition is reintroduced after severe starvation). Or she may become hypermetabolic, which is when the metabolism "wakes up" after having been dormant during a period of starvation and can result in clients requiring four thousand calories or more per day simply to maintain their weight. In short, once a body is in full starvation mode, it is a tricky business to safely get it out again, and the body is both vulnerable to collapse and resistant to intervention.

Many women diagnosed with eating disorders express ambivalent feelings about the fragility of their bodies. Some women diagnosed with anorexia report enjoying the "waif look" they can cultivate when deep in their illness. But the reasons for this vary. For some, looking sick and frail makes them feel more feminine. For others, it makes them feel *less* feminine. Some are convinced that physical fragility is the only reason other people pay attention to them or express concern for their well-being. Still others feel that bodily fragility helps them avoid notice by dissolving into the background, where they are more comfortable.

Whatever their associations with the *appearance* of physical fragility, most women diagnosed with eating disorders that I've encountered (and here I include women diagnosed with bulimia as well as women diagnosed with anorexia) also seem to hold tightly to an *experience* of their bodies as extremely tough and resilient—many of them would say maddeningly stubborn—and capable of sustaining extreme degrees of self-punishment. Carly, for example, may recognize that she is at 78 percent of her ideal body weight and understand that her labs indicate she is deficient in certain vital nutrients; yet she may not believe, despite the medical evidence, that she is at risk for major organ failure. Or Sheila may acknowledge that she throws up blood every day when she purges yet still deny that this could indicate any sort of serious medical problem. For *other* people, maybe. But not *her*. Her body is a different sort of force to be reckoned with than other people's bodies. This sense of sturdy embodiment is both a positive and a negative. While Sheila may on one level be glad she is not acutely medically compromised, it is also frustrating for her when she is bent on self-destruction. Her body is more stubborn, more obstinate, and more resistant to her attempted interventions than it "should" be, in her estimation, which is why she must continually step up her destructive regimen.

In other words, there is often a tension between fragility and resistance in the experiences of people diagnosed with eating disorders, a tension that emerges in interesting counterpoints in the psychological realm. Here, the point is that the same bodies that are construed from a medical perspective as being highly at risk for a range of complications are often experienced by clients themselves as stubbornly robust, despite their best efforts to destroy them.

This tension also comes into play interpersonally as family members and loved ones interact with a person in the throes of an eating disorder. This is perhaps most clearly seen in anorexia, where a person's dwindling frame can generate intense concern from others, who become increasingly fearful for her health. In these cases, parents, partners, and friends often describe the person as looking "fragile," "like a little bird," or "like you could break her in two." They become afraid to touch or hug the person with an eating disorder, fearful of hurting her. At the same time, as noted above, they often experience the person with the eating disorder as being extremely rigid and fixed in her ways. She can be fiery in her reactions to others who try to talk to her about food or persuade her to eat, and she often protests that she is "just fine, thank you," and rejects attempts to care for her. Although she may be fragile in many ways, then, she is also fiercely resistant to the will of others.

The fragile/resistant theme shows up somewhat differently in feminist/ cultural interpretations of eating disorders. According to this view, anorexia functions as a kind of corseting from the inside, a way for women to reduce the amount of space (physical, interpersonal, political, social) they inhabit in order to make themselves more acceptable to patriarchal demands.[19] By inhabiting a body (and sets of body practices) associated with fragility, dependence, and weakness, the eating-disordered person replicates—albeit in extreme form—the demands of patriarchal culture on women's flesh. On the other hand—yet at the same time—self-starvation or preoccupation with thinness may be a way of enacting a "hunger strike,"[20] pushing back against such expectations by eradicating the very markers of femininity that are the currency of subjugation. This figuring of eating disorders as either capitulation to or resistance against patriarchal pressures (or both) highlights the critical importance such theorists place on questions of agency and autonomy in their understandings of health, an issue I will return to throughout this ethnography.

While different approaches to eating disorders take somewhat different positions on the fragile/resistant dynamic, they all engage it in substantial ways. Ego fragility and interpersonal resistance go hand in hand in the psychodynamic perspective. Susceptibility to cognitive distortions and resistance to change are paired in the cognitive-behavioral view. In the feminist perspective, resistance is framed somewhat differently, as a political stance that is to be cultivated and redirected away from the self and toward the cultural beliefs and practices that sustain eating-disordered attitudes. In all cases, the theme of fragility versus resistance becomes an organizing one. In terms of relationships of care, the fragile/resistant dynamic, like the others, sets up a double bind for clients to be stronger and more independent while simultaneously being more compliant with treatment interventions.

REFLECTIONS

These three themes that predominate in theories of eating disorders and their treatment—dynamics of control, depletion, and resistance—can be read not just as descriptions of clinical or interpersonal phenomena but also as *sites of contestation about who is considered to be a legitimate subject and what kinds of claims that subject is authorized to make on others and on the world around them.* In addition to the practical double binds these issues generate, it is imperative that we recognize these themes as *deeply gendered* formulations of (de)legitimation that structure not only how health and pathology are understood but also how relationships of care are elaborated accordingly.

What, then, are some alternatives? How can we rethink eating disorders in a way that gets us out of these double binds and centers these core issues regarding legitimate subjectivity? This is the focus of the next chapter.

Little Debbie

APRIL 1979

I love Little Debbie Star Clusters. *Love* them. Those things are *delicious.*
Mom puts one in my lunch every day, and it's my favorite part.

As I go to sneak another one—my third one this afternoon—my dad's
voice echoes in my head. "Linda, she's getting chubby," my dad said to my
mom the night before. "You really need to limit her snacks."

Reaching for the Star Cluster, my hand freezes. What was it that I'd
heard? That if you imagine something really gross on the food you want, you
won't be as tempted by it anymore. What could I imagine on the Little
Debbie Star Clusters? I pick one up and look at its chocolaty, caramelly good-
ness through the crinkly cellophane wrapper. It's brown and gooey with
those crunchy Rice Krispy things on top. What do I hate more than anything? Roaches. Yes, that's it. I'm going to imagine that there are smashed
dead roaches baked into the Little Debbie Star Clusters and that I can see
their mushed bodies and legs just underneath the chocolate coating. I stare
at the Star Cluster, willing myself to see dead roaches in it, and after a few
moments I can almost see a hairy little leg here, a smashed-up body there.

I throw the package back in the box, thoroughly grossed out. Just to show
that I can do it, I decide I'm not going to eat the one Mom puts in my lunch
tomorrow.

THREE

Eating Disorders as Technologies of Presence

I exist, that is all, and I find it nauseating.

—JEAN PAUL SARTRE,
Nausea

Absence, the highest form of Presence.

—JAMES JOYCE,
A Portrait of the Artist as a Young Man

Anthropological theories and methods are uniquely suited to engaging the sorts of thorny issues raised in the last chapter. By combining engaged qualitative research on the phenomenology of self-starvation, bingeing, and purging with critical cultural analyses of the systems through which that phenomenology is articulated and shaped, an anthropologically informed perspective can lend a constructive voice to understanding eating disorders and developing more effective forms of care.

Anthropological writing on eating disorders stretches back many decades. As the consummate culture-bound syndrome,[1] eating disorders have long been a focus of inquiry in both anthropology and cross-cultural psychiatry. Early studies of culture and eating disorders[2] centered around questions of why women (until recently, men were thought to be "protected" from eating disorders) in postindustrial Western societies seemed especially prone to developing these conditions, whereas their counterparts in non-Western settings seemed not to be at risk.

Beginning in the 1990s, in part reflecting disciplinary wrestling with the culture concept and a growing interest in processes of globalization, scholarly attention regarding culture and eating disorders turned to questions of how to explain the rise of these supposedly Western, supposedly culture-bound syndromes in other places, like Japan, Fiji, and Iran.[3] The most common explanation was that they were a result of the "Westernization" or "moderni-zation" of the society in question. The basic proposition in this literature is that as societies become more Western or more modern (or both, as the two were generally seen to be linked), the specific behaviors associated with eating disorders (e.g., self-starvation, bingeing and purging, body image distur-bances, intense fear of gaining weight) become meaningful expressions of particular cultural features: heightened consumerism, media saturation, an ethos of independence, an idealization of self-discipline, and the constant seduction to "supersize" everything, from fries to TVs to SUVs.

From this perspective, the appearance of eating disorders in a given society was read as evidence of social change, a clear sign that Westernization and modernization were underway and that individuals in these societies were becoming increasingly acculturated to modern Western values. This perspec-tive has been hotly debated in the literature and remains a point of conten-tion today, with some holding fast to the "acculturation hypothesis" and others calling for a radical re-engagement with the concept of culture in the field of eating disorders.[4]

In the wake of these cross-cultural explorations, anthropological interest in eating disorders has intensified in the past fifteen years, with theorists productively complicating understandings of culture, practice, and embodi-ment.[5] What these more recent engagements share is a complex view of cul-ture as constituted by and constitutive of interpersonal practices that emerge and assume meaning within sometimes shifting and multiple epistemological and moral universes. That is, they consider how disordered eating is figured as an object of concern within different moral and social worlds, and exam-ine the specific kinds of affective, interpersonal, and pragmatic work such practices do. In this way, recent anthropological work on eating disorders resonates with projects in medical anthropology more generally that grapple with questions of ontology, or how illnesses—as categories of knowledge and practice, and as lived experiences—are generated in the context of social interaction.[6] This enables anthropologists to examine how illness simultane-ously generates, reflects, and anchors local patterns of relatedness, material-izing commitments of care.

In my own understanding of eating disorders, I build on ontological approaches, structural approaches, phenomenological perspectives, and cross-cultural studies of eating disorders. But my view also differs from these perspectives in important ways.[7] My aim is to extend the excellent works my colleagues and interlocutors have produced and thereby offer a contribution to an ongoing conversation.

I get at these issues by approaching care as *an intersubjective, constitutional process*[8] and by considering eating disorders as a very particular sort of practice that I call technologies of presence.

TECHNOLOGIES OF PRESENCE

A technology of presence is a suite of culturally informed bodily, affective, cognitive, psychological, and interpersonal practices that work together to conjure a form of being that has two distinct features: (1) it involves an experience of immediate, grounded, and engaged connection to the world—a subjective sense of "being there"; and (2) it renders one perceptible and intelligible to others as a legitimate subject in local terms—a relational sense of "being there." In other words, "presencing" in this context means *coming into being* or *becoming real in ways that are locally recognized as mattering.* This is an existential project, as it entails questions of the meaning of existence and the purpose of being. It is a metaphysical project, as it speaks to the ways bodily and nonbodily dimensions of existence are thought to relate in a given setting. It is a social project, in that what kinds of subjects and existence are recognized as real and legitimate are variable and locally and culturally shaped. It is an interpersonal project, as practices of recognition and acknowledgement occur (or are withheld) between people. And it is also a moral project, in that our "presence" always emerges within social life and in the context of relationships, where some forms of presence become possible or impossible and some forms are valued over others. We might say, then, that *a technology of presence is a sort of practical metaphysics through which a person comes to experience her or his existence within local relational worlds and through which he or she becomes perceptible to others.*

Eating disorders are a technology of presence in that they become a way for individuals to modulate the degree, intensity, and contours of their presence in the world, both in terms of the felt sense of "being there" and in terms of how they appear (physically and otherwise) to others. They also become a way for societies to draw lines around behaviors, affects, and ways of interacting that are deemed acceptable from certain kinds of subjects.

Allow me now to unpack all of this a bit further. My use of the term "technology" borrows from French philosopher Michel Foucault's notion of "technologies of the self"[9] in that eating disorders are culturally available bodily practices that, over time, shape the way a person experiences herself and the world around her in fairly systematic and predictable ways, and this transformation is tied to broader social and cultural values about what it means to be a good or valuable person. But I do not use this term without some reservation. Foucault's work has been productively critiqued within academic circles,[10] and I do not want my use of the term "technology" to be mistaken for an endorsement of all aspects of Foucault's approach. I also struggled a bit with whether "technology" conveyed too mechanistic of a sense that would obscure or minimize the messy, chaotic, fear-driven panic and desperation that characterizes so much of life with an eating disorder. In the end, however, I decided that it was the term that best captured the complexity and multiscalar nature of eating disorder practices and the way they function together to accomplish various tasks.

My understanding of "presence" brings together contributions from existential philosophy,[11] psychoanalysis,[12] and religion,[13] as well as recent work on virtual reality.[14] By "presence," I mean the lived experience of "being there," being alive in the world, *and* being perceptible and recognizable as such to others as well as to oneself. In this regard, presence is not simply an experience or condition of being, as philosophers might have it. Nor is it a purely subjective state, as many psychological theories suggest. It is not simply a matter of representation, linguistic or otherwise, either. Rather, presence is always an *intersubjective* process. That is, the experience of presence is qualitatively dependent on others perceiving us and recognizing our right to exist, which in turn is dependent on us making ourselves perceptible and recognizable in particular ways that may or may not resonate with our actual experiences of who we are. I can *feel* fully present, for example, yet be interpersonally invisible or only partly visible to those around me for reasons having to do with race, sex, gender, sexual or political orientation, or some other facet of who I am, who they are, or the circumstances in which we interact. In such a situation, my "presence" is contested, and ultimately, if parts of who I am remain invisible to others or are denied the right to exist, it will become increasingly difficult for me to feel "present" in them as well.

I want to stress that this perspective does not presume a prerelational "self" and "other" as bounded, autonomous entities that then come into contact and engage in representational negotiations. Instead, it concerns the emergence of "being" *within* relationships, even as it acknowledges that some forms of presencing will be experienced by participants as more or less sincere or persuasive than others. That is, it is not a matter of a dichotomous subject versus object or presence versus absence but rather a spectrum or range, akin to bringing a camera into focus or tuning a radio receiver to pick up a station. Presencing, therefore, does not place sole responsibility on the subject to render herself knowable in the terms of intelligibility with which she is confronted, though this is part of the story (a radio station must transmit via the airwaves on a recognized frequency or it will not be detected, at least not by radios). Nor does it place sole responsibility on others to perceive or understand her, no matter how obscured or submerged she might make herself, though this too is important (a radio must have the ability to intercept and interpret transmissions on a range of frequencies). Rather, presencing is an ongoing process of *attunement* through which *being comes to be*.[15]

To use a somewhat different metaphor, virtual reality (VR) uses the term "presencing" to refer to both the experience of being present or immersed in a virtual world and one's virtual self-representation becoming present to others—via an avatar, for example. Presencing in the first sense—feeling immersed—is largely dependent on the quality of the VR technology as what Giuseppe Riva and his colleagues[16] call *affective mediation*—that is, on the degree to which the technologies of engagement (the computer itself, the VR code that generates the virtual world, etc.) facilitate and mediate experience while at the same time receding into the background so that they become imperceptible as mediators. The more natural such technologies feel, the more they facilitate experiences of presence.

Extending this metaphor, we can say that eating disorders are a technology (like computer equipment or computer code) that *mediates presencing,* both in the sense of how immersed one feels in the (virtual) world and how effectively one can generate a self-representation that others perceive as "being there." What happens for the person with an eating disorder is that the "affective technology" of the eating disorder comes to feel so natural that it disappears from view *as* a technology—that is, it becomes a lived, embodied way of experiencing that facilitates a form of presencing that the person can learn to modulate as needed, often without being consciously aware of this process. Indeed, in the course of treatment, one of the first tasks for both clients and therapists is to identify the eating disorder as an affective technology (though they don't use this term at Cedar Grove) and then to remove it as an option. Clients are frequently admonished for "listening to their eating disorder" or "letting their eating disorder be in control" instead of perceiving and acting within the world in a more immediate and less mediated way (see chapter 8). At the same time, the eating disorder becomes a way for others to identify and make sense of the person who is struggling, particularly when their modes of relating are fraught, conflicted, or disjointed. In other words, eating disorders are technologies of presence in both directions, as sufferers struggle to make themselves known and others struggle to know them. What is problematic, however (as we saw in chapter 2), is that our contemporary notions of what eating disorders are and what their symptoms mean are conditioned by centuries of received wisdom about gender, sexuality, and "the self" that renders the legitimacy of some subjects impossible.

Importantly, eating disorders are not simply strategies for experiencing oneself as alive in the world, but also for *honing* that experience in very particular ways. The specifics are different for everyone, but in their entanglement of physiological, affective, psychological, behavioral, interpersonal, social, and cultural experiences and meanings, eating disorders—as daily practices—enable the struggling out of complex and difficult to articulate issues regarding what it means to exist—physically, psychologically, socially, and even spiritually—in a given social and interpersonal context. Eating disorders are everyday, mundane practices whose stakes are the fundamental elements of being.

PRESENCE/ABSENCE

A core feature of eating disorders that renders them powerful as existential techniques is that they are simultaneously technologies of *presence* and technologies of *absence*. That is, they make some things visible, but they also obscure, distort, and interfere with being seen, heard, known, and understood. They can also numb sensation and engagement, acting as a safety valve for modulating presence by allowing one to "turn down the volume" on living when it is too loud, too intense, too raucous, too discordant.

Eating disorders, at heart, are strategies for manifesting and working through existential, metaphysical, moral, social, political, and interpersonal issues of presence and absence. They both enact and attempt to resolve experiences of fundamental misrecognition and misattunement. These are profoundly interpersonal processes, depending not only on local cultural categories of intelligibility but also, most importantly, on ongoing dynamics of intersubjective recognition.[17]

I want to be clear that when I say eating disorders are technologies of presence, I don't mean that they are particularly good ones. They are not especially successful, because they presence forms of being—and nonbeing—that are traumatized and tormented, although they are also attempts to presence forms of being that are otherwise.

Thinking of eating disorders in this way helps us understand why people cling so tenaciously to them, even when they are miserable and claim (often quite truthfully) to want to get better. It is not just that they are stubborn, resistant, or lying. Rather, over time, people come to *presence through* their eating disorders, even when that presencing involves forms of absence. It is how they come to inhabit the world and how they become materialized, perceptible, and recognizable to others (and themselves), although this perception and recognition is fraught with blind spots, misalignments, and blurred edges. The loss of the eating disorder means the loss of presencing. It is an existential death.

EATING DISORDERS, PRESENCING, AND AFFECT

One could engage the issue of presencing from a range of angles. In thinking about these issues, I have found the recent scholarly literature on affect to be especially useful. But before diving in, let me say a bit more about what I mean by "affect" in this context and why it matters. In everyday language and therapeutic discourse, the terms "affect" and "emotion" are often used interchangeably. But they actually mean quite different things, depending on context. In the simplest of terms, affect refers to an animating force of bodily, cognitive, and imaginative excitation to which thoughts, feelings, sensations, and behaviors accrue. What distinguishes affect from emotion is that emotion is a discrete, demarcated bundle of thoughts, feelings, sensations, and behaviors that are given semantic significance within a given social, cultural, and interpersonal context. For example, if I can feel my heart racing, my thoughts scattered, my breathing increased, and my palms sweaty, that is affect. But whether I demarcate this bundle of things as hanging together to form a distinct "experience," and whether I attach any specific meaning to is (e.g., nervousness, anger, infatuation) depends on a second-order process. That is emotion.

Affect theorists have a range of ways of thinking about what affect is, where it comes from, how it moves, and how it relates to the body, the self, and to other people. As I develop more below, when I talk about affect I do not mean it in the sense of sedimented emotional states, like sadness, anger, or depression, though these may be temporary manifestations of the kinds of affect I want to describe. Nor do I mean the impersonal, nonrepresentational affect described by Brian Massumi, Nigel Thrift, and other Deleuze-inspired theorists that pulses, leaks, and circulates largely independently of human interest or investment, though that, too, may be a feature of what I hope to capture.[18] Rather, I am interested in the *in between space* approached by such theorists as Sara Ahmed, Lisa Blackman, and Margaret Wetherell, who attempt to capture *affect as the broker of the material and the immaterial,* who consider *how matter is animated* (or is seen to be animated, or conversely, to be stagnated or fixed), and who speculate about *how interpersonal connections are forged, mediated, and undone* in and through these intensities.[19]

Affect, then, is the push, force, or "oomph" of being, what cultural theorists might call the qualia of life. It can be positive or negative or neutral; it can be high intensity or low intensity or in between; its inputs can be stitched closely together or basted far apart or located somewhere in the middle. *Affect is the saturation of life with life.* It is inherently social, interpersonal, and intersubjective, even when at its most personal and intimate. I understand affect as an interpersonal, mediating, translating force that threads through different levels of analysis and abstraction, from the material to the social to the ideological. What I mean, and what this has to do with eating disorders, will hopefully become clear in the following pages. For now, we can see how, in each of the three domains identified in the last chapter—regulated/dysregulated, depleted/depleting, fragile/resistant—the focus of concern is the modulation of intensity, of unformed and unstructured potential, which is the very definition of affect. That is, if eating disorder theories are theories of embodiment (of how the material and immaterial aspects of being interact), affect is the energy that animates these dynamics. By entailing propositions about the patterning (regulated/dysregulated), flow (depleted/depleting), or amplitude (fragile/resistant) of affect, we might say that different eating disorder theories are *cultural models of affective embodiment.*

While I draw on recent developments in affect theory in thinking through contemporary models of eating disorders, I differ from other theorists of affect in that I want to bring in perspectives from anthropology that situate local understandings of affect within broader social and cultural economies of meaning and consider affect not as wholly separate from regimes of power, nor as simply products of them, but as complexly entangled with local instantiations of subjectivity, agency, and interrelationship. That is, I am interested in how local understandings of affect—what it is, where it lives, how it moves, and what it does—constitute a core feature of life at Cedar Grove, and how this, in turn, tells us important things not only about contemporary American psychiatry as a cultural system but also about how people make and find meaning in the world. I want to be clear that I am not interested in presenting a new model of affect per se but rather in illuminating how, in the context of Cedar Grove, affect can help us understand what it means to be sick, what it means to be in treatment, and what it means to recover, as well as what it means to be a person, to be in relationship with others, and to change.

The domain of affect is not foreign to scholars of eating disorders. Eating disorders have long been constituted as psychological disorders centering on "distorted" thoughts, feelings, and self-perceptions, perhaps arising from pathological feeling states. Traditional theorizing suggests that emotions such as sadness, anger, shame, longing, or grief become enacted or sublimated through disordered eating practices, which "speak" these emotions when clients don't have the words to do so. The term "affect" is commonly used in the clinical arena to characterize a client's overall state of being and the kind of energy she manifests in interpersonal interactions; for example, eating disorder clients are generally perceived as having restricted, dissociated, or dysregulated affect.

But eating disorders are not simply somatic enactments of underlying or preexisting emotions; rather, they also *enable* one to cultivate, suppress, and/ or modulate a range of different *affective states,* which coordinate physiological arousal, interpersonal exchange, and social engagement. That is, eating disorders don't just encode internal affective states and express them in outward behaviors—the behaviors themselves *create* and *coordinate* affective states. This is an important departure from earlier thinking about eating disorders, and it makes recent theoretical engagements with affect particularly fruitful for thinking about how and why eating disorders develop and persist. These theories also give us some critical tools for thinking about how eating disorders are (re)produced in and through interpersonal relationships, social arrangements, and institutional contexts, which fertilize them as affective strategies.

In the remainder of this book, I draw on three concepts from affect theory in thinking about affect and presencing at Cedar Grove. First, cultural geographer Ben Anderson's notion of "affective atmospheres" speaks to the ways in which places such as cities (and, in this case, a clinic) both generate and are generated by particular affective energies and characteristics.[20] They have a "feel" to them that infuses people and practices within them. Second, cultural theorist Sarah Ahmed's concept of "affective economies" concerns how affect circulates through and accrues in and around particular objects and subjects (like eating disorders and eating disorder patients), materializing them through the very imbuing of affective potential.[21] That is (although she doesn't use this language), she is interested in how affective atmospheres generate certain kinds of realities within them. And, finally, Margaret Wetherell's formulation of "affective practices" enables us to look more carefully at how this affective materializing occurs within and through everyday practices (such as structured mealtimes or therapy groups), while also allowing (or requiring) us to grapple with questions of subjectivity and agency.[22] That is, she is interested in how individual people participate in creating and maintaining their own experiences of affect within different affective atmospheres and affective economies.

In considering these three concepts in conjunction, we have some tools for thinking about how the clinic itself functions as an affective space, how affect circulates and creates objects and subjects within it, and how such affective effects are (re)produced—and sometimes challenged—in the context of everyday practice. A key argument of the book is that the particular orchestration of these affective technologies in the eating disorders clinic renders healthy or effective subjectivity impossible for patients, catching people in paradoxes that keep them unwell, figure them as "failed" patients, or both.

EATING DISORDERS AS AFFECTIVE PRACTICES

Eating disorders are affective and affecting in a number of ways. At a fundamental level, eating disorders emerge as a means for tinkering with affect, emotion, physiological arousal, and sensation. Molly, a twenty-year-old woman diagnosed with anorexia nervosa, had a lot to say on this subject:

> There are a lot of misconceptions about eating disorders that need to be changed. The main one is, why don't you just eat? Why don't you just eat a candy bar and you'll be cured. Or when you put on weight or you're at a

healthy weight, they think you're fine. Because that's definitely not the case. You can be really doing really unhealthy things and be really unstable emotionally and still be at a healthy weight.

I think eating disorders are a way to deal with the pain. People don't get that. People will say to you, "You're so, so skinny. I don't understand why you think you're fat." . . . But at the same time the eating disorder once again is kind of like your pain medication. And you get to that point where you're so fragile looking, and nobody wants to be around you. And you become more isolated and more depressed, and you feel even worse about your body because you think you look disgusting because of all these bones sticking out. And people give you weird looks. And you feel like a complete freak. And so you're like, "Wow, I'm just really isolated."

As Molly's comments make clear, eating disorders both are and are not about thinness. They both are and are not about vanity. But importantly, the "vanity" of eating disorders is not that people think they look wonderful. Rather, it comes in not wanting one's core repulsiveness to be visible to others. Ironically, an eating disorder often leads to a materialization of the "repulsiveness" many clients feel. Molly continued, "The only friend I have left is my eating disorder, so it's going to comfort me." For Molly, an eating disorder functioned as her "pain medication," but it also isolated her and interfered with her relationships to the point that connections with others became painful to her. While the eating disorder helped block emotional pain in some areas, it generated new kinds of pain in others. It shifted, as it were, the affective load.

Like Molly, Kelly, a twenty-seven-year-old woman diagnosed with anorexia, understood her eating disorder as part of an affective strategy:

We never talked about feelings in my family. Never. So I didn't know what to do with any of that, with my emotions. When I would restrict I wouldn't feel things anymore. I just kind of numbed out. It helped me cope, turned down the intensity. Of course, I had other things come up, like fear of eating in front of others, or fear of calories and gaining weight. So now that I think about it, maybe it didn't numb me out so much as just make me feel anxious and depressed about different things.

For Kelly, like Molly, the eating disorder became a way of tinkering not only with emotions but also with affect, lessening it in some areas while intensifying it in others.[23]

Before moving on to how affect and presencing are engaged in the clinic, I want to spend a bit more time with this dimension of eating disorders, as it is absolutely fundamental to understanding their hold on people as well as the challenges clients encounter in treatment.

What Molly and Kelly describe resonates with what anthropologist Ken MacLeish calls the "ambivalent anesthesia" of American combat soldiers, with whom he conducted extended ethnographic research.[24] While it may seem odd to compare having an eating disorder to being a combat soldier, there are actually a significant number of similarities in how people going through both experiences systematically capacitate the body to withstand extreme hardship and deprivation in the service of a larger goal. One of the most impressive contributions of MacLeish's work is that he was able to document the everyday micropractices that enable soldiers to develop these abilities, as well as the contradictions and paradoxes often entailed in such practices.

On the one hand, MacLeish observes, soldiers are highly regimented, disciplined, and invulnerable; yet they are also acutely aware of vulnerability and the fact that they are, at every moment, a split second away from death or grievous injury, not simply from enemy fire but also from the very materials (tank metal, body armor) that are in place to protect them. In this way, MacLeish says, "the line between what is harming and wearing out the thirsty, chapped body on the one hand, and what is keeping it alive, on the other hand, blurs and folds in on itself," and "what saves the body is wrapped up with what harms it."[25] Soldiers become inured to pain and discomfort and able to endure extreme conditions of deprivation and exertion even as they acquire a heightened awareness of their vulnerability to harm.

Importantly, MacLeish notes that anesthesia and sensation are not fait accompli but rather must be constantly produced through what he calls soldiers' "sensory everydayness,"[26] a kind of tactility that is, as anthropologist Michael Taussig puts it, "an embodied and somewhat automatic 'knowledge' that functions like peripheral vision, not studied contemplation."[27] Within this "involuntary dimension" of the senses,[28] MacLeish argues that "what heat and weight reveal is the fraying, nervous edge where anesthesia has not fully taken hold, where it is challenged by ungovernable sensory impingements and must be reasserted by discipline."[29] In this way, invincibility and vulnerability are not pure states but "signposts around which . . . experience is organized."[30]

A similar dynamic occurs in eating disorders. A main goal of someone with an eating disorder is to produce oneself as an anesthetic subject, to numb out, to feel less, or to feel nothing at all. But the practices of an eating disorder also *hurt,* and they heighten one's senses in other ways. The more you discipline yourself into anesthesia, the more you become aware of how vulnerable you are to sensation, which generates a dynamic that must be constantly managed. One key strategy for managing sensation and affect in eating disorders involves paying careful attention to feelings of hunger and fullness.

HUNGER AND FULLNESS

Hunger and fullness are overdetermined sensations in people with eating disorders and can mean different things for different people at different times. Generally speaking, however, both hunger and fullness are experienced as that "fraying, nervous edge" described by MacLeish, the moment when sensation breaks through the anesthetized mode of being and plunges the person into the experience of acute vulnerability, panic, and pain. Sometimes, these sensations can be harnessed for "thinspiration," such as when, as I saw on a pro-anorexia website, hunger pains are reframed as "your stomach applauding." Similarly, fullness can be experienced by some people (usually those struggling with bulimia or binge eating disorder, although not all people with these diagnoses feel this way) as comforting. For the vast majority of people I spoke with, however, both hunger *and* fullness could be acutely triggering of overwhelming affect in different ways and at different times. There is often a narrow band of not-exactly-hungry-but-definitely-not-full within which people with eating disorders prefer to exist and where they describe feeling "safe" and "comfortable." Anything on either side of that divide could trigger panic and urges to engage in eating disorder behaviors (restricting, bingeing, purging, overexercising) or self-harm behaviors in order to regain the anesthetized state.

But more than this, hunger and fullness are often deeply moralized in eating disorders, with hunger and deprivation almost uniformly valued over and above fullness and satiety, even when the latter contains elements of physical or emotional comfort. Remember that a key common theme in eating disorders is a core, pervasive, corrosive *shame* of existing and of needing or wanting *anything.* Given this, hunger, like other kinds of bodily discomfort, can become moralized as evidence that one is "doing good" by denying oneself what one "clearly" does not deserve. Fullness, similarly, can be experienced as evidence that one has *taken* (and perhaps, God forbid, *enjoyed*) that to which one is not entitled.

In this way, eating disorders become what Bernard Williams calls a "ground project"—a set of ethical commitments that come to frame the subject's own conception of "the good" and that constitute what someone feels their life is about.[31] They become the fundamental mechanism through which someone enacts and experiences *integrity*—morally, yes, but also psychologically and physically. The eating disorder becomes the gravity that holds a person together. Without it, the center does not hold, and she falls apart emotionally, psychologically, and existentially.

Olivia's case is an exemplar of how an eating disorder can function in this way.

OLIVIA: A CASE STUDY

Olivia, who was thirty-one years old at the time, sat perched on the edge of the sofa, leaning forward with her elbows on her knees, looking tense and acutely uncomfortable. It was her first day at Cedar Grove, and we were beginning our initial therapy session. After I explained my research and obtained consent, Olivia dived right in. "OK, let me give you my history," she said, matter-of-factly. Olivia was a medical resident at a prestigious university in another state, and she knew how these things worked.

Olivia identified her main diagnosis as bulimia, which she traced to when she was age fourteen and had just moved to a new high school. She remembers being painfully lonely, and she was embarrassed to eat alone, so she would eat in a bathroom stall during lunch period. She was a "nerd" and recalled feeling like she needed to make some changes; she wanted to become athletic and lean. She learned about purging in health class and, after some practice, found she could do it relatively easily. In the beginning, she would purge just after meals. But soon she began bingeing and then purging. Around this time, she also started jogging three to four hours per day. At some point, her parents found vomit in the toilet and "freaked out." She promised them she would stop, but instead she started throwing up in bags in her room and then taking them to school to dump in the dumpsters. This went on through sophomore and junior year. In her senior year, she was caught dumping the bags at school, and her parents involved her in outpatient treatment. Olivia reports that it went well and that the behaviors stopped.

College, she said, was a "honeymoon period" for the first two years. Then, at one point, she noticed her clothes getting tighter and weighed herself. "I completely freaked out," she said, and she went back to bingeing and purging. As a college student, her funds were limited, so she would steal food from different dorms for binges. "I felt horrible about it, but I didn't know what else to do."

By the time she got to medical school, things were "completely out of control." There were no more dorms, so she began to shoplift food for her binges. She was caught several times at her favorite grocery store and told not to come back. "So, I got a haircut and went back the next day," she recalled. "No one noticed me."

The shoplifting continued until her first year of medical residency, when she got arrested. She stopped stealing, but around this time, alcohol became a problem. It started with wine—a glass or two here and there. It turned into several shots of vodka, which she would put in a water bottle so her boyfriend wouldn't know. "I drank because it kept me from bingeing," she said. "That's the only way I could keep from doing it—to get so drunk I was out of it." Olivia survived two different fires that occurred when she left the oven on after passing out from taking Benadryl and drinking alcohol to avoid bingeing. In one case, she ended up in the ER. Eventually, she was outed by another resident in her program and suspended from her residency for alcohol abuse. Around this time, she was also hospitalized for pancreatitis. She was allowed to resume her residency when she vowed to stop drinking, and she did stop for a while, but she eventually started again. Her residency program told her that she had to pursue treatment or she would be kicked out of the program. Recognizing that her primary issue was actually an eating disorder, and knowing the excellent reputation of Cedar Grove, she sought treatment at the clinic. Her residency program helped facilitate the process, but her insurance would not cover her treatment. She paid out of pocket. Olivia and I worked together for three months, meeting three times a week for individual therapy, and she also engaged actively in other facets of the clinic's program.

Olivia's "ground project," or orienting ethos, was one of *streamlining*. "I hate wasting anything," she said. "Time. Energy. Money. Resources. I want it all as lean as possible." She used an economic filter on her eating disorder and her relationships, thinking of both food and relationships in terms of "debt" and "saving things up." She would "save up" calories until the end of the day to "spend" on a binge or on some kind of food of "quality." She felt that she needed to repay gifts of attention and care from others by performing certain actions—such as excelling in school, working, or giving gifts. She reported feeling intense guilt if she received something from someone and did not feel she had at least equally compensated the person who had given it to her.

Olivia traced her preoccupation with efficiency and cost-effectiveness to the influence of her father, who grew up quite poor in his home country (both her parents were immigrants). He also worked in the environmental sciences and was extremely resource conscious. Olivia remembered embracing this ethos with particular gusto as a child. She recalled going to the store as a little girl with her mother and enjoying helping her economize, or even one-upping her mom by seeing who could save more. Although her family was financially comfortable, and despite knowing she would be teased by other kids, Olivia insisted on getting her shoes at Payless as a child. She remembered a time when she was given one dollar for a treat when she was in kindergarten. She used only fifty cents of it and savored the treat all day, feeling proud of herself for saving half her money. When she got little packages of M&M's or Skittles at a birthday party, she would open them but limit herself to eating one candy a day, feeling that she was building her moral fortitude. Despite this austerity, she also remembered stealing books from the library as a child, which led her to talk in therapy about the similarities between books and food for her. Both offered sustenance that she needed and that could also be very enjoyable. She felt guilty for enjoying the nonessential features of both, and she wondered in therapy if stealing books and food somehow bypassed the economic circuit for her and allowed her to feel permission to simply take pleasure in them.

Olivia's relationship with food was similarly economic and value driven. She often didn't keep "American" food in (that is, she would purge after eating it) because she thought of it as low quality, empty, and not worth the expenditure of calories. She considered herself a "foodie"—dishes should have the right ingredients, be at the right temperature, be plated artfully, and so forth. If these conditions were met, she would allow herself to keep the food in. Even so, she struggled with the fact that food was her only source of sensual pleasure and yet was also deeply associated with guilt and shame.[32]

In terms of her body image, Olivia experienced herself as "far too large" and described this as "feeling like a sweater that needs a sweater shaver." There was "overflow" and "excess," and she felt "unkempt," in contrast to the lean, tight, smooth, and efficient body she desired. Being lean, she said, is "clean and pure." She identified actresses with her ideal body type as Linda Hamilton, Jody Foster, and Hilary Swank—"strong, smart, immovable, and androgynous."

Olivia often described her emotional self in similar terms—that is, she desired to be emotionally lean, clean, and pure. One day she noted, "I want to be contained. I want people to see only what I let them see. It's important to me to present myself that way. I don't want anything to leak out." By this point in our relationship we had built a good alliance, and I felt comfortable pushing and challenging her a bit. I responded as compassionately as I could that she actually "leaks" all over the place all the time and that what she "leaks" is so much more remarkable and beautiful than any packaged self she could present. This statement took her aback, and she began to cry. "You leak because you're human," I said softly. "And it's in connecting on that really human level that people can care for you." "I don't want to be human," she said through her tears. "Recognizing that people care for me means I'm leaking, and that's really not OK with me."

This discussion led Olivia to talk about an aspiration she has had since childhood to surpass or overcome mundane human existence and achieve "some sort of almost mystical understanding of the way the world works." She described being continually frustrated by her human desires and the fact that she needs human connections. She used to model herself on characters from books who were "islands unto themselves" and "didn't need anyone or anything." She modeled herself especially on John Galt, the antagonist of Ayn Rand's *Atlas Shrugged,* who lived by an individualist, utilitarian ethos.[33]

Olivia always felt as if she were failing at this goal, however. If she felt good about getting a compliment or was hurt by a criticism, she would immediately feel "utter disgust" for herself for caring one way or another what anyone thought of her. To mitigate this vulnerability, she would try to preempt any possible criticism from others by lobbing it at herself first, telling herself constantly that she was a failure and a disappointment. She likened this to a practice she developed as a child of pinching herself really, really hard right before getting a shot so the shot would feel less painful in comparison.

As an adult, Olivia was extremely competent at her work and described herself as "on top of things, organized, and professional." At home, however, things were completely different. Despite having a solid income and a good deal of savings, her furnishings consisted of a plastic shelving unit from Target and a bare mattress on the floor. She kept nothing in her fridge, and sometimes her electricity would get shut off because she had neglected to pay the bill. She didn't have real dishes but instead ate off paper plates. She described herself as "resistant to adulthood"—not because she wanted to regress to childhood but because she didn't "want to think that who I am is who I'm going to be."[34] She explained: "As long as I keep things temporary, I'm still in the process of 'becoming,' and I don't need to worry about the difficulties in 'being.'" At the same time, she said, she didn't want to be grounded, didn't want to be human: "I want to be more than human and to touch things beyond human understanding." In reflecting on this, she noted her love of science fiction and her affinity for characters unfettered by human emotion. I observed that this struck me as a bit sad, and I wondered what was so distasteful for her about human experience. I noted that she had missed out on a lot by not being a "messy human"—by not allowing herself to accept her humanity, she avoids (but also can never embrace) human passions and emotions. This leads to a very deadened existence. "I know," she responded. "That's kind of the point." At the same time, this disengaged existence contributed to a sense of artificiality for Olivia. "I always wanted to be solid and confident," she said, "but I actually feel like an onion—you peel back all the layers and there's nothing at the center. It's the classic postmodern dilemma," she sighed, rolling her eyes.

Olivia was at Cedar Grove for just over three months. During that time, we worked on a number of issues, including the feelings that came up for her when she was forced in the clinic to eat "American" (or nonfoodie) food and keep it down, and when she was not able to binge and purge. In both cases, anxiety was the primary feeling that arose, along with a sense of dissolution or fragmentation. "I don't know what to do with myself and all these feelings," she said. "The more I feel them, the more I'm afraid I'm 'leaking,' and then I want to binge and purge even more, and I can't."

To help her develop alternative ways of dealing with the "leaking" (i.e., having human emotions and feelings), we worked on how Olivia related to the other clients in the clinic. In the early part of treatment, she (as a medical student) identified primarily with the clinical staff and took a somewhat disdainful view of the other clients. She didn't socialize with them (which is actually hard to do when you live with people twenty-four hours a day), and they experienced her as aloof and condescending. By the midpoint of her treatment, however, there was a shift, and she began to spend more time with others in the community and even sided with them against the staff in some complaints that were voiced at a community meeting. This was a pivotal point in many ways, as it signaled the loosening of her clinging to a particular identity or status and the start of a more genuine engagement with what she wanted and needed in the moment.

Similarly, Olivia's sense of herself gradually changed over time. She moved from a polarized view (where needs were bad and denial was good) to a tentative acceptance of her own humanity. "I guess I have to accept that I am human. I'm made of clay. Just like everyone else," she told me about two months into her time at Cedar Grove. "I don't like it, but I do have to accept it and figure out how to live with it." She also gradually became more practiced at allowing herself "extras" or "creature comforts." It began with small things—putting on a sweater when she was chilly instead of just "toughing it out," or allowing herself to turn in early if she was tired. These were brand new experiences for her, and they represented a significant shift. By the time she was discharged from the clinic, she had even ordered a dining room table and a couch from Ikea to be delivered shortly after her return.

REFLECTIONS ABOUT OLIVIA

We can see here how Olivia's eating disorder is part and parcel of a larger ground project or ethos of living, one predicated on conservation, efficiency, and the prevention (or correction) of excess. Now, this might seem counterintuitive at first glance given that she struggled primarily with bulimia and not anorexia, since bulimia is characterized precisely by a form of excess in the practice of binging and with the "messiness" of purging. But this is part of the point. Olivia tries to avoid excess at all costs. But whenever it emerges, she feels she *must* eradicate it. Part of her struggle was precisely around the fact that, unlike John Galt in *Atlas Shrugged,* she could not control her humanity to the degree that she wanted to, and it "leaked" out, not only in her food practices but also in her relationships with others.

But I want to be very careful here not to play into what in the eating disorders world is a very blatant moralizing of anorexia as somehow "better" than bulimia, or of people with anorexia as somehow "more disciplined" or "more successful" at their eating disorder than those with bulimia or binge eating disorder. *This is patently untrue.* Two points bear mentioning here. Having struggled with anorexia, bulimia, and binge eating myself at different points, in addition to engaging in decades of research with people with these conditions, I can say with complete confidence that a person with anorexia is just as out of control around food as a person with bulimia or binge eating disorder. Maybe even more so—to the extent that she feels she has to shut down practically all access to food to prevent an anticipated frenzy. But this point aside, something more important is at stake: engaging in such comparisons continues to support a moralization of desire and need that casts these feelings as somehow negative or "bad" and depriving oneself of them as somehow morally good or laudable. *It is precisely this mindset that we need to combat.* The problem is not need or desire. The problem is that we don't know how to genuinely nourish ourselves—with food, yes, but more so with relationships and within ourselves. And more than this, the problem is that we don't know that *nourishing ourselves is OK* and even constitutes its own "good."

Returning to Olivia, it is clear that while her bulimia enacts her ground project (when she purges), it also continually threatens to destroy it (when she binges). That is, her bulimic behavior is the continual subverting and reasserting of a particular ethos of living. It becomes an ethical practice in and of itself. We can understand, then, how something as seemingly basic as eating sufficient amounts of food and not purging it would take this away from her.

WHAT'S THE PAYOFF?

So, what do we get by viewing eating disorders as a technology of presence animated by issues of affect, sensation, and becoming? I want to end this chapter by gesturing to a few issues that will be taken up in more detail later in the book.

Conceptualizing eating disorders as technologies of presence not only helps us understand the lived experiences of these conditions, their associated features, and their relational expressions but also opens up questions about what eating disorders might presence (and/or conceal) at the social and cultural levels. That is, what do eating disorders—as culturally defined phenomena—presence or elide in the current American cultural landscape?

One core argument in this book is that disordered eating practices such as self-starvation, bingeing, and purging collectively play a particular, though complex, role in human societies in that they become sites where culturally specific anxieties about relatedness, dependence, vulnerability, and morality accrue. In this regard, disordered eating may be "about" a variety of things, depending on the specific historical context and how an individual person makes meaning of it within her or his life circumstances. It might be about God. Or modesty. Or thinness. Or shame. Or some combination of these. Or something else. Whatever the specific content, disordered eating cracks open social and interpersonal bonds, exposing local understandings of the "how" and "why" of human existence.

This is not a straightforward process. Eating disorders are, in many ways, trickster conditions. This is not because people who have them are duplicitous or untruthful (in fact, I argue vehemently against this view). Rather, eating disorders—as culturally and historically constituted phenomena and as collections of very real practices and experiences—are tricksters in that *they reveal what they conceal, and they hide what they show.* They can, however, become potent and constructive interlocutors once you understand some basic premises.

In the context of contemporary American culture, we will see how eating disorders make visible cultural ambiguities and contradictions about such things as autonomy and relatedness, strength and vulnerability, trust and deception, and the nature of the real. They do not fit neatly into our categories of biological versus psychological illness. They do not clearly adhere to our dominant cultural understandings of independence and dependence. They challenge notions about what constitutes strength and what counts as vulnerability. They raise questions about who owns "truth" and where claims to reality should be staked. In the context of American managed care, eating disorders come to inhabit a place of "dirt," in anthropologist Mary Douglas's sense of "matter out of place."[35] This renders them as "polluting" and as targets for incorporative attempts to subsume them into existing categories. Thus, much like an individual with an eating disorder, eating disorders themselves trouble existing regimes of knowledge and perception, presencing an "otherwise" that necessitates new forms of recognition.

Eating disorders as social and cultural phenomena parallel people with eating disorders in another way as well. In family systems theory, the "identified patient," or "scapegoat," is the person in the family system who is explicitly targeted as the "sick one"—the (only) one in need of help—which allows the rest of the family to preserve the fantasy that they are healthy and fine and doing great. In the case of eating disorders, for example, this might show up as a family demanding that their daughter get treatment for "her" problem while refusing to participate in any family therapy or denying that family dynamics may have anything at all to do with the development of the illness. In a parallel process, eating disorders as conditions hold the role of the "identified patient" in the contemporary American healthcare landscape, they are cast as the "problem child," the one who is sick and in need of fixing, when in reality they are "carrying the symptom" of larger systemic dysfunction.

In the next section, we turn to these processes of identification as they unfold in practice, considering how eating disorders become real within clinical, research, and insurance company practices, how Cedar Grove programming constitutes the objects of intervention, and how understandings of recovery and chronicity set the parameters and horizons of care.

For the Ladies

Daddy says I'm getting chubby. He brings me a copy of a diet plan that he gives his "ladies" at work—his patients—for after they've had their babies. Eight hundred calories a day. I'm so excited!

I want him to be proud.

Frameworks

How do eating disorders become real?

In section 1, we considered how eating disorder theories constitute various bodily, emotional, cognitive, and interpersonal experiences and proclivities as problematic, and seek to provide a synthetic explanation of their relationships to one another. That is, these theories are not just about specific illness conditions—they also assert understandings of what the psyche and soma are, how they interact, why it matters, and how people can (or cannot) change. In this way, they serve not only as practical philosophies of the person, but also as a sort of projective repository for the dominant anxieties and concerns of a given society in a given historical moment around such issues as dependency, moral responsibility, and care. How a society understands *who* risks developing disordered eating (and who doesn't), *why* they develop it, *what kind* of "sick" this represents, and *how* to make them "better" tells us a great deal about how these anxieties and concerns take shape in the real world and what kinds of remedies the society has devised for addressing them.

In this section, we look at three frameworks and accompanying practices through which conceptual and theoretical understandings of eating disorders enter into and affect the material world. First, we consider the apparatuses that are used to identify and diagnose eating disorders in clients and the circulations of knowledge and priorities among these structures. Then, we turn to Cedar Grove's treatment program and examine how eating disorders are (re)constituted in the everyday life of the clinic's treatment approach. Finally, we consider recovery and chronicity as structuring horizons that situate the process of treatment within developmental narratives, sometimes with dire results.

FOUR

Identifying the Problem

WHEN IS AN EATING DISORDER (NOT) AN EATING DISORDER?

In chapter 2, we traced how contemporary approaches to eating disorders retain and amplify a core set of culturally informed tensions regarding how the "mind" and the "body" are conceptualized and how they are thought to interact, as well as how these tensions articulate with larger cultural concerns regarding relationality and care. Specifically, we saw that concerns about the boundary, flow, and amplitude of affect are shared across different models, which crystalizes these cultural tensions and anxieties and affords them a sense of legitimacy. Chapter 3 introduced the notion of eating disorders as technologies of presence across the multiple domains of the affective, the interpersonal, the social, and the structural. We learned how eating disorders facilitate different sorts of presence while simultaneously creating conspicuous absences.

Building on this idea of eating disorders as sites for articulating and struggling out tensions around presence, absence, and legitimacy, this chapter looks at how the structures of managed care, eating disorder research agendas, and clinical practice coincide to render eating disorders as particular sorts of objects of concern within certain epistemological and practical frameworks that, in turn, dictate access to care, what that care will look like, and how the horizons of "recovery" are imagined. Along the way, these healthcare structures generate relationships of care that are fraught with mistrust and suspicion for both patients and clinicians alike. To this end, I look closely at three interrelated practices: processes of intake and diagnosis, determinations of medical necessity, and appeals to evidence-based practice. Taken together, these practices create the reality of what an eating disorder is at Cedar Grove, who a given client is thought to be, and how relationships of care are structured and managed.

The first task in treating a client with an eating disorder is defining what an eating disorder is and then determining whether or not the client has one. Unlike diabetes, thyroid disease, or a broken bone, an eating disorder cannot be diagnosed definitively by a simple blood test or x-ray. Instead, a lengthy intake assessment must be performed by a trained clinician (see box 1; this process is detailed in chapter 7). This structured interview, which usually takes approximately two hours, enables the intake coordinator to collect detailed information about the client's background, family dynamics, family history of mental illness and/or addictions, previous treatments, current stressors, possible comorbid conditions (such as depression, anxiety, or self-harm), the history of her eating disorder, and her current reasons for seeking treatment. Once the assessment is done, the intake coordinator recommends a level of care for the client: residential program, partial hospital program (PHP), or intensive outpatient program (IOP). Whether a client enters treatment, and at which level, almost always depends on whether her insurance will cover the hefty cost: $1100 per day for residential care, $875 per day for ten-hour PHP, $675 per day for six-hour PHP, and $475 per day for IOP at the time of my research.

Given the cost of treatment, the vast majority of clients—even those who are financially well-off—depend on insurance benefits to pay for their care, and the trajectories and lengths of their treatment stays are often directly determined by decisions made by insurance care managers (many of whom have no specialized education in mental health issues, let alone eating disorders). Dotty, the utilization review manager at Cedar Grove, was responsible for obtaining the initial certification of insurance benefits for each client. This would often be the deciding factor for whether someone got treatment.

Clients almost universally described the intake process as terrifying. Most didn't even entertain the possibility of treatment until they felt they had absolutely no other option and it had become a choice between life and death. "People were telling me, you have to choose to be alive or you have to choose to give up," Karma, a twenty-two-year-old woman diagnosed with bulimia told me about her decision to schedule an intake assessment. Marjorie, a twenty-six-year-old woman diagnosed with anorexia, had a similar story. "I don't have a choice. I mean, the weight I'm at now, it's not healthy," she said. "I will eventually die. I don't want to die." "Really, any purge right now could give me a heart attack," said Dannilyn, a thirty-four-year-old woman diagnosed with bulimia, "so I knew I had to get help." "Right now, well, I don't

Clinician: Brooke Kennerly

Client: Priya Evanston

Date: xx/xx/xx

Intake with client. Brought in food rules. Discussed rigidity in all areas of life—plans out day in 15-min increments, cleans "obsessively" w/ritual aspects (certain chores certain times of day). Very controlled in all areas. Does not deviate. Mentioned that she enjoys amusement parks because of the "adrenaline rush." Only other place she gets that is from refereeing lacrosse. Notes that it's a "power trip" for her and helps her feel like she's imposing structure/control on a situation that's potentially out of control. Talked about super-high standards, how she's only fallen short of them with dance and volleyball. Did well @ practice, but wouldn't do well in competition. Attributed this to wanting to do well so badly that she just didn't. Was able to see parallels with "healthy" eating. Does not see a middle ground with food or anything else. Fearful of going back to the way she was when overweight. Hated the way she looked. Parents didn't like it, talked about it constantly—able to do so well in so many things, why not that? Priya would become defensive, but says she agreed with them. Got lots of positive feedback from them when she started to lose weight. Doesn't want to disappoint them. Mom doesn't understand why she can't just sit down and eat a cookie. Pressure to "get it together" and get on with school. Parallels with parents' disappointment when she wouldn't do well at competitions—she "should" be able to succeed, implication that it's a choice or a failing not to. She has really internalized this voice and made it her own. Asked her what she wants to get out of treatment—not sure. Gave her the assignment of developing 3 goals for treatment, stressed importance of them coming from her. Noted that she would like to be more flexible in some areas (e.g., food) but can't envision having a "normal" relationship to food. At the end of the session, Priya asked about standards for moving out of residential. Does not feel comfortable in the residential house, feels she connects with staff but not clients because they seem really "young." I told her it was different for every person, but that we'd first and foremost need to make sure she was medically stable. I encouraged her to give it some more time. She also asked for Internet password for Cedar Grove so she can work on assignments during breaks. Provisional diagnosis of obsessive-compulsive personality disorder, eating disorder not otherwise specified. She does not think she has an eating disorder per se—more orthorexia (her words). Seems invested in being "unique" and "different" from other eating disorder clients (mom seemed to stress this, too). Recommend residential.

really care if I pass away," Abby, a twenty-three-year-old woman diagnosed with anorexia, noted. "So, I have to let other people control that, I guess. And hopefully make me care for myself."

Lilia's account of her decision to schedule an intake assessment (for treatment for bulimia) is particularly harrowing:

> LILIA: It's like I'm eating like a cyclone, totally out of control, and my husband doesn't say anything. He sees me eat, but he doesn't say anything because he thinks I'm too skinny and he wants me to eat. He didn't know I was puking. But I get up in the morning and then I open up the trash and I go, "Oh my god, I couldn't have, I didn't." But then I know because my stomach is out to here.
>
> REBECCA: But you don't remember it?
>
> LILIA: Sometimes I do, but then I'll see crumbs on the counter, and I think, "God, what did I eat?" That part's scary, the blackouts. I mean, I'm afraid I'm going to get in the car and hurt somebody.
>
> REBECCA: So, coming into treatment, what motivated you to schedule your intake? What was the catalyst?
>
> LILIA: Well, I've been puking seven days a week, and my body's just had it. But what really scared me was probably about a month ago, I had a blackout, and my husband found me on the kitchen floor lying in a puddle of puke, and I got up the next day and he said, "I can't believe you're up," and I said, "What do you mean?" He says, "Don't you remember?" "Remember what?" "Last night." And I didn't, and that really scared me. I realized, if I don't do something, I'm going to die.

Some clients had tried to get better on their own, outside of treatment, without success. "It was worse right before I came in," Julia, a thirty-six-year-old woman diagnosed with anorexia, recounted about three days into her stay. "Because I tried to get better on my own, and it didn't—you can't. It's not possible to gain weight by yourself, not when you're that low." Whatever path they took to get to the intake, clients uniformly reported that they came to the appointment hoping for answers, clarity, and direction.

HARD DIAGNOSIS, SOFT DIAGNOSIS

As we've seen, the diagnosis of an eating disorder is based on the definitions given in the *Diagnostic and Statistical Manual of Mental Disorders,* which is now in its fifth edition. For each of the eating disorders, criteria must be met regarding behavioral, emotional, and cognitive features along axes of both amplitude and temporality; that is, symptoms must be present to the extent that they cause significant impairment in daily functioning (amplitude), and they must do so for a specified duration (temporality) for the person to be diagnosed with one of the eating disorders. Clinicians then distill their intake notes, like those on Priya (see box 1), into summations to share with the rest of the team (see box 2). The challenge for clinicians is how to render complex behaviors, feelings, and physical states in standardized terms that insurance companies will see as valid.

Given the specificity and clarity of diagnostic parameters in the *DSM* and the kinds of florid behaviors clients report, arriving at a diagnosis and recommendation for treatment might seem like it would be a straightforward task: a prospective client does or does not exhibit a particular behavior for the required duration. But whether a client actually gets approved by her insurance company for treatment involves yet another negotiation. As the following conversation with Patricia (a Cedar Grove intake coordinator) demonstrates, generating an official diagnosis and persuading an insurance company to cover care are entangled processes:

> What is always on my mind throughout an intake is, "What are the client's [financial] resources? What's their insurance?" That weighs heavy on my assessment of what level of care is most appropriate. I *diagnose* according to the *DSM,* of course. But, honestly, I can't fully separate that from the insurance situation, because I have to keep in mind that what I see in the client and what's on paper or in the *DSM* are not always going to match up. I may know very well that someone has anorexia or bulimia, but these are messy illnesses. They don't always fit the cookie-cutter mold of the diagnosis. So you have to get creative in how you ask questions and what you write down. You're not falsifying things, but just trying to help the client give you a picture you know the insurance company is going to understand.

The assessment and intake process at Cedar Grove, then, is a multilayered one. Clinicians first gather the client's narrative of what is going on. Then, they evaluate this narrative to determine the potential client's eating disorder pathology according to the *DSM*. Finally, they have to figure out how to *package*[1] the client so she will have the best chance of obtaining insurance coverage, all the while engaging in what anthropologist Erica James calls "bureaucraft" to get coverage for clients for care they need.[2] As Susan, a Cedar Grove therapist, told me, "It's hard when the person on the other end of the phone [the insurance company representative] is basically a bean

Current level of care: none

Admit date: xx/xx/xx

Age: 23

Admit weight: xxx

Height: 5'3"

Discharge goal weight: +/– 5 pounds from admission weight

Current calorie level: xxxx–xxxx

Cedar Grove therapist: Brooke Kennerly, LPC

Cedar Grove dietitian: Angie Carlson, RD, LD

Cedar Grove psychiatrist: Dr. Valerie Casey, MD

Outpatient therapist: John Palmeretto

Outpatient dietician: n/a

Outpatient psychiatrist: n/a

Primary care physician: n/a

Estimated length of stay: 4–6 weeks

DSM **diagnosis**

I. Eating disorder not otherwise specified

II. Deferred

III. Fatigue, chest pains, bradycardia

IV. Problems with primary support group, occupational problems

GAF score [general assessment of functioning]: V.34

Patient's long-term goals: Wants to be able to have a "normal" meal without "freaking out" about calories and exercise. Wants a "normal" relationship with food.

Patient's strengths: determined, focused, knowledgeable.

Patient's needs: permission and safety/containment to access authentic feelings.

Patient's abilities: sports, music.

Patient's preferences: "learn how to eat a normal meal"; "deal with people better."

Needs beyond the scope of Cedar Grove: will need long-term outpatient follow-up with therapist, dietician, psychiatrist.

Referrals for such needs: Will refer patient to Marsha O'Neill for therapy and continue with Angie Carlson as dietician and Dr. Casey as psychiatrist.

counter and you're here with a really sick patient in your office, and you're desperately trying to get them treatment. So you have to learn how to talk to them [the insurance case managers] to find out what they're looking for and what their priorities are, and then you try to fit the client's story into that mold." In other words, clinicians have to learn how to massage the information they get from clients into a form that is recognizable to case managers.

To do this, specialists at Cedar Grove continually tack back and forth across different registers, crafting and refining the "eating disorder" and the "eating disorder patient" through the interplay of attention to visual, interpersonal, biometric, verbal, social, and historical cues that are deemed meaningful and significant, either in isolation or in conjunction with one another.

For example, in a Cedar Grove therapists training session we learned that if a potential client reports that she eats 1600 calories a day but is at only 80 percent of her ideal body weight, we (clinicians) should not simply assume the client is lying (though that may be the case). Rather, we should build an understanding of this apparent incongruity by triangulating other information. What is the person's weight history? Is she purging? Overexercising? Has she experienced any recent losses or traumas that might help make sense of any recent drop in weight? Does she present with heightened anxiety about weight and shape issues? What is her interpersonal presentation? Does she make eye contact? Are her answers evasive or direct? What are her relationships like with her family and significant other? This sort of information is gathered in the assessment and must be continually and alternately isolated as "data" on the one hand and contextualized within the patient's life story on the other.

Information gained in the intake must also be explicitly "quotation marked," in the sense that patients are thought to not be reliable reporters of their own histories of behaviors, as they often minimize the severity of their illnesses. "If someone tells you she purges three times a week, multiply that by at least two, probably more like three," Janet, an intake coordinator, told me. "Same with the restrictors. If they tell you they eat eight hundred calories a day, divide that in half and you probably have a better sense of what's really going on. It's not that they are purposefully lying—not necessarily," she clarified. "It's just that there's just so much shame around this disease. Or they don't want to believe they're as sick as they really are. Or they're terrified of giving up the eating disorder, so they don't want you to know how bad it is. Unfortunately," she added, "we can only go by what they tell us in terms of trying to get insurance coverage. So, if they say they only purge three times a week, but we suspect it's more like three times a *day*, we're still stuck with not being able to get benefits for that client."

This movement between "hard diagnoses" (diagnoses according to the *DSM*) and "soft diagnoses" (what the clinician actually thinks is going on with the patient) affects both the care a clinician can deliver and the relationships that form as a result. Janet went on to describe a recent encounter: "[A client] walked through the door of my office, and I immediately knew that she was chronic, most likely bulimic, and was going to need a lot more than outpatient [treatment]. She sat down, we did the assessment, but I'm already thinking, 'What level of insurance does she have? How long could she really get in a treatment center?' Maybe outpatient [treatment] is all it's going to take. But I know that's not what she needs. She needs twenty-four-hour supervised care to break the cycle of binge eating."

"What happened?" I asked. "In this case, the insurance would only cert[ify] outpatient [treatment]," she replied. "I heard later that the client died. She's not the first, and she won't be the last."

Trying to get a patient covered for the level of care the clinician believes she needs often involves creating a narrative of the patient's struggles that portrays her as a certain kind of subject, specifically one who is *sick enough* to warrant care but *not too sick* to benefit from it. Janet continued:

> One of the things that really frustrates me is insurance companies needing to know—and this was the language that they use—that clients have *failed* a lower level of care. "Failed" is the word that they use. So, obviously, clinicians, we know what that means. That means that the intervention at the lower level of care was not effective and they need more support. But when you say that to a client, it sounds terrible. They come in saying, "I really want to go into residential [treatment]," and you tell the insurance company, "These are my patient's issues, I think they need residential." Then the insurance comes back and says, "Well, why are we going to residential? They need to fail at a lower level of care." So sometimes, I put these really acute people in PHP or even IOP when I know, ultimately, based on my professional experience, it is not going to be an effective intervention.

In other words, clinicians sometimes placed clients in lower levels of care than they needed specifically *so that they would fail* and therefore demonstrate to the insurance company the need for a higher level of care. While this makes some sense if we are talking about antibiotics, it is a different thing all together when we are talking about a deadly condition that is framed as a problem of the self or the will and when those suffering from it are historically perceived as resistant to getting well. Such "failures" further reinforce these stereotypes as well as narratives of chronicity (see chapter 6). "In that sense," Janet continued, "we are wasting resources, wasting time, putting a client at risk, often not capitalizing on the current level of motivation to change. Ultimately, [this] frustrates the family and further burns the family out."

But even while intake coordinators have to demonstrate that their client is *too sick* to succeed at a lower level of care, they also have to demonstrate that she is *sick enough* for a higher level of care. As Janet explains:

> The other issue that I have a lot is [the insurance company saying], "Your client isn't sick enough for this level of care." That language is really difficult to stomach and even more difficult to try and explain to the client without them thinking, you know, the thoughts that perpetuate eating disorders: "I'm inadequate, not good enough, undeserving, worthless, unlovable"—you go down the list of faulty core beliefs, they have it. And then they come in, finally seeking treatment, maybe having some infinitesimal amount of hope, and I have to come back and say, "You're just not sick enough to get the treatment that you're looking for."

When I asked Janet how she manages such situations, we had the following exchange:

JANET: I remember getting trained by Cathy [the person who served as intake coordinator before Janet]. She's such a riot. She would tell me, when she was training me, "This is going to happen, you're going to be frustrated about these things, and all you can do is really hope that they're cutting."

REBECCA: That they're *cutting?*

JANET: Yes. Cathy said, "If you can pull"—she would call it "the cutting card"—"If you can pull the cutting card, then they will get a higher level of care." And I think that that's clearly illustrating what a difficult place insurance has put everyone on the treatment side in. I'm thinking, "OK, they want PHP, they want residential, they're really motivated, but they're not going to get approved for anything but intensive outpatient." But if you realize, "Wow, they're cutting," you can definitely get them on a higher level of care. It is difficult. People that I really know need a higher level of care, and I am worried they wouldn't get it, I find myself thinking about how I can explain their case effectively. I feel like I am the Zen master with insurance companies.

It didn't always work, however. "There are plenty of times when people really need care but insurance just isn't going to come through," Janet said. "That is probably one of the most difficult parts of my job." When I asked her how she deals with situations like this, she told me:

> I ultimately, and I have no shame about this, throw the insurance company under the bus. First, I would try and help the patient understand that when you've got a bad heart, you're not going to immediately need to do open-heart surgery. That you might try some medicine or you may even have to put a pacemaker in before we want to actually do a bypass or something like that. I try and soften the blow a little bit. But at the same time, I tell them that this is an insurance decision and not a medical one, and it's not what the clinical team recommends. And I alert the [treatment] team that the patient will eventually end up in a higher level of care, sicker than she was before. But we have to play the game.

As we can see, these, clinicians are caught in a difficult bind. In such cases, they must explain to the patient why she is not able to get services she might need, want, and be entitled to, while at the same time trying to keep her invested in the *idea* of treatment and recovery. They must also advocate for the client when dealing with the insurance company, knowing that the insurance company doesn't want to pay for care and that even if it does, the client might not follow through.

In such situations, the eating disorder as the identified problem to be tackled takes on different contours and substance within different interactions. To the client, the eating disorder is presented as a serious, chronic, deadly condition that will require a massive life transformation to address. To the insurance company, the eating disorder is configured as a set of behavioral and medical issues that can, with the right type of treatment, be corrected. Both of these figurings are "true," but each tells a particular kind of story about what is wrong with the patient and what kinds of care are necessary to help her get well, and each banks on different kinds of information in constituting this narrative.

The eating disorder that requires treatment at any level (outpatient, IOP, PHP, or residential) is therefore a composite object.[3] Diagnosis entails integrating various elements—behaviors, thoughts, feelings, history, level of functioning—into a composite whole around which epistemological and practical lines are drawn. However, while these lines may be clear in many ways, they are not the end-all, be-all of how eating disorders are conceptualized at Cedar Grove; a number of other factors contribute to determining what is "wrong" with a client and how to best intervene to help her (see also the discussion of halo features in chapter 10).

In fact, diagnosis is just the first step in getting a client into treatment. It is here that the issue of "medical necessity" comes to the fore.

MEDICAL NECESSITY

To obtain insurance coverage for treatment at Cedar Grove, a potential client not only has to meet diagnostic criteria for an eating disorder but must also be demonstrably medically compromised and meet the "medical necessity" criteria defined by her particular insurance plan. This generally means that she must have documented symptoms such as severe bradycardia (slow heartbeat), marked postural hypotension (change in blood pressure on standing, indicating that the heart may be compromised), and/or labs that show a dangerous electrolyte imbalance or damage to the kidneys, pancreas, or liver. Clients are generally not admitted to treatment based on their eating disorder diagnosis or behavioral symptoms alone, no matter how severe these may be. If clinicians can't also demonstrate medical necessity for treatment, clients are unlikely to get insurance approval for care. This can be extremely frustrating for staff and clients alike and can put clients at significant risk.

I want to unpack this issue of "medical necessity" a bit. Medical organizations like the American Medical Association and the American Psychiatric Association determine the diagnostic criteria for different illness conditions (what constitutes appendicitis, hypertension, or schizophrenia, for example), and they also publish treatment guidelines that indicate the generally agreed upon interventions to be used at different stages of the illness process. This biomedical meaning-making is a separate process from how insurance companies function. While insurance companies recognize (for the most part) the legitimacy of biomedical illness categories and the diagnostic criteria that define them, they retain the authority to determine what, under their various plans, constitutes "medical necessity" for a given intervention, and this may—or may not—map onto medical understandings. For example, the American Medical Association recognizes certain diagnostic criteria for myocardial infarction (commonly known as a heart attack) and publishes practice guidelines for what interventions to employ at different points in the illness process. Insurance companies do generally abide by these guidelines, but technically they don't *have* to, and even if they choose to do so, they may require significant documentation in the form of lab or EKG results before determining that a certain intervention is, indeed, "medically necessary."

Managed care companies, then, have a direct hand in determining what constitutes a "problem" that requires medical intervention, what counts as "treatment," what qualifies as a medically relevant "illness," and what "health" looks like. Such authority enables them to control (and in some cases manipulate) the relationship of supply (health) and demand (illness) through certain kinds of boundary work, what sociologists Steve Woolgar and Dorothy Pawluch call "ontological gerrymandering," to maximize company profits.[4]

Such issues become even more fraught in the context of mental health, where there are no lab tests or x-rays that can definitively validate the "medical necessity" of an intervention and there is significant disagreement among clinicians about what constitutes best practices for the treatment of different conditions (this will be discussed in detail later in the chapter). Instead of depending on biological tests, mental health clinicians rely primarily on patients' self reports, the accounts of loved ones, and observed behaviors. A skilled clinician learns how to triangulate this information and, drawing on her or his own clinical expertise, use it to build a largely reliable assessment of what kind of intervention is needed. But this is a far cry from the kinds of clear-cut thresholds favored by insurance companies. What results, then, is a strategic negotiation among interested parties to determine the "reality" of the patient's condition, whether clinical intervention is warranted, and if so, what *kind* of intervention is most expedient.

FELICIA

Take the case of Felicia, for example, who was a twenty-year-old student when she entered treatment at Cedar Grove. She was not notably underweight, yet she had an eating disorder history that stretched back to when she was fourteen. At the time of admission, she was purging up to fifteen times per day, restricting her food intake, and using laxatives. Additionally, she struggled with acute depression. She had experienced difficulty getting treatment approvals due to her weight (she was not considered medically at risk in this regard), and so her only eating disorder care had been going to an outpatient group once a week.

Felicia's parents were angry at her for continuing to struggle with her eating disorder and were at the end of their rope. She had been on practically every medication and had gone through several rounds of intensive outpatient treatment with psychiatrists and dieticians. She had briefly been in another residential treatment facility but had been sent home for being "resistant." Felicia, for her part, was angry at her parents as well. She had been doing OK, she noted, but then she discovered that her father was using an online dating site behind her mother's back, and her weight began to plummet. This downturn was facilitated by her mother, a nurse, who gave Felicia diet pills (her mother had dieted her whole life and was perpetually worried about Felicia's weight).

Felicia acknowledged that, on one level, she "got her parents' attention" with her eating disorder. After they found out about it, her mom had stayed home from work to support her, and her dad was kinder. "[Her] dad shows his frustration by getting angry," Danya, the dietician, observed. "I've seen him get enraged firsthand. And he's in law enforcement. It's pretty scary." But then they would get fed up and angry and throw up their hands in sometimes harmful ways (for example, they left her home alone all weekend before she came to Cedar Grove, and she binged and purged nonstop). Dr. Casey stressed that Felicia had been ill for over six years and had come close to death more than once. "It's understandable that the parents might feel both significantly concerned and utterly exhausted," she said. "We should cut them some slack."

The team found themselves facing a serious dilemma. Felicia's insurance covered only acute inpatient hospital treatment (she had been to the hospital twice for low potassium and dehydration) and some partial hospital treatment (six hours a day), but not twenty-four-hour residential care, which is what the team felt she needed. She had been admitted to partial care, but it was not providing enough support. Her purging continued and seemed to have worsened.[5]

"The big question," Dr. Casey posed at the treatment team meeting the week before Felicia was admitted, "is whether this level of care [PHP] is going to work for her or not. Or will it stir [her] up more, so she'll go home and binge and purge?"

The following week's team meeting offered some insight into these issues. Cheryl, Felicia's therapist, said Felicia reported a very difficult weekend, with violent purging where she threw up blood. On hearing this, Dr. Casey expressed frustration with, rather than support for, the family, particularly with Felicia's mother. "The parents don't show up for family meetings and leave her alone all weekend," she reported. "She's only in PHP rather than a higher level of care because Mom said she was going to support her. So, it's reasonable to expect Mom to be there."

Dr. Arnold, a psychiatrist who worked part-time at the clinic, echoed this frustration. "My sense in meeting with the parents is that neither is particularly invested in her getting better," he observed.

"Do we think she's using her eating disorder to get close to [her] mom?" asked Dr. Casey.

"Yes," Dr. Arnold affirmed. "But Felicia wants exclusivity. She wants her mom to herself without her sister. And this is backfiring. Mom is showing she's not really able to support her. Mom and Dad have basically been checked out for the past six years. Dad is angry."

"So what can we do to help the outpatient therapist?" asked Dr. Casey.

"Well," said Brianna, a dietician, "she's still not following her meal plan. She restricts, then binges and purges."

"The research says that PHP or outpatient [treatment] is the best level to use for bulimia," Joan, an advanced practice nurse and the assistant director of Cedar Grove, observed, "so the insurance company is not going to pay for residential [care]. Period."

"Should we just discharge her, then?" asked Dr. Casey. "Because she needs a higher level of care. She is in PHP, and she is failing. She doesn't have supports. She needs twenty-four-hour care, but insurance won't pay."

Cheryl chimed in, "The problem is trying to break the cycle. We can cert[ify] her via medical benefits for a hospital, but then she wouldn't have mental healthcare, and it would cost insurance and the family more. *She* wants a higher level of care. That's part of what's so frustrating here."

Dr. Arnold had a different perspective. "The problem with twenty-four-hour care is that then we're doing it *for* her," he said. "It may also be hard to then get her *out* of twenty-four-hour care. She might really regress."

"OK," concluded Dr. Casey. "So we tell the family that if they can't go to a higher level of care because of insurance, we will do a medical evaluation and management plan and discharge her, rather than waste their resources."

A number of things are going on in these conversations that illustrate how the boundaries of eating disorders are drawn, so let me unpack them. The upshot is that Felicia, a very sick young woman who wants care and has insurance that covers eating disorders, is nevertheless not able to get the level of care her treatment team fervently believes she needs—twenty-four-hour residential care—because her insurance company does not think it is medically necessary. Her insurance will cover inpatient hospital treatment for acute medical emergencies (usually three to five days, with no mental health treatment) or day treatment, which the treatment team has seen actually exacerbates, rather than helps, Felicia's eating disorder. Or Felicia can be discharged and continue her downward spiral.

Why were inpatient hospital treatment and outpatient care the only two available options? In Felicia's case—and this is common—her insurance company's threshold for "medical necessity" was so high that she would have to be literally at death's door and need emergency hospital care to avoid impending death to access the benefits. Anything less than that, and the company mandated partial hospital treatment or outpatient treatment for maintenance. *The entire middle zone of care*—residential care, for people who need significant, round-the-clock support to *avoid* becoming acutely medically endangered—was simply not available to her unless she was willing and able to self-pay at a cost of over a thousand dollars a day.

What, then, should the clinicians at Cedar Grove do? In the end, the team opted to refer Felicia for medical evaluation and monitoring and to forego therapeutic support; that is, they decided that if the family could not afford to pay out of pocket for residential care, Felicia would be kicked out of the program. This is not as callous as it sounds. The team feared that being in day treatment was both making Felicia worse *and* depleting the family's resources. If residential care was not an option, they determined that, in this case, *withdrawing* care and referring Felicia to medical management was a way of, ironically, caring for her the best they could under the circumstances.

Of course, the team was doing more here than simply strategizing about insurance benefits. In the process of trying to determine their actions regarding care, the clinicians were also crafting understandings of Felicia and her parents (and the eating disorder) that were directly relevant to how that care would be delivered. On the one hand, Felicia and her parents were faulted for not taking recovery seriously and not being committed to doing what needed to be done for Felicia to get better. Her parents were portrayed as distant, disinterested, or angry, and Felicia was configured as a sort of passive victim, as someone who needed to be saved. Yet on the other hand, Felicia was portrayed as "grasping" in various ways. She wanted, they concluded, exclusivity with her mom, a desire that echoes traditional views of eating disorders as manifesting enmeshment. She also wanted residential care, which was seen by some of the clinicians as a good thing (indicating a desire for recovery), but was viewed by Dr. Arnold as possibly expressing an unhealthy dependency. What emerged were portrayals of Felicia's parents as inconsistent and unempathic, and of Felicia as clingy and needy. *This matters,* because it also affects how both clinicians and insurance company personnel evaluate what constitutes the best care for Felicia under the circumstances. Significantly, it offers the clinical team a way to make clinical sense of having to adhere to treatment restrictions imposed by nonclinicians at the insurance company. By viewing Felicia as potentially too dependent and at risk of becoming "regressed" in residential treatment, the team was eventually able to rationalize that fighting for residential treatment would not make healthy sense and that the removal of care was actually the "better" option for her.

Clinicians are not always able to rationalize such decisions, however, and they often directly challenged insurance rulings. "Sometimes, the [insurance] person on the other end of the phone just doesn't have experience with eating disorders," Brooke, a therapist, told me. "Or sometimes they do, but they have a different assessment of what's going on or what should be done. You have to pick your battles—you can't fight them on everything every time. But sometimes, if you really think a decision is unfair or is going to put a patient at risk, you have to." In the event that the clinic wishes to challenge an insurance company decision, the case goes to a phase called "peer-to-peer," where Dr. Casey consults directly by phone with a psychiatrist or other medical doctor at the insurance company to discuss the case in depth. The insurance company physician makes a final determination about the issue. "It goes our way about 50 percent of the time," Dr. Casey told me. "It's impossible to predict what will happen."

In such negotiations, healthcare professionals and insurance companies generally view each other with mutual suspicion. This is built into the system and is part of the history of managed care itself. Healthcare professionals were key targets of the healthcare reforms in the 1970s and 1980s that generated the current managed care environment, and they were portrayed as major causes of waste, inefficiency, and needless expense.[6] This negative characterization of clinicians was used to justify the transfer of control and decision-making authority from clinicians to the managed health plans. To promote the view that they are neutral third parties interested in patient welfare over profits, insurance companies developed increasingly specific rules (e.g., medical necessity criteria, guidelines, standards, practice parameters, best practices) to govern the provision of care.[7] The underlying claim was that healthcare costs would decrease if clinicians would adhere to such "objective" measures and use "research-based" treatments to devise appropriate treatment strategies.[8] Despite the fact that this reduction in costs hasn't materialized, the domain of "evidence" and "evidence-based practice" has emerged as a key space of negotiation for both clinicians and insurance companies in determining patient care, and it continues to function as a provisional "neutral zone."

EVIDENCE-BASED PRACTICE

In the 1990s, as managed care companies were raking in record profits while increasingly restricting access to care, "evidence-based practice" or EBP, gained purchase as what public health scholar Sandra J. Tanenbaum calls a "public idea."[9] A public idea distills complex and multidetermined phenomena into something that can provide the gratification of action without necessarily significantly addressing the underlying causes of a problem, such as focusing on arresting drunk drivers to reduce automobile accidents or requiring background checks to reduce gun violence. These types of interventions may be helpful, but they don't take on the deeper structural and cultural issues that give rise to the problems in the first place. EBP, argues Tanenbaum, is one such public idea that functioned to focus consumer anger about rising healthcare costs on providers rather than insurance companies. As psychiatrist Geoffrey Reed and psychologist Elena Eisman note, "The American public has been offered the idea that the essential problem with the health care system is uninformed practice, which could be resolved if health care professionals practiced in ways more consistent with research findings."[10] This perspective was legitimated by academically based clinical researchers, who suggested that the core problem in healthcare services was the inappropriate application of their research by clinicians. In other words, skyrocketing healthcare costs were increasingly attributed not to the greed of managed care companies but to the inefficient practice of care, which could be remedied (supposedly) by requiring clinicians to employ EBP. This was a powerful rhetorical move because after all, as Tanenbaum notes, "Who can argue with evidence?"[11]

Importantly, however, not all "evidence" is created equal. There is what David Sackett (widely recognized as the father of EBP) calls a "hierarchy of evidence" that frames what the EBP movement considers as legitimate.[12] At its most basic, to be considered "evidence-based," an intervention must have been shown to be "effective" in several published peer-reviewed research studies. The epitome of such studies is the randomized controlled trial, or RCT.[13]

In RCTs, strict participation parameters constitute largely homogenous sample populations based on selected criteria. Participants are randomly assigned to one of two or more interventions that are being investigated for efficacy. Conditions outside the test variable are carefully controlled.

RCTs are the gold standard in medical research, but they have some unique problems when deployed in the domain of mental or behavioral health. Controlling the experimental conditions and measuring relevant variables is tricky when the boundaries of the target of study (mental illness) are not easily discerned amid everyday life activities and when forms of suffering are not easily quantifiable. These concerns are compounded in the case of eating disorders, where the mental illness in question not only causes significant distress to those suffering from it but also can be physically damaging or even fatal if left untreated. The ethics of designating a control group (a group that does not receive the intervention being studied) in eating disorder research, then, must be very carefully considered and managed. This challenge has been a significant part of why there are so few RCTs for eating disorders, and this in turn further contributes to insurance companies' reluctance to fund treatments for these conditions.

To meet the highest standards of EBP, an intervention must not only have been studied using multiple RCTs but also be accompanied by a standardized treatment manual that can (in theory) be taken up and utilized by any clinician with the appropriate training. "Care," then, becomes abstracted out from the particulars of the therapeutic relationship and conceptualized as something that can be contained within a manual. This leads, as Reed and Eisman observe, to "a view of treatment manuals as constitutive of psychological treatments rather than as exemplars or laboratory analogues of them."[14] What such a "pharmaceutical" model of therapy[15] misses is the importance of the therapeutic relationship, which repeatedly has been found to be among the strongest and most consistent predictors of treatment outcome.[16]

Indeed, while the use of EBP is appealing to clinicians and funders alike,[17] Reed and Eisman argue that "there is virtually no evidence to support the underlying assumption that the implementation of EBP will improve health care services and outcomes or reduce health care costs, except to the extent that it serves to restrict access to care."[18] That is, the main reason the focus on EBP saves money may not be that it provides *better* care but that it *limits* care. This is for a very simple reason: insurance companies are more likely to pay for evidence-based treatments than those that are not evidence-based, and they often exclude coverage for any interventions that are not explicitly evidence-based. As a result, the main cost savings that derive from the implementation of EBP practices may come from decreased access to treatment rather than improved care services.

This provocative claim gains traction when we consider that less than one third of patients with mental health disorders receive treatment that meets even minimal standards for treatment adequacy.[19] This situation is especially pronounced among people with eating disorders. Only 10 percent receive any care at all, and only a fraction of *those* receive specialized care.[20] And as we saw in Felicia's case, appeals to evidence may mean a client receives no care at all.

CIRCUITS: INSURANCE, RESEARCH, AND TREATMENT

What I want to highlight with this discussion is the looping effect of the relationships among insurance reimbursements, research studies, and evidence-based care, and the resulting implications this has for eating disorders treatment. Insurance companies pay for treatments that are "proven" to "work" for an "identified" problem. To document that treatments work (what counts as "proof" and what counts as "success" is often tied to economics), treatment outcomes must be measurable. This means that the identified problem must itself be rendered in quantified terms. In the case of eating disorders, this means that understandings of the "problem" come to hinge on biometrics—weight, blood pressure, pulse, lab values such as liver and pancreatic functioning—which then serve as proxies for the eating disorder of which they are thought to be indicators. And because of the centrality of insurance company decisions in the provision of care, biometrics assume center stage in both eating disorder research and eating disorders treatment.[21] This is what philosopher Ulrike Hahn calls the "problem of circularity"—that is, the way researchers conceive of rigorous research necessarily affects how they define symptom, illness, treatment goals, and effectiveness.[22]

What emerges in treatment practice, then, is a form of "teaching to the test," where research and treatments become tethered to insurance companies' economic priorities in ways that have dramatically shifted how eating disorders are understood over the past thirty years. This shift has had many consequences. Some have been positive: more people have access to care than before, and clinics and doctors are incentivized to use treatment practices that seem to be efficacious, at least according to some measures of symptom reduction. Others, however, have been disastrous: clients are regularly discharged long before they are ready, and clinicians often find themselves blocked from delivering interventions they believe are needed.

In tracing these circuits among managed care priorities, research design and funding, and treatment practices, we can see that what constitutes an eating disorder is continually negotiated within interactions between different stakeholders. More than this, what an eating disorder *is* is a shifting, fluid assemblage rather than a stable and discrete disease entity. Through processes of diagnosis, determinations of medical necessity, and appeals to EBP, clinicians and insurance companies generate provisional understandings of what an eating disorder is, what a given client needs, and how care should be managed. Yet disagreements, frictions, and contradictions are common. And when it comes to actual practice, many of these provisional understandings are wrong. Nevertheless, they hold powerful sway over determinations about care.

In the next chapter, we turn to how these provisional understandings inform the structure and content of the Cedar Grove program.

Spinning

AUGUST 1980

"Mom, something is really wrong with me," I say shakily, plopping myself down in the mustard yellow vinyl chair in the sunroom. My mother is sitting at the kitchen table in her blue bathrobe, reading the morning paper and smoking a cigarette, her second cup of coffee by her elbow.

She looks up at me, perplexed. "What are you talking about?" she asks.

"Look at me!" I stand up. "No matter what I do I stay fat!" I pound the outsides of my thighs with my fists. "See? Do you see that? I can't get rid of it! Do you see it?" I insist, hitting myself harder.

"I see what you're talking about, but it's not fat, honey," Mom says, clearly not sure how to respond to my increasing panic.

"I ride the stationary bike ten miles every morning and ten miles every night. I'm following the diet dad gave me, and no matter what I do I stay *fat* and *disgusting*. Something's *wrong* with me! I'm not like everyone else. What is *WRONG* with me?" I plead.

FIVE

A Hell That Saves You

CEDAR GROVE'S STAFF AND PROGRAMS

Being here is hell. Absolute hell. The staff try to make it better—
as best they can, anyway. They are really good, and they actually
care about the patients. Not like some other places I've been. But
honestly, treatment is miserable. It's physically painful and just
emotionally brutal. It's absolute hell. A hell that saves you.

—KENDALL

If contemporary models of eating disorders enfold and legitimate a set of
paradoxical subjectivities (as we saw in chapter 2), and circuits of insurance
funding, research priorities and diagnostic practices determine the boundaries of health and pathology (as we saw in chapter 4), then the obvious next
questions are: How does this affect the process of treatment? What kinds of
"healthy subjects" are cultivated at Cedar Grove, and how does this happen?
In this chapter, we begin to answer these questions by looking more closely
at Cedar Grove as a particular kind of microculture, what I call an *affective
institution,* whose purpose is to reshape the emotional, behavioral, sensory,
and interpersonal lives of participants. It does this through a number of strategies, both explicit (like rules, regulations, and consequences) and implicit
(like the organization of space, the tone of interpersonal interactions, the
rhythms of daily life, and responses to emotional expression). The goal of
affective institutions like Cedar Grove is to reshape the affective lives of
participants—to teach them how to feel, relate, and socialize in new and,
presumably, healthier ways.

In addition to reshaping the explicit targets of intervention (clients, in the
case of Cedar Grove), affective institutions like Cedar Grove also bank on and
reshape the emotional lives of their employees. Affective institutions function
by relying on the emotion work (shaping their own emotions) and emotional
labor (using their emotions in the service of caring for others) of their employees, who create and manage the organizational environment so as to facilitate

certain kinds of emotional experiences for clients and for themselves. To do this effectively, employees must continually work on their own emotions in order to present themselves as calm, confident, clear, and therapeutically oriented (see chapter 12). These institutions, then, are affective in multiple, overlapping ways and work on and through different participants differently. To understand this process, let us look at Cedar Grove more closely.

THE CLINICAL SETTING

At the time of my research, Cedar Grove was comprised of three separate buildings: a residential house with eleven beds for clients needing twenty-four-hour care, a transitional house with six beds for clients ready to practice more independent living skills prior to discharge, and the main program facility, where most therapeutic and clinical activities for residential and non-residential clients took place. Clients from the residential and transitional houses, as well as those in outpatient care (usually between ten and twenty clients), converged at the treatment location for programming, which ran from 7:30 a.m. to 7:30 p.m. seven days a week (though clients not in residential care sometimes attended fewer programming hours). During program hours, the treatment suite was full and lively, with anywhere from twenty to thirty patients present, plus the staff.

The residential and transitional houses were, at the time of my research, private houses, located in a moderately upscale residential neighborhood about a ten-minute drive from the program facility (clients were transported between the houses and the program facility in a clinic van). The interiors of the houses were colorfully yet tastefully decorated to create a sense of cozy and slightly zany domesticity—a balance of serenity and originality—with brightly colored throw pillows on the soft couches and fresh flowers in vases. The walls were covered with inspirational quotes and art pieces made by former clients. Each bedroom had two or three beds, and roommate assignments were based on personality and primary clinical issue. "You don't want a bunch of restricting anorexics together," Denise, a nurse, told me. "Too much competition. It's best to mix it up." Bedrooms and bathrooms were kept locked when not in use to prevent clients from disappearing into them to exercise, purge, or simply isolate.

The main treatment suite was housed in a stately old building that had been rehabbed so that the outer exterior of old-timey grandeur felt somewhat at odds with the high-tech provisions such as networked computers, security keypads, and the portable medical equipment necessary for running a contemporary healthcare facility. At the time of my research, Cedar Grove took up most of the second floor of this building, with the first floor rather incongruously occupied by two restaurants, a fitness center, and a beauty salon.

The main treatment suite of Cedar Grove (which is now the adult unit, but at the time housed all programming) was set up like a rectangle, with one side being a wall of windows. The large central common area was framed on one side by the facility kitchen and on the other by a substantial marble fireplace. In front of the fireplace sat a long, curved sectional couch, where clients lounged and slept between activities. Several large wooden tables filled the remainder of the common space, where clients ate all their meals and snacks and also did crafts, worked on homework, and participated in other activities when they weren't in therapy. A long marble counter and glass door separated this dining area from the kitchen. At no time were clients permitted to enter the kitchen.

The spaces off the main common area were divided by function. To the south were the clinical offices, where the therapists and dieticians met with clients (Cedar Grove has expanded since the time of my research, and the clinical offices now also populate the north side of the space). This area also had two large group rooms for group therapy sessions. To the north of the common area were the administrative offices, where the intake coordinator, medical coordinator, program director, and utilization review (insurance) manager had their offices. The nursing station was located on the north side as well. It was comprised of two small rooms—one with a sliding glass window looking out onto the common area, and one with no windows, where charts and medications were kept and where staff could speak out of earshot and eyesight of clients. An electronic keypad limited access from the common room to the administrative offices.

Aside from the keypad restricting access to administrative areas (where confidential patient records were housed), Cedar Grove was not a locked psychiatric facility. Anyone could leave the facility at any time, although doing so without written permission was patently against program rules. Due to the nature of eating disorders and clients' urges to binge, purge, and/or exercise when not supervised, all bathrooms were kept locked and all food-stuffs and drinks were kept in locked cabinets. Clients were required to relinquish their cell phones at the beginning of programming each day, and computer and internet use was limited to certain times in the evenings, mornings, and weekends, when programming was not in session.

Running an eating disorders clinic requires a full, interdisciplinary staff. During the bulk of my research period, Cedar Grove employed one full-time and two part-time psychiatrists, two part-time adolescent medicine specialists, eight nurses, five therapists, three dieticians, fifteen direct care staff, two intake coordinators, a utilization review manager, two administrative assistants, and a small kitchen staff. Direct care staff and nurses worked around the clock in three eight-hour shifts. Doctors, dieticians, and therapists generally worked from 9:00 a.m. to 6:00 p.m. on weekdays and provided on-call coverage as needed in the evenings and on weekends. Irrespective of their areas of expertise, all employees underwent additional specialized training at Cedar Grove to learn the clinic's view of eating disorders and its strategies and policies for working with clients.

Cedar Grove organized its staff into three main lines: medical, therapeutic, and dietary—which mirrored the three prongs of the treatment program. The medical line included the nurses, medical doctors, and psychiatrists. The therapeutic line contained the direct care staff and therapists. The dietary line encompassed the kitchen staff and dietitians. Despite these functional divisions, the clinic program was holistic and integrative in its vision. When a client was admitted to Cedar Grove, she was assigned a "mini-team" made up of a dietician, a therapist, and a psychiatrist, who worked together to coordinate her care. Direct care staff and nurses all worked with all clients, but one of each was assigned to specially attend to particular clients and serve as a liaison with the mini-team.

The mini-team was assigned by the intake coordinator prior to a client's admission based on her assessment of both the incoming client's needs and a given team's availability. The client's therapist led the team, serving as the point person and coordinator. She or he was responsible for overseeing the client's treatment, liaising with the insurance company, communicating with the family, and conveying team decisions to the client. Getting a good fit between client and therapist was therefore a key concern during the admissions and intake process. "I try to match people [with therapists] based on personalities and who I think will work well together," Janet, an intake coordinator, told me. "For example, Susan works really well with bulimics who have been in multiple treatments because she doesn't take any shit and because she's really experienced in CBT, which is the first-line therapy for bulimia. Brenda works better with the more timid anorexics because she's really maternal and they trust her. They would be totally scared and put off by Susan. So I try to match people based on things like that. Usually, it works, but sometimes not. Sometimes it's a disaster." Clients met with their psychiatrist and medical doctor once a week, their dietician twice a week, their therapist three times a week (for residential clients; twice a week for day treatment clients), and had daily, ongoing contact with nurses and direct care staff. The idea was that professionals in these three domains would work together in a coordinated fashion to provide complete and seamless care for clients. Despite the best of intentions, however, this was not always the case.

THE MEDICAL DOMAIN

Nurses

Nurses at Cedar Grove were responsible for the routine medical care of clients, including monitoring weights and vitals, distributing medications, attending to minor scrapes or injuries, and placing feeding tubes. All had specialized training in treating eating disorders, though not as much as the therapeutic staff, an issue that sometimes led to problems (such as when a nurse invited a client to live with her and her family after an early insurance discharge—a flagrant boundary violation). Most nurses were regular RNs, but Joan, the assistant director of the clinic, was an advanced practice nurse, meaning she could prescribe medications and perform procedures above and beyond those permitted for regular RNs.

In the case of Cedar Grove, the specific personalities of the nurses mattered greatly in terms of the overall affective tenor of the place on any given day. All of the nurses were extremely caring, though most also had a take-no-nonsense orientation. This blend of care and limit setting is generally seen to be ideal in working with this population. As Claire, one of the nurses, noted, "You have to be firm but kind with [eating disorder clients]. Many of them have experienced a lot of trauma, so they're hypersensitive to people getting angry at them or being too strict. But they also need clear limits or they're going to push and manipulate and find ways around the rules. It's a delicate balance, and it takes practice to get it right." In particular, nurses had to be comfortable setting and holding firm limits with clients when it came to issues of medical safety or medical procedures. In the event that a medical issue arose that a nurse couldn't handle directly, however, she (they were all women) accessed the next level of expertise, the physicians, which included psychiatrists, adolescent medicine specialists, endocrinologists, and other specialists as needed.

Psychiatrists

Psychiatrists are medical doctors who specialize in psychiatric issues. Psychiatrists who are eating disorder specialists have additional training and knowledge about the particular psychological features, medical risks, and complications associated with these illnesses. They could therefore handle many of the medical issues that arose in the clinic, and they attended to most concerns, with a few exceptions (addressed later in this chapter). Dr. Casey, the clinic director, is a psychiatrist, and several other psychiatrists worked at the clinic on a part-time basis, seeing clients, consulting on cases, and participating in clinical team meetings. Psychiatrists were responsible for the integration of therapeutic and medical care with an eye toward clinical psychiatric concerns that required medical intervention in the form of psychotropic medications. They were also usually the ones who would go "peer-to-peer" with insurance company physicians when an insurance decision was under appeal.

Although psychiatrists in many mental health settings are afforded the highest level of authority and respect,[1] this was not necessarily the case at Cedar Grove. Dr. Casey worked hard to cultivate a sense of equity and balance among the medical, therapeutic, and dietary programs. As will become evident throughout this book, there were many occasions when psychiatrists, therapists, and dietitians disagreed about how to proceed with given clients. In such cases, Dr. Casey's strategy fostered an inclusive view that took all expertise seriously. This sometimes led to excruciatingly extended treatment team meetings that would last five hours or more. But the end result was that each member of a client's treatment team participated in devising a way forward and thus felt heard and respected, even if the outcome was something other than what she or he originally wanted.

In cases where a client required more specialized medical care than what Dr. Casey or the nurses could provide, additional physicians were consulted, either on an ad hoc basis or to follow a client's entire treatment course.

Other Medical Doctors

Unlike therapists, psychiatrists, dietitians, nurses, and direct care staff, medical doctors (aside from Dr. Casey) were not in full-time residence at Cedar Grove. During my research period, two adolescent medicine doctors affiliated with the clinic came to see patients a few times a week or as needed if an acute issue arose (e.g., an endocrinologist consulted on cases involving patients with diabetes). For any other medical issues that required a physician, clients were transported by Cedar Grove direct care staff to appointments or procedures offsite.

THE DIETARY DOMAIN

Kitchen Staff

I had relatively little interaction with the kitchen staff, which mirrored the clients' level of contact with them. Kitchen staff were hired by the lead dietician in consultation with the lead chef, and they mostly kept out of sight. Of note, however, is the fact that, aside from one night nurse, the only individuals of color on the Cedar Grove staff during the time I worked there were those who worked in the kitchen.

In many ways, the kitchen staff had both the most important and the most thankless jobs at the clinic. Taking the premise that "food is medicine"[2] seriously (see chapter 10), the kitchen staff were in charge of preparing and "dosing" (apportioning) the "medicine" that would make or break a client's health and recovery. Yet even so (or, in fact, because of this), they were also the targets of a great deal of suspicion and even hostility from the clients, who often perceived kitchen staff (rightly or not) as not being careful enough with portioning or even of purposefully altering meal plans or calorie content in order to "fatten them up." "I think they're jealous of us," Molly, a twenty-year-old woman diagnosed with anorexia, complained one day in a community meeting. "I wouldn't be surprised if they wanted to do things to mess with us, just because they can."

Because of the potential for clients to vent their frustration at kitchen staff and the fact that, unlike other employees, kitchen staff were not clinicians of any kind, the dietitians ran interference and ultimately bore the brunt of clients' anxieties about food.

Dieticians

Dieticians at Cedar Grove were responsible for the nutritional well-being of clients, a challenging and delicate matter in the context of eating disorders. When a patient was admitted to Cedar Grove, she was assigned a dietician as part of her care team. The dietician's role was to evaluate the patient's current nutritional status based on weight and height, recent eating patterns, lab results, and growth charts. She then developed a personalized meal plan to help the client meet weight gain (usually two to three pounds per week) or stabilization goals while also carefully monitoring and adjusting for the client's unique metabolic response to increased or regularized food intake. Of particular concern is a condition called "refeeding syndrome," a potentially fatal imbalance in fluids and electrolytes that can develop when nutrition is reintroduced after a period of acute starvation, and it can be fatal if not properly addressed.

Dieticians were also responsible for designing and managing clients' meal plans (determining the number of overall calories and their distribution across meals and snacks), including making decisions about when and how meal plans would be increased, decreased, or maintained. They set clients' goal weights, which were articulated as a range and were generally (for clients diagnosed with anorexia or underweight clients diagnosed with bulimia nervosa or other specified feeding or eating disorder) around 90 to 100 percent of their ideal body weight, as determined from childhood or adolescent growth charts plus other factors, such as build and level of activity. Clients who came in at over 100 percent of their ideal body weight were not assigned lower goal weights.

Dieticians met with clients two times per week, and these sessions were often very difficult. "This is the crux of the disorder," Nadia, a dietician, told me. "At least, it's what clients are most fixated on and most anxious about. Our job is to make them do the one thing they are most terrified of doing: eat consistently and gain weight. So of course they're going to see us as the bad guy. That's OK. I can handle that. I don't take it personally. I know it's the fear talking."

Direct Care Staff

Direct care staff at Cedar Grove, as in most mental health settings, were the frontline workers at the clinic. They were the ones with the most consistent contact with clients, those responsible for the everyday tasks of clinical care. Direct care staff woke clients up in the morning, served meals and snacks, sat with clients while they ate, monitored bathroom visits, ensured clients were where they were supposed to be at any given time of the day, transported clients to and from offsite doctor appointments, and administered tube feedings. Staff that had the appropriate training and certification also distributed medications. Direct care staff also served important therapeutic functions, acting as the de facto therapeutic arm of the clinic when clients were not in group or individual therapy sessions. This entailed attending to clients' mood swings and panic attacks, helping them navigate prickly relationships with other clients or staff, coaching them through difficult visits with family, comforting them when they were overrun with guilt for complying with a meal plan increase or dealing with panicky urges to purge, and encouraging them when they were feeling hopeless about recovery. Direct care staff were also responsible for documenting in detail each and every one of these encounters in client charts, and they were expected to update each client's chart during each shift, noting any significant events as well as the client's overall mood, degree of compliance or noncompliance with the program, and any concerns.

Direct care staff were required to have a bachelor's degree in psychology, social work, or a related field, and many were working on advanced degrees in social work or professional counseling. The overwhelming majority of direct care staff at Cedar Grove were female. During my seven years of affiliation at the clinic, I knew of only three direct care staff who were men.[3]

Like anthropologist Paul Brodwin's descriptions of frontline community psychiatry workers,[4] direct care staff at Cedar Grove had both the most immediate patient responsibility and the least authority. They had to deal with panic attacks, accusations of indifference, impatience for bathrooms to be unlocked, meal rechecks (when clients wanted food portions to be remeasured to ensure they got the correct amounts), complaints about therapists, crying, and refusals to attend group therapy. Yet their actual authority to make decisions was limited. If a situation arose that required a clinical decision or a change of protocol, direct care staff had to contact a client's therapist, nurse, or psychiatrist before taking any action.

This doesn't mean that direct care staff had no power, however. On the contrary, they had a great deal of power that could be exercised in any number of ways. They could drag their feet in announcing a smoke break. They could refuse to allow a recheck of a client's meal portions. They could bend rules or choose to enforce them with strict meticulousness. They could decide if or when to take an issue up the chain of command. Because of their numbers and the frequency and significance of their contact with patients, direct care staff, more than any other staff members, shaped the overall "vibe" of the clinic during any given shift.

Direct care staff supported and facilitated all aspects of the Cedar Grove program (medical, dietary, therapeutic), but they reported most directly to the therapists.

Therapists

In addition to providing group and individual therapy (discussed in more detail in chapter 7), therapists functioned as case managers at Cedar Grove and coordinated clients' care while they were in treatment. When a client was admitted, she was assigned an individual therapist who would be responsible for coordinating her care. Residential clients saw their individual therapists for one-on-one therapy (fifty minutes per session) three times a week. Day treatment clients had individual therapy twice a week. Group therapy formed the bulk of the Cedar Grove program.

Becoming a Cedar Grove therapist required levels of training and practice above and beyond standard social work, counseling, clinical psychology, or other therapy training, and therapists were not hired at Cedar Grove unless they had some sort of background or experience working with eating disorders. Many therapists gained this type of experience by working as direct care staff at Cedar Grove or another facility for a number of years. "It's important for therapists to understand what eating disorders are about," Dr. Casey explained to me. "This is a very challenging population. You need to know what you're getting into, and you need to know what to expect. It's different than working with other kinds of issues. These girls are sick in ways that are not always immediately apparent, and you need to be skilled and practiced enough as a clinician to be able to see and work with those dynamics." In

The prevailing understanding is that working with eating disorders is a skilled specialty for which not everyone is suited.

And in fact, therapeutic capacity is not the only kind of skill needed for this work. During the course of my research, the expectations placed on the therapists changed, and they became responsible for handling insurance reviews (previously done by the Dotty, the utilization review manager), meaning that in addition to all of their therapeutic duties, it became their job to call clients' case managers at the insurance company, provide updates about treatment, and obtain authorization for additional treatment days as needed.

On the one hand, having therapists do insurance reviews makes sense— the therapists knew more than anyone else about what was going on with a given client and could therefore, in theory, present the strongest case to the insurance company. But this change also added an enormous burden to therapists' already overfull plates.

Even before they were assigned insurance duties, the therapists were seriously overtaxed. Each residential client required a minimum of seven hours of work per week, between leading three individual sessions per week, communicating with the family, keeping up with documentation, creating treatment plans, and managing day-to-day issues. With four clients considered a full load, that's twenty-eight hours of just individual therapy work. Add to this five to six group therapy sessions per week (sixty to ninety minutes each, plus the time spent filling out documentation on each client in the group, requiring a total of approximately six to ten hours per week), treatment team meetings (two to three hours per week), mini-team meetings (thirty minutes per day, adding up to two and a half hours per week), and you have a very full schedule. And that is if everything goes smoothly, no one has a crisis or needs anything outside of their allotted time, no new clients are admitted, and everything runs as it is supposed to. In reality, crises are common, issues arise, and things rarely run on time. It was not at all uncommon for therapists to work forty-five to fifty hours a week or more, even before they were charged with carrying out the insurance work, and even then to feel like there was not enough time to get everything done. Many were frazzled, harried, and stressed, conditions that were exacerbated by working with a challenging patient population who often resented (or appeared to resent) attempts to be led toward health.

Nevertheless, there was remarkably little turnover of the therapeutic staff at Cedar Grove during the time I was there. This is notable because eating disorders clinicians have among the highest rates of burnout of any clinical specialty.[5] When I asked Cedar Grove therapists why they thought turnover was so low, they uniformly credited Dr. Casey's expertise in the eating disorders field as well as her personal management style, which made them feel valued and important even in the midst of increasing demands and diminishing resources for meeting them.

My experience of the therapists at Cedar Grove was that they were highly skilled and extremely dedicated clinicians who cared deeply about their patients and did everything they possibly could to get them the care they needed. They were not infallible, and there were plenty of instances where they might have chosen to do something differently in retrospect. They were under phenomenal pressure from all sides—from the requirements of their jobs, from insurance companies, and from clients themselves—to "get it right." How and when missteps occurred, then, were telling. In navigating these pressures, therapists (and, indeed, all Cedar Grove staff) found guidance in the clinic's philosophy of eating disorders, which provided a framework for ethical action.

CEDAR GROVE'S VIEW OF EATING DISORDERS

Borrowing from the proliferation of models of eating disorders and philosophies of treatment discussed in chapter 2, the Cedar Grove program staff, under the direction of Dr. Casey, crafted the clinic's program from best practice research in a range of therapeutic modalities. Specifically, the Cedar Grove program incorporates components of cognitive behavioral therapy, dialectical behavior therapy, interpersonal therapy, acceptance and commitment therapy, and Internal Family Systems Therapy,[6] while also privileging a biomedical paradigm. Cedar Grove augments these various therapeutic modalities with authentic movement (dance therapy), yoga, mindfulness, supervised exercise, and art therapy groups, while maintaining a central focus on biomedical management and weight restoration. In drawing on the components of each of these modalities, in conjunction with biomedical models of eating disorders, Cedar Grove has fashioned a program designed to adhere to current best practice standards and yet be flexible enough to be accommodated to individual patient needs.

In brief, the Cedar Grove philosophy views eating disorders as complex, biologically anchored responses to problematic family environments or other dysregulating or traumatic circumstances. Eating disorder symptoms—

bingeing, purging, restricting, overexercising, obsessing about food, weight, and calories—are thought to originate as protective coping mechanisms that can "speak" the pain, hurt, rage, confusion, and other affective dimensions of subjective experience that clients have often been forced to muffle and keep silent to survive.

Eating disorders can also provide a means of affective or physiological regulation in the absence of other skills for doing so. People who are genetically and temperamentally primed for high levels of anxiety or hypervigilance are thought to be particularly susceptible to reaching to eating disorders to help them self-medicate. "It's like an engine idling at a higher speed than normal," Dr. Arnold, a psychiatrist, explained to me. "They are more reactive to change, and small alterations will have more noticeable effects. They need something to help them calibrate. Add to this life events such as attachment challenges or traumas, and their systems can be thrown into overdrive, along with their efforts to regulate. They will reach to what works." In fact, as the Cedar Grove website notes, "Eating disorders are a powerful neuromodulator"—they literally change the way the body and brain process and encode information, enabling people to alter their arousal, their attention, their sensory sensitivity, and even their motor capacity and memory.[7] Once an eating disorder is established, it can quickly eclipse a person's sense of self so that they fear they cannot exist in the world without the eating disorder to function as a buffer or filter. And the longer someone has an eating disorder, the more accurate this fear becomes.

But a biological predisposition is not enough to cause an eating disorder, according to this view. "Genetics loads the gun," Dr. Casey is fond of saying, "but culture pulls the trigger." That is, when a person with such predispositions lives in a social and cultural universe that conditions women (and increasingly men) to feel bad about their bodies and appetites and to "take charge" of their lives through dieting,[8] an eating disorder is a fairly unsurprising outcome.

Over time, the use of such strategies for self-regulation and emotional management can become cognitively and behaviorally ingrained, attaining the force of obsessions and compulsions (or even addictions), particularly as the body becomes more depleted through restriction or bingeing and purging and the person develops what the clinic calls "hungry brain," identified on the Cedar Grove website as "a state of deprivation and toxicity." Living with a hungry brain, according to this view, is like being constantly drunk: "Sufferers become deskilled and unable to manage emotions, caught in the past or ruminating about the future. Patients lack autonomy when in this state and need structure and supported meals to recover." The program philosophy holds that the malnutrition associated with hungry brain must be corrected before other kinds of recovery can occur.

Therapeutically, a key part of treatment at Cedar Grove is helping the client understand how and why her eating disorder originally developed and what it was (and still is) doing for her in her life. Once she is able to understand how her eating disorder speaks her needs (e.g., for empathy, to be taken seriously) and helps regulate her affect (e.g., by numbing her out or enlivening her), she is better able to recognize how, as it progresses, the eating disorder actually *undermines* those very processes (e.g., her parents are frustrated with her rather than empathetic; she is viewed as "crazy" rather than as having legitimate complaints; she is increasingly affectively *dys*regulated rather than soothed). Treatment then focuses on helping her develop new ways of recognizing and articulating these needs and getting them met productively. As a client increasingly is able to use her own voice (rather than speaking through the eating disorder) and manage her affect constructively (rather than using the eating disorder to regulate her feelings), it is believed that the eating disorder symptoms will abate. This is a lengthy and difficult process, however, and it is expected that a client may reach back to her eating disorder as a familiar communication and affect regulation mechanism during periods of stress or vulnerability. She must then work to regain her footing and remobilize her new communication and affect modulation skills. Relapse, then, is considered part and parcel of the healing process at Cedar Grove and is generally viewed by clinicians as an opportunity for continued growth rather than as a failure of the treatment itself.

Cedar Grove therefore sees eating disorders as having three primary dimensions—medical/biological, cognitive/behavioral, and affective/psychological—each of which is targeted in the clinic's treatment program. In addressing these domains, treatment entails a full-scale recalibration of the entire person and her experience of herself in the world—her behaviors, her relationships, and how she lives in her body. To do this, treatment engages an array of sensory, affective, and embodied experiences, including touch, taste, movement, intensity, and temporality. Programming is built around these interventions, targeting the physiological, behavioral, and affective domains of an eating disorder and its effects. The phenomenological, affective, and embodied dimensions of this process are profound, as clients gradually come to experience their own beings—material as well as nonmaterial—in new ways.

Official programming at Cedar Grove during the time of my research followed three main tracks corresponding to the different levels of care offered: residential program (twenty-four-hour care), partial hospital program (PHP, either six or ten hours of programming per day), and intensive outpatient program (IOP, four hours per day). Each track was further subdivided into adolescent, young adult, and adult sections. Clients were expected to attend all therapy groups for their treatment level and age category unless specifically exempted, and schedules for each were posted on a bulletin board outside the nurse's station in the common area. At the time of my research, a typical day for a client in the residential program looked like this:

6:30 a.m.	Wake up; weight and vitals measured and recorded
7:30 a.m.	Transportation from the residential house to the treatment site
8:15–8:45 a.m.	Breakfast
8:45–9:45 a.m.	Unstructured time for therapy sessions, meetings with doctors, etc.
9:45 a.m.	Vitals measured and recorded
10:00 a.m.	Snack
10:30–11:15 a.m.	Group therapy (agenda group)
11:15 a.m.–12:30 p.m.	Group therapy (dance movement)
12:30–1:15 p.m.	Lunch
1:15–1:45 p.m.	Break
1:45–3:00 p.m.	Group therapy (positive femininity)
3:00 p.m.	Snack
3:30–4:30 p.m.	Group therapy (art therapy)
4:30–5:30 p.m.	Group therapy (boundaries)
5:30–6:00 p.m.	Walk
6:15 p.m.	Vitals
6:15–7:00 p.m.	Dinner
7:00–7:30 p.m.	Wrap-up group

7:30–8:00 p.m.	Transportation back to the residential house
8:00–9:00 p.m.	Free time (for laundry, homework, crafts, etc.)
9:00–9:30 p.m.	Snack
9:30–10:30 p.m.	Free time
10:30 p.m.	Lights out

PHP clients arrived at 9:30 a.m. and remained until either 3:30 p.m. (for those enrolled in the six-hour program) or 7:30 p.m. (for those in the ten-hour program). IOP clients attended programming from 3:30 to 7:30 p.m.

The day was organized around three key activities: recording weight and vitals, meal times, and therapy. These three practices were emblematic of the three prongs of the Cedar Grove program: medical, behavioral, and therapeutic. Each of these prongs focused on key tasks or sets of concerns: stabilization (medical), containment (behavioral), and flow (therapeutic). Taken together, these three dynamics constituted a model of the "healthy" affective subject, the cultivation of which is the goal of the Cedar Grove program.

I present these aspects of the program in a particular order—medical, behavioral, and therapeutic—because this is the order of urgency with which they were addressed in the clinic. That is, clinicians were under the weight of constant uncertainty, knowing that treatment could be ended by the insurance company at any point, so they had to take a triage approach to treatment, targeting the most directly health-damaging issues first and doing as much work as they could in as little time as they could. They started with getting clients medically stable so they were not at risk of imminent death. They then focused on behavioral changes so that clients could maintain health outside of the clinic structures. Therapeutic concerns came last, not because they were thought to be unimportant—on the contrary, Cedar Grove clinicians saw them as vitally important—but so that in the event that treatment coverage were lost, clients would be medically and behaviorally stable and could, at least in theory, continue to work on the psychological dimensions of their eating disorder in outpatient therapy. In reality, these three domains are not fully separable, and clients began behavioral and therapeutic work as soon as they entered the clinic. It is believed, though, that clients can't fully engage in psychotherapy until they are medically stable because their brains simply are not nourished enough to be able to do the work. Whether or not this is the case, this belief exemplifies the way the clinic thought about the temporal ordering of treatment focus.

Clients tend to obsess about numbers, so we don't tell them anything with numerical value unless absolutely necessary. No weights, no blood pressure, nothing. If we do, they fixate on it. Even things you wouldn't think they would focus on, like potassium levels. But they do. They obsess about numbers. It's part of the disorder.

—DENISE,
Cedar Grove nurse

They tell us that numbers shouldn't matter, that obsessing about them is all part of the eating disorder. But then they weigh and measure us constantly here. *Constantly.* So how can you not think about it? I mean, seriously. *They* obviously care about numbers. And the numbers *do* matter in terms of getting passes or insurance cutting out. So it's kind of like a mind fuck.

—PEMA,
a thirty-two-year-old woman diagnosed with bulimia

Eating disorders are deadly. As we saw in chapter 4, medical compromise (e.g., electrolyte instability, kidney failure, reduced heart volume) is the primary criteria insurance companies use to authorize clients for residential treatment (rather than outpatient care), as these clients need intensive medical supervision and intervention along with behavioral oversight. Because medical instability was the principal factor on which insurance admissions to Cedar Grove were based, establishing and closely tracking medical status was a primary function of the medical program in the clinic.

Clients, as a result, were constantly surveilled in the clinic (see chapter 7), and this surveillance was tied to multiple forms of knowledge mining and documentation. This scrutiny existed in part to ensure clients' safety and in part to enforce accountability for the clinic in providing treatment that actually "works." As we saw in chapter 4, what this means is a complex issue and is bound up with other interests (e.g., cost-effectiveness, profitability) that often have little to do with "health" itself or what clinicians on the ground deem to be good care. To justify the delivery of services to insurance companies, the clinicians documented the effects of their interventions on a number of key medical "problem areas," including weight, blood pressure, heart rate, lab values, and calorie intake, and the taking of these measurements structured much of the everyday life of the clinic (see chapter 7).

One of the most important indicators of medical status in the clinic (at least for underweight clients) was body weight. Clients were generally weighed once a day, just after waking up in the morning, in a hospital gown (so they could not augment their weight by, for example, hiding things in pockets or socks) and with their back facing the scale so they could not see the number.[9] The weights were recorded in a ledger, which was an important document in the evaluation of a patient's progress toward recovery goals. Clients who were underweight were expected to gain, on average, two to three pounds per week, with a goal of reaching at least 90 percent of their ideal body weight before discharge, as determined based on childhood growth charts and body type.[10]

Weight, however, was just one of the many ways that the body was measured, quantified, and evaluated in the course of treatment. After weigh-ins came vitals—temperature, pulse, and blood pressure—the latter two taken both sitting and standing because variations in blood pressure due to postural changes can indicate cardiac instability and overall physiological dysregulation. All of these data were carefully recorded in a logbook that was consulted in treatment team meetings and in discussions with insurance providers.

Blood work done on admission checked heart, liver, kidney, and metabolic function and was usually repeated weekly to track progress, although the frequency varied depending on the client's situation. Labs were especially critical for clients with bulimia, since dysregulation of electrolytes puts people at high risk for cardiac arrest, but they were also important for those with anorexia, binge eating disorder, and other specified feeding and eating disorder.

The medical program was focused on stabilizing clients' indicators of medical status and returning all measurements to the "normal" range. This was tricky, though, because the sooner patients stabilized medically, the sooner insurance would discharge them, even if Cedar Grove clinicians felt they were not ready from a behavioral or therapeutic standpoint.

One way clinicians dealt with this challenge was by continually endeavoring to educate insurance company case managers about the interplay *among* the three domains of medical, behavioral, and psychological concerns. This was not merely a strategy to get insurance to pay for more care: it is, in fact, true that if someone is medically stable but behaviorally unstable (e.g., she is likely to binge and purge if discharged), her medical stability is genuinely in jeopardy. Insurance company resistance to such logic, however, sometimes led clinicians to take risks they otherwise wouldn't take, like giving a client a pass when they knew she wasn't ready behaviorally or therapeutically and was likely to binge and purge while away from treatment, and then using this return to eating-disordered behavior to demonstrate to the insurance company that the client was not yet ready for discharge, despite being medically stable while in treatment. In some cases, however, this strategy backfired (see, for example, the case of Suzanna in chapter 9); insurance companies were just as likely to view such "lapses" as evidence that treatment was *not* working and/or that clients were not really motivated to get better, and to deny further certification as a result.

The goal of the medical program, then, was *stabilization*—to return the body to an equilibrium so that its outputs in terms of lab results, weight, and functioning were predictable and "normal." The theme of this part of the program was *balance,* a concept that is often very hard for many people with eating disorders to understand, let alone embody. Eating disorders are conditions of extremes—radical starvation, frenetic bingeing, violent purging, compulsive exercise, furious self-recriminations, dramatic mood swings, a deadening of the soul that leaves one flat and empty. The notion of balance, then, was both fundamental and largely elusive for clients, and helping them achieve physiological equilibrium was seen as a critical first step in this process. Once a client was medically stable, treatment focused on the next step: behavioral containment.

THE BEHAVIORAL PROGRAM: CONTAINMENT AND DISTRESS TOLERANCE

In the eating disorders treatment world, the term "behaviors" is used as a shorthand for any practices thought to be endemic to eating disorders, such as food rituals, overexercising, calorie counting, body checking, hiding food, restricting, bingeing, and purging. The focus of this aspect of the program was to help clients "contain" their behaviors, affects, and thoughts, but there was also an explicit concern that this not lead to rigidity or inhibition, which are considered common pathological features of eating disorders, particularly anorexia. Containment must be secure but not repressive. The clinic taught this kind of containment through rules and regulations, with the goal being that clients would progressively internalize and eventually be able to perform techniques of containment for themselves.

Within the firm embrace of this containment, clients at Cedar Grove were continuously surveilled for any engagement in "behaviors" while in treatment, but by far the most intense and fraught times were those having to do with food and eating. It is here that we get a sense of how Cedar Grove approached the behavioral dimensions of eating disorders in the course of treatment and how containment functions in the context of everyday life.

Mealtimes at Cedar Grove were a potent mix of frenetic anxiety and deadly solemnity. Tension built as mealtime approached. Patients checked their watches again and again or glanced up at the big clock on the wall. People paced. They fidgeted. A palpable mixture of expectation and dread hung in the atmosphere. Though many had to restrain themselves from hurrying to their chairs, no one wanted to be the first to the table. No one wanted to look too hungry. Too greedy. Too human.

Before every meal, direct care staff would set the four square wooden tables and put place markers with clients' names on them (which the clients had decorated with glitter, plastic gems, feathers, and other embellishments) at assigned spots, taking care to seat people who do not get along at different tables. Each table had seats for three clients and one direct care staff member or therapist (who rotate meal duty each week). The kitchen staff plated food according to each client's meal plan at a percentage of 100 percent (this is equivalent to the full complement of calories needed for a healthy adult per day; so being plated at 50 percent would yield one half that amount), with "add ons" when necessary if a client required more calories per day or needed more of a particular nutrient.[11] Kitchen staff carefully weighed and measured the portions, covered each plate with plastic wrap, and then wrote the appropriate client's name on top in permanent marker. Direct care staff put the plates at the appropriate places. There was a pitcher of water at each table, and clients were expected to drink two four-ounce glasses of water during the meal (but not more, as that might allow a client to fill up on liquid rather than food or make it easier to purge).

Apart from breakfast, meals consisted of three courses: appetizer, main course, and dessert. When clients finished a course, they needed to ask direct care staff for the next one, and she or he would then ask kitchen staff to bring it out on a per person basis. Clients were not to engage directly with kitchen staff. "This is to protect the kitchen staff from harassment," Amelia, a direct care staff member, explained to me. "It's too easy for these girls to want to argue with kitchen staff about what's on their plate. [Having them go through direct care staff] adds a layer of mediation." If clients wanted a meal reportioned (to ensure it matched their meal plan), reheated, or otherwise altered, they likewise needed to go through direct care staff, who determined the appropriateness of the request (Is it motivated by the eating disorder?) before asking kitchen staff to take action.

During meals, music played quietly in the background, and clients and direct care staff socialized and talked, though anything that touched on topics deemed to be potentially triggering (weight, calories, body shape, sex, food, violence) was "redirected" by staff. Direct care staff also carefully observed clients to ensure they were eating all of what they were served and that nothing had been left or hidden (sometimes clients hid food to avoid eating it; sometimes they hid it to save to binge and purge on later).

Staff were also alert to make sure that clients were not engaging in food rituals.[12] People with eating disorders often develop elaborate rituals around food—a testament, we might surmise, to the overwhelming anxiety and distress they feel at the prospect of eating. Rituals can help people with eating disorders feel safe, as if they have some degree of control over the power of food, rather than the other way around. According to a Cedar Grove policy document, rituals can include such things as pulling sandwiches apart for consumption; spreading out fats, sauces, and cheeses to appear as if they have been eaten; hiding food; diluting or soaking food; consuming excessive amounts of fluids at meals; eating sandwiches with silverware; cutting food into small pieces, taking small bites or shredding food; mixing foods together inappropriately; using condiments excessively or inappropriately; and using utensils inappropriately or eating inappropriately with fingers. It is notable that many of these behaviors were deemed rituals at the discretion of the clinician, who decided what constitutes "inappropriate" or "excessive" practices on a case-by-case basis.

Rituals were disallowed for a few reasons. First, they could be triggering for other clients, heightening their own anxieties about eating. But the main reason was that rituals were thought to be distractions from feeling the feelings that came up around food and eating. "If they don't feel the feelings, they can't learn to work through them," Jennifer, a direct care staff member, explained to me. "It's also just not normal behavior," she added. "We want them to be able to function in the real world."

Once the meal was done (clients had thirty minutes to eat), clients had a post-meal check in, where each person around the table reflected on how the meal went for her, what fears or urges came up, and how she navigated them. Sometimes, clients also set goals for future meals.

While all meals were charged events, the most challenging by far for most clients was the first meal after admission. Since new clients had not been present the week before to fill out menus (requesting selections from available options) and had not yet met with the dietician to determine their meal plan, they were provided with one of the current day's selections, plated at 100 percent. This was generally terrifying for them. It is like asking someone with a fear of heights to bungee jump off the Empire State building. "I hadn't eaten any fat for over a year," Edie, a twenty-eight-year-old woman diagnosed with anorexia, told me, "and there was this pat of butter on my plate. I was like, 'Ew! Get it off of there!' I didn't want it anywhere near my food. I was willing to eat the carrots but not with the butter sitting so close. And there was no way I was going to eat that sandwich." "I was only drinking liquids by that point when I came in," Carly, a twenty-year-old woman diagnosed with anorexia, said, "and hadn't eaten solid food in a month or so. It was really overwhelming to see all of that food in front of me. I was glad when they said I could supplement."

"Supplement" means drinking Ensure or Boost (liquid nutrition) in place of eating food. Usually, supplementing was used if a client couldn't complete her meal in the allotted time, in which case she would be expected to supplement for the remainder. Only rarely would clients ask to supplement for an entire meal, and this was usually when they simply didn't like any of the menu options offered that day, though occasionally supplements were requested when a particularly emotionally difficult event had occurred. In most cases, however, supplementing was meant to be an occasional aid to completing what was, for many clients, a significant meal plan of anywhere from 2500 to 4500 calories a day. Even with three meals and three snacks per day, it could be challenging to get all the needed calories in. Given that most clients had stomachs that were shrunken from months or years of restricting, and/or digestive systems that were malfunctioning and not digesting food at the normal rate, food and eating could cause significant physical as well as emotional discomfort. "I'm just feeling really, really, really overfull all the time, and it's getting kind of old being so full all the time," Theresa, a thirty-two-year-old woman diagnosed with bulimia, told me. Lilia, a twenty-four-year-old woman diagnosed with other specified feeding or eating disorder, shared a similar experience: "My body has difficult time adjusting to eating all this food. I'm having a lot of terrible stomach pains that I'm not used to, putting so much food in my body. I'm having trouble keeping it down, trouble pushing it through. I have a lot of bloating and discomfort, and it's been a really tough week. That's the worst part."

Karen, a twenty-eight-year-old woman diagnosed with anorexia, had a particularly challenging experience, as she told me in an interview about two weeks into her treatment:

KAREN: I'm just really nervous about all the stomach problems I've been having.

REBECCA: Is it pain? Or GI stuff?

KAREN: It's a lot of that. Like in the past I've had trouble with just digesting food. Like a few years ago I had tests run and it showed I have severe delayed gastric emptying. And it's really, really gross. I eat things and there's filth coming up a day later. And twelve hours later it's just—food doesn't go through my system, and it's really, really painful. And it's just like it all piles on top of each other and it doesn't move. Two days ago, before breakfast I took some of my medicine, and at 4:00 in the afternoon, it came back up, whole, and I told one of the nurses, and they said that's a sign that something's really wrong. And if that isn't digesting, how do they know if my other medicine is digesting? If it's not, that would explain why sometimes I feel the way I do.

Sometimes, the difficulty is not the food but the fluids, as Anita, a thirty-three-year-old woman diagnosed with other specified feeding or eating disorder, told me about two weeks into her treatment stay:

REBECCA: How has the food piece been going for you?

ANITA: Well, I am kind of mad right now. The food is not that bad, but they have me on extra fluids, which makes it hard to get the food in. So I literally feel like I am going to pop.

REBECCA: Do you know what the fluid thing is about?

ANITA: It's something about my labs. They don't really explain it to me, which also makes me kind of angry.

REBECCA: And so how do they deliver that kind of thing to you, just like, "Oh, by the way, you have extra fluids?"

ANITA: Yeah. Like one day, they came to me and said, "You're supposed to drink extra fluids." They're supposed to tell you that stuff in advance, but it doesn't always happen.

A few days later, we reconnected, and I asked how things were going.

ANITA: I hate the damn fluids. I'm really mad about them.

REBECCA: What makes you mad about it?

ANITA: It's because it's hard if they increase your meal plan *and* increase your fluids. It is a lot at once. It's hard, like I have more trouble with fluids than I do actual food.

REBECCA: Is it because of the volume, or how it makes you feel?

ANITA: It's how it makes me feel, like it's hard to focus and have good body image when you just feel so full all the time. And right now, I guess all the weight just goes to your stomach. I mean, I know eventually everything will proportion out, but it's hard because all that food just sits in your stomach. So that's all you see.

REBECCA: So how do you deal with that feeling and the thoughts that go along with it?

ANITA: I just tell myself that I'm getting better, I don't know. I just go with it I guess. There's nothing I can do.

As we can see, the meal portion of the program is not simply about getting calories into bodies; it's about helping clients adjust to new sensations and tolerate feelings—notably fullness—that they experienced as completely intolerable before coming into treatment.

I want to pause here for just a moment, because this goes to the heart of the issue of containment that is the focus of this dimension of treatment. It's important to note that "fullness" in this context is not just the sensation of having a lot of food or fluid in one's stomach but, as we will see in chapter 10, can also apply to the sensation of "containing" swelling amounts of other things, like anxiety, anger, sadness, or other kinds of affects (including, even, hope and joy). That is, "feeling full" is a sensation of expanding to the limits (whatever those may be), feeling the self press against those limits, and feeling the limits press back. It is this feeling of "reaching capacity" and the risk of exceeding limits that so many people with eating disorders experience as extremely distressful. This is not because they are childish or undisciplined or like to think they are "special," as so many eating disorder theories and popular conceptions suggest. Rather, my sense is that this discomfort centers primarily on the resonance of this feeling with being told that and treated as if they were always "too much" for others: too loud, too needy, too demanding, too difficult—too *there*. Often, such injunctions are accompanied by either implicit or explicit messages that they should be less vocal, less stalwart, less capacious, less present—simply *less*. People with eating disorders have internalized these messages about being too much and have amplified them to a deafening roar, such that it is hard for them to hear anything else.

Given such experiences, feeling "full" (of food, fluid, or even feelings) can trigger the same feelings of shame about "overflowing" one's allotted space and place, and an internal backlash demanding that one *do something* to rectify the situation. We might think of the theme of behavioral interventions in the Cedar Grove program, then, to be *sitting with fullness* and *distress tolerance*.

In this way, the food aspect of Cedar Grove's behavioral program is emblematic of other forms of containment, like the daily schedule, the maintenance of locked spaces, or keeping clients under visual observation. Each of these mechanisms is intended to keep clients safe—from their eating disorders and from themselves—as well as to make them easier to surveil and measure (see chapter 7). "It's like holding a toddler who's having a temper tantrum," Claire, a nurse, explained to me. "We provide the containment for them, and they may strain against it, but it also helps them feel safe, like this is something bigger than their feelings, bigger than their eating disorder. Eventually, they can do it on their own." Because they focus on containment, practices like meals at Cedar Grove and other behavioral interventions are considered to be both medical *and* therapeutic events. They set the groundwork for the more explicitly psychotherapeutic activities of the program.

THE THERAPEUTIC PROGRAM: RELEASE AND FLOW

Sitting in tension with the stabilization practices of the medical program (which promotes balance) and the containment dynamics of the behavioral program (which promotes distress tolerance) are the therapeutic dimensions of treatment, which encourage *dynamics of release and flow*. Cedar Grove's therapeutic program is built on individual, group, and milieu therapies and promotes a transtheoretical approach to understanding and treating eating disorders that incorporates perspectives and techniques from psychodynamic psychotherapy, cognitive behavioral therapy, interpersonal therapy, dialectical behavior therapy, and Internal Family Systems Therapy, as interpreted through a combination of medical model and recovery model orientations (see chapter 6).

While one-on-one therapy comprises an important part of treatment at Cedar Grove, the heart of the Cedar Grove program is group therapy, which clients attend for many hours each day. Groups are on topics such as positive femininity, body image, mindfulness, and art therapy and follow a set schedule that repeats weekly. Clients are expected to attend all groups unless they are specifically excused from them due to the subject matter or because they have a therapy, doctor, or lab appointment.

Group Therapy

During my research, groups were held in the two group rooms on the north side of the treatment suite and were run by clinic therapists, clinical interns, or outside clinicians hired on an as-needed basis. They lasted from sixty to ninety minutes, depending on the group, and the topic or specific group exercise for the day was left up to the group leader to decide. Participants sat on "foofs" (enormous beanbags) rather than chairs, as they were thought to encourage more openness and were also more comfortable for underweight bodies than hard chairs.

While in group therapy, clients were expected to be attentive and engaged, to share (offer their thoughts, opinions, and feelings), and to give feedback (reflect constructively on the thoughts, opinions, and feelings of others). However, some clients curled up on the foofs and fell asleep, or wrapped themselves tightly in blankets and disengaged from what was going on in the session. Therapists were instructed to encourage engagement but not to ask clients that weren't participating to leave group unless they were being significantly disruptive, as it was thought they might gain something from listening to the group discussion, even if they did so passively. Most clients actually did engage, albeit with varying levels of enthusiasm and capacity. Sometimes this depended on the specific group or the specific time of day. "I hate community group," Pema told me. "It's always so stressful, and people get really upset with each other." "Positive femininity is right after lunch, and I'm always in so much physical pain," Carly groaned. "It's hard to pay attention to what's going on when you're literally in agony." Whether and to what degree each client participated in a group was recorded by the group leader in a logbook after each group therapy session.

Homework

In addition to having clients participate via sharing and feedback, therapists assigned homework as one of the principle methods of getting the therapeutic messages to sink in. Cedar Grove maintains a collection of over one hundred "assignments" derived from different therapeutic modalities, and each client was provided with copies of them in their patient handbook, which they received on admission to the clinic. The client's primary therapist then assigned specific activities that were to be done outside of group sessions and then brought into groups to share and receive feedback. Homework assignments were meant to help clients internalize and practice new ways of viewing themselves and the world.

Three assignments in particular were seen to be absolutely pivotal to recovery and were prioritized temporally and in terms of how much importance was placed on them in the treatment process: "Timeline," "Pros and Cons of Having an Eating Disorder," and "Letters to and from Your Eating Disorder." These assignments were completed by the client during the first two weeks of treatment, reviewed in therapy with the client's individual therapist, and then presented in agenda group, a daily group session designed for this purpose. A closer look at these assignments will give us some additional information about the clinic's therapeutic priorities.

Timeline "Timeline" is an exercise where a client traces her past from the time of her birth to the present, noting key events in the development of her eating disorder. It is not a holistic "this is your life" exercise but rather a very purposeful and intentional reconstruction of the client's life story that figures the eating disorder as an organic entity whose roots reach back into the past, long before any "behaviors" appeared, and whose origin and development can be discerned from the standpoint of the current self. For example, Darcy, a thirty-two-year-old woman diagnosed with anorexia, noted that when she was ten years old, a babysitter told her that she "had a nice shape" but "was a little thick" and her face was "too round." Although Kelly did not blame the babysitter for her eating disorder, this event was emblematic for her of a time in her life when she started to become aware of her body shape and how she was perceived by others. Similarly, Bethany, a twenty-year-old woman diagnosed with anorexia, recalled June of the summer between her freshman and sophomore years of high school as the time when she increased her exercise and started to become compulsive about running. In reviewing their pasts and flagging such incidents for special attention, clients learn to trace the development of their eating disorders as embedded within their autobiographies and emergent within their own developmental trajectories.

The "Timeline" serves a number of important therapeutic functions. By constructing and presenting their timelines in group therapy, clients learn to draw lines around the eating disorder, both temporally (distinguishing between before the eating disorder and after it) and experientially ("this is when my eating disorder was getting stronger"; "my eating disorder had taken over by this point"), while at the same time seeing their eating disorder as inseparable from other events and relationships in their lives. It encourages an ecological perspective that helps clients separate themselves from their eating disorder and see it as something other and different from who they really are, while also highlighting the conditions under which it developed and thrived. The "Timeline," then, positions clients temporally and relationally in new ways (more on this in chapter 6).

Pros and Cons of Having an Eating Disorder The "Pros and Cons of Having an Eating Disorder" exercise, based on cognitive behavioral therapy principles, is designed to unveil underlying beliefs and cognitions that may be fueling a client's eating disorder, as well as reasons that can be capitalized on for engaging in recovery. For example, pros of an eating disorder could be, "It keeps my parents focused on me instead of fighting with each other," or, "I don't have to feel my feelings."[13] Cons could be, "My eating disorder isolates me from family and friends," or, "I feel tired and sick all the time." Clients write their personal pros and cons down and share them with their individual therapists and also in group.

If used in a strict cognitive behavioral therapy sense, this exercise would be leveraged to challenge the pro beliefs and shift clients clearly toward the con view of having an eating disorder. But at Cedar Grove, it was primarily used to elicit details from clients about their relationships and family or social dynamics. It provided important information about how clients experienced themselves agentically in relation to their eating disorders as well as to other people in their lives. It encouraged them to see how the eating disorder had enabled them to accomplish certain goals (such as numbing out) but blocked them from accomplishing others (such as being present in social situations rather than distracted by thoughts of food). By encouraging clients to reflect on these factors, this exercise positioned the client agentically in her social context as well as in relation to her eating disorder, the pros and cons of which could be evaluated from a place of at least provisional remove.

Letters to and from Your Eating Disorder For this exercise, the client writes two letters: a letter from herself to her eating disorder, and a letter from her eating disorder to herself. The point of this exercise is to further explore the relational aspects between the client and her eating disorder (how her sense of self is bound up with the eating disorder and/or being sick), examine what is keeping them bonded together, and identify points of friction or leverage where therapy might help with a separation.

For example, in her letter to her eating disorder (which she shared with me), Shelly, a twenty-seven-year-old woman diagnosed with other specified feeding or eating disorder, wrote, "You have always been there for me. When I'm alone, you're there to comfort me, to keep me company, to help me feel less isolated." But she also wrote, "You get in the way of my social relationships. You make me feel ashamed and ugly and disgusting." In her letter from her eating disorder, she wrote, "Shelly, you don't know how to cope with your feelings, so I'm there to take care of them for you," and, "If you leave me, I will cease to exist." In working with her individual therapist, and by presenting and discussing these letters in group, Shelly was able to pinpoint challenges with intimacy as a key factor in the development and maintenance of her eating disorder and to identify the ways her eating disorder both helped her navigate this (by giving her comfort and managing her feelings) and also exacerbated the problem (by getting in the way of social relationships). In other words, the exercise helped Shelly see beyond her food and eating behaviors to the deeper dynamics that kept the eating disorder alive and well. As a result, developing alternative coping skills and working on her fears of intimacy became primary goals in her individual therapy work. In this way, this exercise positions clients psychodynamically by helping them reflect on different aspects of their selves and how these aspects relate to and interact with one another.

The primacy of these three assignments reflects key aspects of the therapeutic orientation of Cedar Grove and its view of the causes of eating disorders. They also spotlight the core of the clinic's therapeutic program, which is focused on helping clients separate themselves from their eating disorders ("Timeline," "Letters to and from Your Eating Disorder"), helping them see how the eating disorder both helps and hurts them ("Pros and Cons of Having an Eating Disorder," "Letters to and from Your Eating Disorder"), and recognizing the environmental and relational conditions that enabled the eating disorder to arise and thrive (all three). Ideally, clients can then turn their energies to changing these conditions while also developing alternative strategies for getting their needs met.

Significantly, the psychotherapeutic program encourages clients to begin to experiment with "letting go"—letting go of information and feelings in groups, but also letting go of the eating disorder as the primary scaffolding of their identities and senses of self. This becomes a key thread in clients' experiences of treatment.

MILIEU THERAPY: THE WHOLE CLINIC IS THE FRAME

Cedar Grove's program is transtheoretical, interdisciplinary, and integrative. It is designed to attend to the medical, behavioral, and psychological dimensions of eating disorders through a number of structured interventions. Ultimately, however, clinicians believe that what heals are the ways these interventions *knit together* to form a cohesive whole and how the clinic engages eating disorders as a comprehensive phenomenon and eating disorder clients as whole people.

According to the Cedar Grove philosophy, an eating disorder takes over every aspect of a person's life; it controls not just how much she eats or doesn't eat but also her capacity and desire for social engagement, her bodily presence, her energy, her curiosity about the world, and her perspectives on the future. For this reason, treating an eating disorder means treating the whole person, her entire relational system, her being-in-the-world. It means, as Gemini, the dance movement therapist put it, "helping [clients] to inhabit their bodies and lives in a new way."

At Cedar Grove, this task is approached through the use of milieu therapy, in which the entire clinical context is constructed to be the site of therapeutic intervention. This means that each and every thing that happens in the clinic—not just meetings with therapists, dieticians, and doctors, but every minute of the day—is thought to be saturated with therapeutic (and therefore also countertherapeutic) potential. Every interaction counts and is considered to be part of the overall therapeutic intervention. Each meal or snack, each dose of medicine, each exertion, and each social interaction *matters* and is thought to have the potential for profound positive—or negative— impacts on the course of a client's treatment. From how they communicate a concern about choices to whether they permit a client to watch a preferred television show, staff members at Cedar Grove are expected to be "therapeutic" in their interactions with clients, even though they often have only partial, confusing, or conflicting information about what is in the patient's best interest. As we will see in part 3, it is in these everyday interactions and micropractices of care that the contradictions and paradoxes inherent in theories of eating disorders and the American medical system more generally are struggled out.

CULTIVATING THE IDEAL(IZED) SUBJECT

Programming at Cedar Grove attends to the three domains where the eating disorder is thought to be most destructive: medical compromise, behavioral dysregulation, and psychological distress. By focusing on the themes of balance, distress tolerance, and letting go, the three prongs of the treatment program target key capacities that clients need to develop on their path to recovery: namely the capacity to self-regulate, the capacity to tolerate distress, and the capacity to be flexible without falling apart or losing one's sense of self.

The idealized or "healthy" subject cultivated in the process of treatment, then, is stable (but not fixed or fixated), contained (but not constricted), and able to "flow" (but not structureless or unbounded). Getting to this point is an idiosyncratic process, and treatment unfolds differently for each client, depending on what concerns she brings into treatment as well as what issues arise in the process of this transformation. And recovery, according to the Cedar Grove view, does not proceed in a prescribed, linear fashion; rather, it is uneven, looping, and characterized by fits and starts. As stated on the Cedar Grove website:

> The reality is there is no defined or "right" way to view recovery from an eating disorder. Recovery looks different and means different things to each person. Often times, people view recovery on a continuum. That is, some people view themselves to be in recovery if they are refraining from active eating disorder behaviors such as bingeing, purging, compulsive exercise, and food restriction but still struggle greatly with ED [eating disorder] thoughts. Other people view themselves to be in recovery only if they are able to refrain from ED behaviors and report an absence of ED thoughts and beliefs.... Recovery comes in many different shapes and forms and is different for everyone. Although attaining recovery is difficult, it is possible with the right tools, knowledge, and determination.

Cedar Grove views recovery, then, as a dynamic, individualized process that is continual and fluid rather than linear and progressive. Accordingly, treatment is structured to facilitate and accommodate this indeterminacy, and care must be attuned first and foremost to the specific and unique needs of each individual client.

At the same time, however, as we saw in chapter 4, to get insurance company approval and payment, Cedar Grove clinicians must be able to demonstrate that what they do "works" in some sort of objective sense, and they must adhere to "best practice" evidence for a given set of concerns, which is often organized around themes of standardization, efficiency, and predictability. Interventions must be clearly delineated and their outcomes rendered in terms that are unambiguous and measurable. A set of tensions therefore sits at the heart of the Cedar Grove approach and belies deeper issues regarding epistemology and practice. We turn to this topic in the next chapter.

Lettuce Sandwich

SEPTEMBER 1980

I sit, staring down at my sandwich. If you can call two slices of diet bread with some lettuce squeezed in between them a sandwich.

"Is that *lettuce?*" my friend Kyle asks.

"Yeah," I say, somewhat defensively. "I like lettuce."

"Um, sure, OK," he mutters, rolling his eyes at me.

I pick up my lettuce sandwich and look at it. I don't want to eat it. I don't want to eat anything. But I have to eat something or people will notice. They already notice. I take a bite and feel the softness of the bread and the crunch of the lettuce. Chew slowly, I remind myself. Thirty seconds between bites. Don't rush. I feel the calories from the bread begin to accumulate on my thighs, and I feel thoroughly disgusted with myself.

I resolve to do better.

SIX

Fixing Time

CHRONICITY, RECOVERY, AND
TRAJECTORIES OF CARE AT CEDAR GROVE

"She just *stopped*, Rebecca. She *stopped the car*, right in the middle of the highway! You know that place heading south on 170 where it ends and forks into eastbound and westbound 64? You have to make a choice, you know—are you going to go east or west? Because the highway is *ending*. She couldn't decide which way to go, so she just *stopped the freakin' car*. Right there in the road. I thought we were going to get rear-ended and *die*."

Betsy was telling me how bad things had gotten with her teenage daughter Miranda before Miranda went into treatment at Cedar Grove for bulimia. "We didn't know she was sick then," Betsy continued. "If I'd known, I would have never let her get behind the wheel. She was in no shape to drive."

Betsy's account is powerfully emblematic. Eating disorders do stop people dead in their tracks, both literally and figuratively. They are dramatic—even traumatic—events for sufferers and their families. Monumental and life-arresting, eating disorders not only stop people cold, they sever time into a "before" and an "after." Before an eating disorder, one can't possibly imagine what is coming: the depths of misery, the swells of anxiety, and the knots of fear that will make everyday life unbearably awful; the depleted thoughts, tunnel vision, and shaky limbs; the foggy mind and careening emotions; the vigilant body in full, thrashing survival mode. And after a diagnosis of an eating disorder, nothing is ever the same. Things may be fine. They may even be good. But they will never, ever be the same.

Eating disorders structure time in other ways, too, temporalizing everyday life in ways that become deeply, viscerally embodied. In the midst of the illness, the practices of the eating disorder become the metronome for the sufferer's life, parsing out the seconds between when she last ate and when she can eat again, how long it's been since her last meal and whether she can still effectively purge, how long she has to wait between bites, how many reps of leg lifts she must do in what amount of time, how long she has to run, how many hours of the day she needs to spend standing (rather than sitting) because it burns more calories. Eating disorder practices mark time through calories the sufferer consumes (or doesn't consume) during a twenty-four-hour time span, the number of times she steps on the scale and at what time of day, how often she checks the diameter of her thighs. "It dictated my whole day," Marta, a twenty-seven-year-old woman diagnosed with bulimia, recounted to me. "It controlled my every waking moment—when will I eat, when will I *not* eat, when will I find time to binge, how long after that until I can purge, how many times. I structured my whole day around the food." Priya, a twenty-six-year-old woman diagnosed with other specific feeding or eating disorder, had a similar experience. "I scheduled my life in fifteen-minute increments," she said. "And it was all about making sure I had time for my eating disorder. It controlled everything." Whatever else they may be, eating disorders are fundamentally *temporal* practices, not just marking but also actively *creating* time for people who experience them.

Eating disorders also *unmake* time. Once an eating disorder progresses to a critical state, there is a paradoxical stopping in both time and space, coupled with an intense, frenetic, frantic energy that fragments experiences of self and scatters attempts at concentrated action. Like Miranda's freezing on the highway, both extremes are paralyzing and produce what philosopher Guy Debord evocatively calls "coagulated temporality."[1] Life potential is diverted from school, work, and social relationships into ever-intensifying frenzies of self-destruction until, ultimately, the bypass is complete. The sufferer withers, while the eating disorder flourishes.

In over 20 percent of diagnosed cases, this coagulated temporality converts into a "chronic" eating disorder,[2] defined as consistently meeting diagnostic criteria for an eating disorder for more than seven years, and showing a "lack of response" to available evidence-based treatments.[3] While receiving a diagnosis of a chronic mental illness like schizophrenia or bipolar disorder makes a person eligible for additional resources like disability benefits, supportive housing options, and Medicare, receiving a diagnosis of a chronic eating disorder is very different. With eating disorders, the designation "chronic" generally results in the *withdrawal* of support, the denial of further care, and increasingly, a referral to hospice to await death.[4] Being diagnosed with a "chronic" eating disorder, then, has profound and potentially life-ending consequences, a performative quality that makes it a unique designation among psychiatric diagnoses.

Recovery and chronicity form the two possible end points of an eating disorder: either the individual recovers or she (by definition) becomes chronic and the condition often ends in death. Eating disorders treatment is meant to intervene in this illness process, prevent a decent into chronicity, and remobilize an eating disorder's coagulated temporality in a particular direction, toward "recovery." Yet in the midst of treatment, the ultimate outcome is as yet unknown; things could go either way.

Given this, eating disorders treatment is what we might call an *anticipatory project;* that is, it is structured not only in response to here-and-now concerns (e.g., an inability to function at school or work, acute depression, or anxiety) but also in relation to a range of imagined possible future outcomes (e.g., the potential for cardiac arrest, the risk of organ failure, the possibility of brittle bones breaking, a life spent incapacitated and ill, or alternatively, recovery and a life filled with joy and promise). The eating disorder becomes a site for imagining and anticipating all *possible* outcomes and attempting to provide just the right intervention, at just the right time, in just the right place, to affect the desired end result. How such anticipatory regimes function at Cedar Grove and how they condition relationships of care tells us much, not only about what is viewed as most important to clinicians, clients, and insurance companies but also about the places where these priorities coincide or come into conflict.

To get at these issues, this chapter considers how the powerful anticipatory constructs of chronicity and recovery function as the epistemological limits within which eating disorders are diagnosed and treated at Cedar Grove and how various anticipatory regimes and practical chronographies—ways of conceptualizing and accounting for time—structure both the intelligibility of suffering and relationships of care within the clinic.

CHRONICITY AND RECOVERY

Our understandings of an illness and its chronicity depend on whether or not we have the ability to treat it effectively. Such designations can change over time, reflecting social, ideological, and financial priorities and investments. A diagnosis of a chronic illness is thus much more than an unproblematic response to a natural disease course—it enfolds information about the current state of medical knowledge, clinical practice, and community commitment. In thinking about chronicity and recovery in eating disorders,

I follow anthropologists Lenore Manderson and Carolyn Smith-Morris's injunction that "we must be critical of the paradigms that govern diagnosis, treatment, and survival, with the imprecision, elisions, and slippages that occur in reference to chronic disease." We need to recognize that the designation "chronic" emphasizes certain states at the expense of others.[5] Indeed, the chronic (ongoing) versus acute (extreme, but temporary) dichotomy is a temporal framework that not only characterizes the nature of an illness but also constitutes individuals as certain kinds of sufferers who merit different kinds of empathy. Importantly, it is also a political and pragmatic distinction, as notions of acuity and chronicity are intimately related to anticipatory regimes[6]—how we envision possible (or impossible) futures—that hinge on our biotechnological capacities to treat a given condition.[7] Promises of recovery are not just about symptom abatement but also enfold imagined ideal futures. Notions of "proper" development and projections of what constitutes a happy, healthy, functional life shape our understandings of what recovery looks like and how possible it is thought to be for a particular patient.

Engaging notions of chronicity and recovery in eating disorders treatment gives us a window into how care practices constitute the objects and subjects of their attention in articulation with broader social, cultural, and economic values. Specifically, I am interested in how strategies of anticipation become critical vectors for the formulation of certain kinds of problems and certain kinds of patients.

THE ANTICIPATORY PROJECT OF TREATMENT

By engaging and remobilizing the coagulated temporality of eating disorders, treatment, like an eating disorder itself, is a distinctly temporal project, with different recovery models constituting an eating disorder as a certain kind of problem, the individual with an eating disorder as a certain kind of person, and change as a certain kind of process. Eating disorders treatment involves not only addressing acute suffering in the present but also *reimagining* the past, present, and future in a narrative arc within which the disruption and repair of an eating disorder makes some sort of sense. Such a re-visioning of time, as political economist Harold Innis argues, is always political, as the way time is organized produces different subjectivities, different moral actors.[8] But more than this, temporal schemes orchestrate experience, relationships, and in-the-world action, creating what communications theorist Sarah Sharma calls "power-chronographies," or certain politics of temporality that come to function as forms of biopolitical social control.[9]

Expanding on this notion of power-chronographies, I am interested in how temporal reckonings in eating disorders treatment at Cedar Grove organize not just physical space (as examined in Sharma's work) but also psychological space and understandings of the "journey" of recovery within the parameters of chronicity and health. Importantly, Sharma notes that multiple chronographies—time reckonings—are often in at play in any given situation and that people must learn to navigate them. This is also true at Cedar Grove—competing chronographies do not only condition how the coagulated time of eating disorders is remobilized in different ways according to different priorities; they also situate the eating disorder client and others around her into particular kinds of relationships. Relationships of care are therefore the enactment of anticipatory logics within which various—and sometimes competing—chronographies operate. This happens through what anthropologists Vincanne Adams, Michelle Murphy, and Adele Clarke call "regimes of anticipation."[10]

REGIMES OF ANTICIPATION

One defining quality of our current historical and cultural moment is its peculiar management of time and its particular "politics of temporality."[11] This instantiation of modernity offers what Adams, Murphy, and Clarke call "both a promise of certainty (that the truth can be known for certain in a way that applies across time, into the future) coexistent with the acknowledgement of an ongoing deferral of truth as ever changing (as more sophisticated ways of knowing it continually emerge)."[12] That is, we can and should be certain about what we know, and yet we should also accept that knowledge itself is tentative, contingent, and always incomplete and must therefore be engaged with skepticism and suspicion. In this view, "the future" as a conceptual possibility plays a crucial role in that it is always knowable in new ways, even while it is elusive, such that "grasping for certainty" about it is an ongoing and persistent process. The future, in other words, must be *anticipated,* so actions in the present both prepare for and presuppose a future that appears both certain and yet, depending on what happens in the present, avoidable.

Eating disorders treatment is structured by such practices of prediction and anticipation, hinging on tensions between what is known in the here and now and what is not yet known about the future. Decisions about care require constant speculation, data gathering, and revision, followed by more speculation, and so on, as clinicians try to anticipate what will happen next—or later, or down the line—all within an imperative to "get it right" so as to provide care in the most cost-efficient manner possible. Will raising a client's meal plan cause her to push back and refuse to eat at all? Will it trigger her into a hypermetabolic state? Or result in refeeding syndrome? Or will it help her finally get over the hump, allowing her brain to get nourishment so that she's able to engage more constructively in therapy? These kinds of uncertainties and calculations characterize the bulk of treatment, as clinicians try to anticipate all possible outcomes and decide which is most likely, which is most potentially dangerous, and whether a given intervention is worth the risk.

For example, the diagnosis and intake process gathers information about a client's past behavior to make predictions about a prognosis. Accounts of previous therapies and treatments serve as anticipatory tools for gauging how treatment might go this time. Medical history becomes the foundation for speculations about potential future complications and what kinds of services might be needed. Once in the clinic, treatment planning and program decisions draw on such predictive technologies as growth charts and weight histories to set target weights, develop food plans, and plot anticipated changes. Treatment plans delineate an anticipated trajectory of progress through various levels of programming and support. In contemplating discharge, clients are asked to predict what their posttreatment lives will be like, what kinds of stressors they are likely to face, and how they will navigate them. They are induced to imagine their future selves back in school, work, romantic relationships, and family situations, and to put supports in place that will help them hold onto the gains they've made while in treatment.[13] From beginning to end, then, treatment is first and foremost a practice in *anticipating* the future and preparing for its eventualities.

Such politics of anticipation, Adams, Murphy, and Clarke argue, are both temporal and affective. Relying on proliferating modes of prediction, anticipation hinges on "the speculative forecast" in ways that combine predictability and uncertainty to produce anticipation as an *"affective state,* an excited forward-looking subjective condition characterized as much by nervous anxiety as a continual refreshing of yearning, of 'needing to know.'"[14] In other words, anticipation carries with it certain kinds of affective affordances (that is, it facilitates or nudges one toward certain affective states more than others). Critically, "*as an affective state, anticipation is not just a reaction, but a way of actively orienting oneself temporally.*"[15] In other words, anticipation is a regime of *being in time,* one that takes you out of the "now" and focuses on the "yet to come" as the domain of concern, while also stressing that what happens now will shape that future.

In terms of eating disorders, this way of being-in-the-world is far from value and politics free. Indeed, such an affective orientation of anticipation not only fits well with the actuarial logics of managed care (which hinge on strategies of anticipating how many people will need what kinds of care at what points in time and for what kind of costs) but also is actively cultivated by the information technologies through which care is delivered. For managed care companies' predictive models to be successful, patients must act more or less as expected. Managed care structures, accordingly, are designed to predispose patients to "choose" to act in ways that fit with the models—that is, to become "rational" actors who are anticipatable because they reliably choose health over illness and efficiency over waste. Such inducements can come in a number of forms, such as, for example, basing subsequent treatment authorizations on the amount of weight a patient gained the previous week or her degree of compliance with meal plans.

The goal of regimes of anticipation like managed care, then, involves the "optimization" of participants through increasingly fine-grained management of the psyche and the body, "anticipatory audits" of accountability,[16] and the simulation of catastrophes (e.g., hurricanes, terrorist attacks, relapses) to preemptively stave off disaster. Whether or not such anticipated calamities come to pass, they have already impacted the present by shaping the ways people engage in their everyday lives with an eye to the future. In this way, the future not only defines the present, but also "creates material trajectories of life that unfold *as anticipated by those speculative processes.*"[17] The present becomes governed by possible futures that are "*lived and felt* as inevitable in the present, rendering hope and fear as important political vectors."[18] That is, possible future outcomes become part of the experienced present and come to order that present through an urgency and anxiety about acting now to protect the future.[19] This involves a telescoping of temporal possibilities and a "forced passage through affect" in the sense that an anticipatory regime achieves its ends by arousing a sense of inevitability about the future that is usually manifest as an entanglement of fear and hope.[20] We see this, for example, in Shelia's question from the preface: What's the point of trying to get better?

Importantly, anticipation as an affective condition is not simply a matter of the anxieties within individual subjects. Rather, "regimes of anticipation are distributed and extensive formations that interpolate, situate, attract and mobilize subjects individually *and* collectively."[21] That is, the affective effects of anticipation are often shared and can emerge as collective structures of feeling that condition the entire atmosphere of an organization or group.[22] In this way, anticipation can be part of what Jackie Orr calls "psychopolitics,"[23] in which states, corporations, and military complexes (and, I would add, clinics) "tactically project and distribute fear and anxiety as a means to interpolate and govern bodies."[24] In terms of Cedar Grove, anxieties about anticipation are not simply idiosyncratic to particular clients or clinicians but come to characterize the entire affective atmosphere of the clinic.

MULTIPLE CHRONOGRAPHIES

Unlike the scenarios described by Adams, Murphy and Clarke, in which a dominant anticipatory regime prevails, at Cedar Grove *two distinct* anticipatory regimes are at play. For the sake of simplicity, we can shorthand these as the medical model and the recovery model of mental illness, while recognizing that these are broad characterizations of what are much more complex perspectives (as I hope will become clear). Each of these models has its own epistemology (theory of knowledge) and chronography (means of accounting and structuring time), and each has its own understanding of what eating disorders are and how to treat them. Both regimes are, at heart, *developmental* schemes that trace how things change over time, and both are concerned with the relationships between illness course (the process and progress of an eating disorder itself) and life course (human development from childhood to adulthood), though they understand the connective tissues between illness and life context in very different ways.

The Medical Model

The medical model of mental illness (broadly conceived) encourages clinicians to approach psychiatric conditions in the same way they would approach a fractured arm—that is, by recognizing that something is broken and needs to be fixed and that the route to doing so is grounded in biology. Psychiatrist George Engel identifies three essential components of the medical model: a concept of disease (disease is biological dysfunction), an ethic (the ethical imperative to cure the disease), and a logic (scientific rationality, epitomized by evidence-based practice; see chapter 4).[25] The medical model relies on scientific proof of a pathological process and treatment interventions that have been replicated in multiple studies.

In terms of psychiatric illnesses, the medical model distinguishes between "sick" and "well" based on *DSM* criteria and, as a result, draws clear boundaries around illness episodes. With practice, one can clearly identify when an illness begins and ends. In synergy with biomedical psychiatry and cognitive behavioral approaches (which enable controlled outcomes research and therefore lend themselves to cost-benefit analyses in ways more psychodynamic approaches do not), the medical model is the approach most favored by managed care companies.

The medical model has become the predominant perspective for treating eating disorders over the past three decades, its prevalence in the field coinciding with the rise of managed care. This view figures eating disorders as episodic biological-cognitive-behavioral dysfunctions that are essentially resolved once the symptoms abate. From this perspective, unlearning an eating disorder rests primarily on interventions targeting the specific behaviors involved (e.g., bingeing, caloric restriction, purging, overexercising), countering problematic cognitions (e.g., a patient believes she doesn't deserve to eat or doesn't deserve to be cared for), and restoring medical stability. Given the model's reliance on the scientific method, its overall orientation is one of skepticism and doubt with regard to patient experiences (which are considered to be part of the disease), relying instead on empirical (generally biological) evidence rather than on subjective accounts. Interventions based on the medical model, such as cognitive behavioral therapy and weight restoration approaches, tend to be structured, time limited, goal oriented, problem focused, and centered on present symptomatology rather than on etiology or course.

As an anticipatory regime, the medical model is structured by what we might think of as a "metronomic chronography," or what I call "managed care time," which is tethered to the structures and priorities of managed care and biomedicine more broadly. Based on the premise that health is the absence of pathology (in the case of eating disorders, the absence of bingeing, purging, or restricting), managed care time is focused on control and regulation. It is linear, ordered, standardized, universalized, and above all, limited. It is measured in daily weights and vitals recorded in logbooks; schedules of meal times, therapy times, and recreation times; and the number of days of treatment approved by managed care case managers. Time, in this view, is money, and it is in short supply. Care in this model involves setting limits, focusing on the here and now, and enforcing change to which a patient is expected to become habituated over time. The point of treatment is to entrain the client's will toward desired behaviors. The arc of transformation is goal-oriented, and pace and progress are predicted through the use of evidence-based practice. Relapse in this discourse represents a failure of the habituation process, which must then begin anew (see chapter 9). The ideal patient is one who is disciplined, self-regulating, efficient, goal directed, and active.

The Recovery Model

Beginning in the 1930s and gaining ascendance in the 1980s and 1990s, the recovery model of mental illness offers a response to the medical model's pessimism regarding the outcome of serious psychiatric conditions. The most commonly accepted definition of recovery within this paradigm is summarized by the psychiatrist William Anthony: "[Recovery is] a deeply personal, unique process of changing one's attitudes, values, feelings, goals, skills, and/or roles. It is a way of living a satisfying, hopeful, and contributing life even with limitations caused by illness. Recovery involves the development of new meaning and purpose in one's life as one grows beyond the catastrophic effects of mental illness."[26] According to this definition, a person may recover without necessarily experiencing symptom remission or a return to premorbid functioning. Similarly, a person may experience symptom remission but still be ill. The main tenets of the recovery model—hope, spirituality, personal responsibility and control, empowerment, connection, purpose, self-identity, symptom management, and overcoming stigma[27]—focus on the whole person rather than on just disease or symptom remission. As an overall philosophy of treatment, the recovery model is not an empirical treatment in and of itself, although elements of it have received empirical support[28] and evidence-based treatments can be used in conjunction with a recovery approach.[29]

In terms of eating disorders, the recovery model draws many of its core concepts from the treatment of alcohol and drug addiction. According to this view, eating disorders, like other addictions, are lifelong predispositions that one must continually manage, even once acute symptoms abate, lest they recur. Recovery, then, is not primarily symptom based but entails a *reorientation to living* that goes far beyond the specific diagnostic expressions of the disorder. Unlike the medical model, which is skeptical of subjective experience, the recovery model views the individual's experience as a source of expertise and privileged knowledge and cultivates an orientation of trust, hope, and community. Healing is holistic and integrative, and its concern is with empowerment, connection, and the building of trust and integrity within clients. Interventions based on this model tend to be organic, time expansive, iterative, process oriented, and focused on how the past informs the present.

While the recovery model is certainly compatible with the treatment of eating disorders, some special considerations require careful attention.[30] Anorexia in particular is different from many other mental illnesses in that it is generally ego-syntonic, meaning that the person experiencing it feels that it is "right" and therefore generally has low motivation to change.[31] Also, unlike symptoms like hearing voices, for example, which can be folded into a recovery strategy for a person suffering from schizophrenia,[32] self-starvation or binging and purging are medically dangerous and cannot easily be accommodated as parts of healing. On the other hand, the recovery model orientation offers a clear counterbalance to the tenor of eating disorders themselves, which are often focused around issues of control, regulation, counting, anticipating outcomes, and so forth. As a capacities-focused approach that values subjective well-being, intuitive forms of knowing, and the empowerment of the client, the recovery model works in a different register than an eating disorder and can therefore be especially therapeutic for someone struggling with one of these conditions.

As an anticipatory project, the recovery model is structured by what I call an "organic chronography," or "recovery time," which is tied to the patient-centered commitments of the recovery movement. Based on the metaphor of recovery as a journey or quest, recovery time is fluid, individualized, and abundant. It is measured in phases that can last weeks, months, or even years as clients take things one day at a time, growing and exploring, moving two steps forward and one step back, until eventually they find themselves "ready to get better." Change is understood as a natural, growth-oriented process, and the arc of transformation is long, with an emphasis on the future and a mantra of "progress, not perfection." In this model, pace and progress cannot be predicted or forced. Care is focused on making the conditions right for change to happen and on keeping the patient oriented toward her desires for the future. Health is determined not by behaviors per se but by one's *orientation* to those behaviors. It is a developmental discourse that hinges on someone being "ready," a state that can be anticipated and welcomed but not mandated or scheduled. Relapse, in this discourse, is part of the process of moving forward, and what matters is how someone orients herself to the relapse—does she move backward or keep moving ahead? The goal is to keep looking forward, to expand the reach of time. The ideal patient, according to this model, is just that: *patient*—attuned, open, pliable, willing to surrender to the process of recovery.

Frictions

The medical model and recovery model both structure care at Cedar Grove. While these perspectives are not in and of themselves diametrically opposed[33] and can even be viewed as complementary,[34] in practice they do sit in tension in ways that produce a number of frictions and ambiguities that shape the unfolding of care at the clinic. As we will see over the following chapters, these contrasting chronographies produce different (yet overlapping) understandings of the client's "will" vis-à-vis recovery—specifically, how the "will" is related to health-seeking behaviors. Such overlaps create contradictions, ambivalences, erasures, and amplifications that have implications not only for how care unfolds but also for how eating disorders themselves—and eating disorder clients—are understood. This matters because it dictates what kinds of resources will be brought to bear—or withheld—in the course of treatment and to whom they will be available.

SHEILA

Sheila's case can help illustrate these frictions and how they play out in the delivery of care. Sheila (whom we met in the preface at Allison's funeral) was a "repeat customer" at Cedar Grove; at the time of this incident, she was in her second treatment stay. The previous year, she had been in residential treatment at Cedar Grove for bulimia. She was also diagnosed with a mood disorder and borderline personality disorder, which is characterized by self-regulatory deficits that often manifest in dramatic behaviors (in Sheila's case, emotional outbursts and cutting herself with razor blades). During her stay the previous year, she was notoriously "noncompliant," ran away from treatment more than once to binge and purge and self-harm, and was generally considered a "difficult case." At the same time, clinicians found her bright, engaging, funny, and likable.

During that previous stay, and despite her struggles in treatment, Sheila was able to make some good progress. After being discharged from residential care the year before, she remained in outpatient therapy with one of Cedar Grove's therapists and seemed to being doing quite well for some months while attending school and working. Eventually, however, she began to relapse and quickly found it difficult to remain in school or keep her job. Her therapist recommended that she return to Cedar Grove and enroll in the partial hospitalization program (PHP) so she could remain in school while pursuing treatment.

When she entered PHP, Sheila reported that she was motivated to recover. And she did well for about a week. Then she began to have more and more difficulty adhering to the limits of the program. She continued to binge and purge every night, and in fact, these symptoms seemed to worsen. Her self-harm activities increased. She dropped out of her classes at college. After the first week, she began to arrive late for programming, which started at 9:30 a.m. She would routinely arrive at 10:00 a.m., sometimes 10:45 a.m., and occasionally even as late as 11:30 a.m. While in programming, Sheila would sometimes refuse to attend groups and would not always complete her meal plan requirements.

About three weeks into her second stay, the treatment team was faced with deciding what to do, and they discussed the situation during a weekly treatment team meeting. It is here that we can see what I call a *practical ethics of uncertainty* at work, as clinicians tried to reconcile medical model and recovery model principles by juxtaposing the known and the unknown to hypothesize different outcomes and then filtering the likelihood of those outcomes through their personal impressions of the client.

ZOË [SHEILA'S THERAPIST]: OK. Sheila [*sighs*]. What do we want to do?

DR. CASEY: Well, let's think this through. She's actually been way more compliant than she's ever been before. She really has been trying to be collaborative in many ways. She just gets so overwhelmed, and those other parts of her kick in.

BROOKE [ANOTHER THERAPIST]: She's in that place she gets to where she just pushes the limits, and pushes them and pushes them until we push back.

ZOË: I'm worried that her coming late and pushing things like that really sets a bad precedent for the other patients.

BROOKE: I agree—it communicates that that kind of behavior is OK. It's really having an effect on the community. The clients need to trust that we are a safe place and that we can contain things for them. We don't feel safe for them if we don't hold our limits.

DR. CASEY: Exactly. We need to be consistent. These are the program parameters. Everyone else can manage to get here on time.

ZOË: It's because she's up late binging and purging, and then she has a hard time getting up in the morning.

DR. CASEY: Well, that's the thing. We definitely shouldn't make accommodations if we know it's for her eating disorder. I wonder why her symptoms get so kicked up in this level of care? This happened last time, too. PHP just doesn't seem to work for her for some reason.

ZOË: But she won't do residential. She's been crystal clear about that.

DR. CASEY: Are you sure?

ZOË: Yeah, she's told me that pretty much every session.

DOTTY [THE UTILIZATION REVIEW MANAGER]: I'm not sure we could even get her certed for residential at this point.

ZOË: Really?!? Why not? Clearly, she's really struggling! If anyone needs residential, it's her!

DOTTY: Yeah, but if she can't adhere to the program limits at PHP, there's no way they're going to say, "Sure, let's put her in residential!" Especially with the kind of track record she's had. I mean, it's possible, but it would be a gamble. It wouldn't be a for sure thing. We'd have to convince them that she was really on board and that she was going to follow the program and do what we ask her to do. And if we move her before the cert comes through, the family would have to be prepared to pay for it if they don't approve it.

ZOË: Well, *that* won't happen. Her parents are against her being in treatment at all.

DR. CASEY: So, here's what we do. I think we need a team recommendation and then a plan B. I think we recommend she come to residential. [*Groans from around the table.*] Even though the insurance thing might be iffy, that is what we think she needs, right? [*Agreement from others.*] So, we give her our clinical recommendation, that she come into residential. Now, we know she won't do that. We also know there are some drawbacks to that. Even if she does come in, if she's not really ready to collaborate with us, it doesn't make much sense. So, what's our plan B?

ZOË: I guess the only other option is to discharge her, but that just makes me really nervous with where her behaviors are right now. It just doesn't make a lot of sense to me to discharge someone because she's struggling.

BROOKE: But we're discharging her because she can't—or won't—follow the limits of the program. That's a separate issue.

ZOË: I guess. But what do we do with the safety issue? We know she's cutting.

BROOKE: Well, the thing about Sheila is that she uses her behaviors to communicate and to get people to jump in and take care of her, and we need to really put the responsibility back on her. We know she's cutting, but we also know she's been able to get herself to the ER for stitches in the past when necessary. So, I think she has a really strong self-preservation part there that is active.

ZOË: That's true.

DR. CASEY: So, I think we recommend residential and, assuming she says no, assess her for safety. If she's not actively suicidal, we have no grounds to commit her against her will, so we ask her to contract for safety and set up the next week or two of outpatient appointments. [*To Zoë*] Are you willing to see her outpatient?

ZOË: I guess so. I mean, yeah. I really care about her, but I'm really worried about her as an outpatient. She's pretty out of control right now. It's a lot to take on. But, yeah, I'll see her.

DR. CASEY: OK. And I'll see her, too, for the medical piece. Can she see Nadia [a Cedar Grove dietician]?

BROOKE: I'm pretty sure Nadia will see her.

DR. CASEY: OK. So that's what we do.

DOTTY: So, discharge will be today, or yesterday? If it's today, we need her to stay a full day or her insurance won't reimburse for today.

DR. CASEY: [*To Zoë*] When do you meet with her?

ZOË: At 11:45, right after this.

DR. CASEY: OK. So, let's try to get her to stay through snack at 3:30 and give her a pass for the rest of the day. That way she'll get support through lunch and snack, and we can count it as a full day.

We can see in this discussion the various ways the treatment team maneuvers around and through the clinical and anecdotal information about Sheila, working to find consensus about anticipation that will clarify the best path of clinical action given the tensions among what the client needs (residential treatment), what she will agree to do (the current level of care, but not the residential program), what is best for the community (discharge), and what insurance is likely to pay for (outpatient treatment).

In talking about Sheila and building an anticipatory logics in this case, we can see how a practical ethics of uncertainty unfolds and is put into play as clinicians navigate between medical model and recovery model views. Through observing and being involved in dozens of cases like Sheila's, I have come to view such practical ethics of uncertainty at Cedar Grove as being sustained by six core propositions, each of which is informed by the particular therapeutic philosophy of the clinic:

1. A client will recover only if and when she is "ready" to recover, and no one (not even the client) can know for sure if or when this might happen.

2. Families are complex systems that operate to sustain homeostasis, even if that homeostasis is unhealthy. Altering one element of the system (e.g., the client) can have unpredictable effects on the rest of the system.

3. A therapeutic community is organic and can be shaped for better or worse by the individuals that constitute it and the dynamics among them. The relative "health" or "toxicity" of the community can shift at any time and can directly impact client treatment.

4. The role of the treatment center in the process of recovery is sometimes a first step, sometimes a last resort, and sometimes one of a series of treatment attempts. This role is often not clear until treatment is underway, or it may not be clear until after discharge.

5. Insurance coverage is tentative at best and can end at any time, prompting immediate discharge. Treatment decisions can affect insurance coverage in unexpected ways in the future.

6. Eating disorders are responses to toxic environments (e.g., family, peer group, society), which may or may not change. The question is not *if* relapse will happen but *when* it will happen, how severe it will be, and if treatment has enabled the client to develop skills to manage setbacks without becoming seriously ill.

Within these fields of uncertainty, clinicians function as "runners" or "brokers" across different epistemological frames, while trying to attend to the (often competing) interests of clients, family members, and insurance companies. This requires them to continually evaluate the known, the unknown, and the range of possible outcomes in any given situation; to draw on both medical model and recovery model anticipatory logics; and to assess all of this information against what their own clinical "guts" tell them in order to decide on a course of clinical action. All this must happen very quickly, as clinicians have only a few minutes once a week (during staff meetings) to sit around a table with the rest of the treatment team to discuss suggestions, as they did with Sheila's case. During the rest of the week, such decisions have to happen within minutes, or hours at most, but more often within seconds.

ABDUCTION

It is here that what Adams, Murphy, and Clarke call "abduction" comes to the fore. Abduction is "the process of tacking back and forth between futures, pasts and presents, framing the life yet to come *and* the life that precedes the present as the unavoidable template for producing the future."[35] In abductive reasoning, "ideas about how to 'move forward' are generated *by tacking back and forth* between nitty-gritty specificities of available empirical information and more abstract ways of thinking about them."[36] In anticipation, abduction also acquires temporal form: it involves "telescoping the future into the present."[37]

In Sheila's case, we can see how clinicians try to reconcile the perspectives of the medical model and the recovery model in charting a path of action. We also see how these two models inform their practices of anticipation. What *did* they know? They knew that Sheila's symptoms were not being contained and were, in fact, worsening. They knew that her adherence to program protocols was becoming poorer. From her previous stay at the clinic, they knew that she had a history of testing boundaries and challenging limits and that she responded well to firm and clear limit-setting. They also knew that Sheila's parents, who lived out of state, were not a source of support for her and that she tended to backslide when they were around. In other words, enlisting her parents' help was not an option. What the clinicians *didn't* know was what would be the best way to increase Sheila's collaboration in the treatment process. They considered three possible interventions—recommend a higher level of care, continue with the current treatment protocol, or discharge her—and looked at the pros and cons of each.

The question looming over the treatment team in this discussion—the big unknown—was: Would Sheila respond to their intervention (whatever it was) by becoming more collaborative with treatment or would she be thrown into crisis? This sort of thing is a gamble. Clinicians must use their best judgment to guess how a client will respond in a given situation, and if they are wrong, the consequences could be deadly.

BASTING

Two different anticipatory schemes and two different processes of abductive reasoning predominate at Cedar Grove, and these must then be somehow integrated into a perspective of the patient and the illness that clinicians can then act on. This happens through a process I call "basting," where clinicians move back and forth between anticipatory regimes and their respective chronographies and logics in trying to make sense of a client's behavior and experiences. Clinicians read across anticipatory regimes of the medical model and the recovery model, and across managed care time and recovery time, when fashioning their understanding of a client's core concerns and how to best intervene. This is an improvisational practice wherein conjectures about the relationships between life course and illness course for a client help clinicians to conjure a particular clinical reality within which they can feel empowered to act.[38]

In Sheila's case, for example, clinicians relied not only on the "factual" information in her chart and progress notes but also on their own sense of where she was in her process of recovery. Despite Sheila's current noncompliance, the team felt that she had made significant progress over her stay and that she was actually "way more compliant than she's been before," which they took as indicating important steps toward recovery. At the same time, they had to balance this interpersonal sense of Sheila with the kinds of information that would be relevant to her managed care company, which was interested less in relative improvements and more in Sheila's ability or inability to make use of treatment in the here and now.

PUCKERS

As a given client's eating disorder takes shape within these divergent anticipatory schemes and trajectories of development, and as abduction and basting happen simultaneously, frictions and ambivalences—or what I call "puckers"—emerge around what it means to be sick, what it means to get well, and what kinds of vulnerabilities are at stake. These puckers trouble, and sometimes disrupt, anticipatory regimes of care.

Returning to Sheila: After the team had debated all the different contingencies and come up with an intervention (recommend residential care) and a plan B (discharge, if deemed safe), the room got quiet. "What's your gut feeling about what she'll do?" Dr. Casey asked Zoë. After a pause, Zoë responded, "Well, I think she'll crash. I think she'll crash hard. But then I think she'll come back. And maybe she'll be more ready next time. But I also think in order for her to be able to use us effectively, we have to show her that we can hold our limits. That's the only way she'll trust us to contain her when she finally really *is* ready." In this case, then, the clinicians' inability to tailor care to Sheila's needs and the lack of concurrence between models of care led them to make a decision that they knew was likely to provoke a crisis.

As it so happened in this particular case, the therapist's gut feeling was right. After Sheila was discharged, her symptoms continued to intensify, and she had a serious (but thankfully unsuccessful) suicide attempt a few months later. But she remained connected to her therapist at Cedar Grove and eventually requested residential treatment.

MEASURING PROGRESS: DIVERGENT AUTHENTICITIES

As we can see, the medical model and the recovery model both orchestrate care at Cedar Grove, but they enfold competing views of what the "problem" is at the heart of a client's eating disorder and how to intervene. At the same time, they also have some similarities. Both endorse the notion of the autonomous individual as the model of health. Both understand *autonomy* in the modern liberal, political, philosophical sense as a form of self-governance, as "acting within a framework of rules one sets for oneself" and having "a kind of authority over oneself as well as the power to act on that authority."[39] They differ, however, in how they formulate *authenticity* and whether authenticity is considered an integral component of autonomy. This is important because it helps us understand puckers and the barriers to their resolution.

In the liberal humanist tradition (and in colloquial usage), *authenticity* often connotes a sense of being true to one's self, of expressing and inhabiting a core existential orientation to the world. But this is only one interpretation, and a very specific one at that. In fact, the philosophical literature is replete with debates about the term and its use. Here, I want to build on philosopher Marina Oshana's distillation of these debates and her distinction between what she calls "procedural authenticity" and "epistemic authenticity" to tease out those contradictions between the medical model and the recovery model that seem most troublesome for eating disorders treatment.[40]

Procedural authenticity has to do with the consonance (or lack thereof) between one's actions and one's stated moral values. Epistemic authenticity is of a different order; it has to do with the degree to which one's internal "radio" is "tuned" to those values. Let us look more closely at how these different formulations of authenticity unfold in medical model and recovery model discourses.

In the medical model, the metric of progress is procedural authenticity, or acting in accordance with one's stated priorities. In this view, authenticity involves the development of *capacities to act* in concert with the values and ideals one endorses, a *consistency of action within a moral system* rather than an expression of intrinsic, essential self. That is, authenticity is grounded in the ability to reason and act in the world unfettered by maladaptive impulses. Whether or not such action reflects the true commitments (in an epistemic sense) of the subject are of little relevance to the exercising of procedural authenticity, which involves bringing a subject's actions in line with the ideological commitments she espouses. The focus here is on the outward manifestations of behavior and whether these "outputs" line up with the stated goals or values. Procedural authenticity in the case of eating disorders treatment is measured through indicators such as weight gain, lab values, and behavioral monitoring. If these are improving, recovery is (supposedly) happening.

In the recovery model, the metric of progress is *epistemic authenticity,* or the internal investment one makes in one's priorities, independent of what is happening behaviorally (though behavior is generally thought to follow naturally from internal commitments). One of the hallmarks of the recovery approach is that idea that the healthy subject develops along a trajectory from enmeshed dependence with caregivers to individuation and autonomy, epitomized by self-mastery and self-efficacy. How and when and to what extent such individuation occurs is a matter of debate across recovery models, but the idea that mental health is characterized by the development and solidification of the self as a seat of largely independent thought, motivation, and action is central to all such approaches. Specifically, the notion that a healthy self is a "true" self forms the core of the recovery model approach. Authenticity, in its *epistemic* sense, then, is necessary for the achievement of healthy autonomy, according to the recovery model view. The focus here is on one's subjective orientation and whether it is consistent with one's stated values. In eating disorders treatment, epistemic authenticity is assessed through such things as a client's relationships and general life orientation and is less amenable to the quantification favored by managed care companies.

Managed care, as a system of healthcare, does not explicitly articulate a theory of human psychological functioning—or at least not self-consciously. One can argue, however, that managed care philosophies rest entirely on propositions about why people do what they do, how well we can predict such behavior, and how economics can be brought to bear on shaping that behavior.

Specifically, the managed care model is built on a notion of autonomy as entailing procedural, as opposed to epistemic, authenticity. Grounded in a rational choice model of human behavior, the managed care approach presumes that patients will make good faith use of treatments as prescribed in order to maximize health and minimize harm. Accordingly, managed care practices emphasize a standardization of the provision of care (the guidelines for which derive from projected cost-outcome analyses), and services are "managed" according to such assumptions about client participation and provider adherence to these guidelines. This model assumes that individuals will freely choose from an array of options and will maximize their health benefits in the service of self-preservation and development. Success, in the managed care framework, is gauged as the degree of correspondence between a client's behavior and the indicators of health outlined by the managed care organization and the service provider, whether or not such behavior reflects the personal values or commitments of the client herself.

Even managed care case managers who were sympathetic to the recovery model view found themselves caught between compassion for clients and the requirements of their jobs. As one generally quite helpful case manager at a major health insurance company told me, "The 'in recovery' view is fine, but what I really need to know is if they are medically compromised and if they meet criteria [for admission]. Saying someone is 'in recovery' doesn't give me much to go on. I need specifics about their weights, vitals, and behaviors in order to make a determination about benefits."

Procedural authenticity and epistemic authenticity are not in and of themselves incompatible, but they differ in important ways. Take, for example, the following: I believe in the value of helping those less fortunate than

I am. Each year in early December, I donate bags of clothes to a local charity. My actions are in line with the values with which I identify, making this action authentic in a procedural sense. But whether or not it is authentic in the epistemic sense depends on my motivations for donating the clothes and the degree to which I am aware of those motivations. I may genuinely wish to help others and feel a moral obligation to share my good fortune. This would lend my act a degree of epistemic authenticity in addition to procedural authenticity. But perhaps what truly motivates me is the tax deduction I can take if I make a large charitable donation before the end of the year. This changes the context of the action, which, although still procedurally authentic, is now epistemically *inauthentic*. I may or may not be aware of this underlying motivation for my charitable act—in fact, I may have convinced myself that my motivations are entirely unselfish and that the tax benefit is of no consequence. Whether or not this is actually true for me, and whether or not I know it, depends on my ability to reflect on my own actions. The determination of epistemic authenticity is predicated, then, on a capacity and desire for critical self-reflection and self-awareness, practices that risk the discovery that one's motives are not necessarily what they seem. Such tensions are far more than just philosophical differences—they lead clinicians and managed care officers to differently evaluate indicators of pathology and recovery in eating disorder clients and thus shape the clinical decisions that follow from such evaluations.

Importantly, in eating disorders treatment, these two kinds of authenticity figure the body in very different ways. If the body is understood to be the bearer of "truth" through biometric indicators, as in the medical model, it can come to assume center stage in diagnosis and treatment and can be relied on in lieu of the client's own accounts of her experience. If, instead, "truth" is sought *despite* the body rather than *by means* of it (that is, if the body is understood to be implicated in the illness experience itself, such that it gives false information through such things as dysregulated hunger cues or distorted body image), as in the recovery model, the body is viewed as a source of deception or dysfunction and is not to be trusted. Both of these metaphysics—the body as a source of truth, and the body as a vehicle of deception—are at play at Cedar Grove, producing tensions and ambivalences that get read back onto clients, who are then labeled as "manipulative" and "sneaky." I will return to this theme in chapter 10.

The Cedar Grove view of eating disorders draws on both medical model and recovery model approaches, attempting to synthesize the two. While most Cedar Grove therapists operated primarily with a recovery model orientation in their day-to-day work with clients, they were constrained by managed care companies, who almost exclusively relied on the medical model in making benefits decisions.

Cedar Grove clinicians and clients, then, are suspended between these two models of the subject and two frameworks of ethical action that share some concerns but that maintain fundamentally different views of the person, the illness of concern, and what constitutes "best practices" treatment. They also facilitate very different sorts of relationships of care.

AUTHENTICITY AND THE ETHICS OF CARE

The two formulations of authenticity in the medical model approach and the recovery model approach lead to different ethical trajectories of care (see table 1). Contrary to the medical model, with its rational choice assumption that an individual's prime directive is self-preservation, the recovery model recognizes that mental illness often entails self-destructive intentions (e.g., suicidal gestures, poor self-care, social isolation), the causes of which are frequently outside an individual's conscious awareness. Given its understanding of psychiatric distress as embedded within an individual's life history, the recovery model approach rejects the medical model's notion of "standardized" care delivered by clinicians acting as technicians and instead privileges individualized treatments and emphasizes the primacy of the therapist-client relationship in the healing process. Similarly, treatment course and length are determined within the context of that relationship in the recovery model, not a priori based on the diagnosis alone, as they are in the medical model. Recovery-oriented treatment also involves an ethos of care predicated on a holistic understanding of the person as made up of complex moods, experiences, thoughts, and behaviors that have developed over time in the context of social relationships with others. From this perspective, a client's present difficulties are both contiguous with her past and hold implications for her future. Her psychiatric distress is part and parcel of who she is as a person. The medical model, in contrast, maintains an ethos of care focused on the isolation and treatment of disease as discrete and separate from the person as a whole. Unlike the recovery model, the medical model understands psychiatric distress as episodic rather than endemic, as a "state" the person is in versus a "trait" that endures.

TABLE 1 Trajectories of Care: The Medical Model versus the Recovery Model

Medical model	Recovery model
Autonomy is predicated on procedural authenticity.	Autonomy is predicated on epistemic authenticity.
Successful treatment: the development of capacities as action as consistent with positive health outcomes.	Successful treatment: the development of critical self-reflection and "owning" one's actions.
Rational choice—people act toward self-preservation.	Stochastic choice—behavior is overdetermined and complex and may include self-destructive intention.
Focus of treatment should be on acute symptoms.	Acute symptoms manifest chronic difficulties. Treatment must attend to both to prevent relapse.
Psychiatric distress is episodic.	Psychiatric distress is often chronic, with periods of flare-ups.
Psychiatric symptoms are discrete, separate from the person.	Psychiatric symptoms are embedded in the person.
Symptoms abate in response to standardized *interventions*.	Symptoms abate through the discovery of the functions of those symptoms for the individual and the development of alternative behaviors. This occurs in the context of a long-term *therapeutic relationship*.
Care should be standardized and time-limited.	Care should be individualized and tailored to each client's particular needs.
Symptom relief indicates the end of the acute episode of distress.	Symptom relief indicates that treatment is *in the process of working,* though several cycles of abatement and intensification of symptoms are expected in the process of healing.
Mental health providers function as technicians, delivering interventions in standardized form.	Mental health providers are specialists. The type and quality of therapeutic relationships they develop are individualized for each client.
The primary ethical imperative is cost-effectiveness.	The primary ethical imperative is client care.

Using a somewhat different theoretical lexicon, we might say that the medical model views recovery as a *technology of action,* whereas the recovery model construes recovery as a *technology of self.*[41] While these two formulations are related, they often come into direct conflict in the context of eating disorders treatment, structuring understandings of why clients do what they do and whether or not it indicates progression toward health.

Caleigh's case illustrates how these different ethics of care become entangled in the clinic and the kinds of consequences this can have. Caleigh was twenty-seven years old when she was admitted to Cedar Grove. She reported a ten-year history of eating disorder that began her senior year in high school, though she traced the roots of the problem back to age ten or eleven. At her lowest point, Caleigh, who was five-foot-seven, weighed 78 percent of her ideal body weight, and she revealed that she had experienced amenorrhea (the cessation of menstruation) for the past three and a half years. She had been hospitalized for dehydration, malnutrition, and low potassium prior to coming to Cedar Grove, and her labs were still dysregulated when she began treatment, showing very low protein and irregular liver enzymes as well as severe osteoporosis. She was admitted with diagnoses of anorexia nervosa, depression, and anxiety. Given her significant medical compromise, her insurance company approved her for eight weeks of inpatient treatment—an unusually long approval—although the company was to be given weekly updates on her progress.

Although her primary diagnosis was anorexia, Caleigh's problem was more than simply not eating enough—it had to do with how her eating disorder had come to structure her life. For four years prior to admission, Caleigh had been restricting her food intake to six to eight zucchini per day. She would meticulously slice, cook, and eat one zucchini per hour from 2:00 a.m. to 8:00 a.m. and then sleep all day until 9:00 p.m. Then she would get up and do it all again. She became unable to work or go to school. She had tried outpatient treatment but was unable to make herself get up on time to go. Caleigh's eating disorder determined her daily rhythms, literally marking the hours and flipping her days and nights. It became the sole focus of her life; eating and not eating regulated her temporal orientation.

One of the very first tasks of residential treatment at Cedar Grove was simply acclimating Caleigh to a regular sleeping, waking, and eating schedule, which took about a week of concentrated behavioral intervention. Adjusting Caleigh's temporal orientation was both a pragmatic and ideological task. Certainly, staff and activity schedules required that Caleigh be awake during the day and asleep at night and that she eat at certain times of the day when the food was prepared. But more than this, "regularizing" Caleigh's temporal rhythms was a way of regularizing *Caleigh*, cultivating in her a disposition to be amenable to institutional management and surveillance. As a strategy of containment and structuring, this temporalizing was productive of a kind of passivity and deference to the biomedical structure.

Although Caleigh was eventually able to adhere to the clinic schedule, this temporal regularizing wreaked havoc on her body. As she began eating more regular food at regular intervals, she developed severe edema (swelling)—a common side effect of "refeeding"[42]—to the point that she could not bend her knees. She gained sixteen pounds of fluid weight in one week, which not only completely freaked her out but also made it very hard for the treatment team to assess what, if any, "real" weight was being added. Caleigh was getting more "regulated" temporally, but her physiology was in full revolt.

Caleigh's insurance company, however, was happy. Although they recognized that the weight gain was largely due to the edema, they were pleased nonetheless that Caleigh was nearing her discharge weight so quickly. For them, it didn't matter that Caleigh was eating only under duress, that most of the pounds were water weight, or that her acute fear of the rapid weight gain would likely trigger subsequent restricting or purging. Their assumption, expressed explicitly to me by her insurance case manager, was that Caleigh would "begin to think more clearly" and become "more rational" as she gained weight and then would simply "naturally" want to get better. Mostly, however, the case manager was pleased that she was "following the rules of the program" by sleeping, waking, eating, and subjecting herself to various forms of monitoring (vitals, etc.) on schedule. For the insurance company, *compliance within a certain chronography* (procedural authenticity) was a principle indicator that recovery was happening.

Caleigh's clinical team, however, was more cautious. Well aware that Caleigh was eating only because she was in twenty-four-hour care, and knowing that she was in full panic mode about her precipitous weight gain, the treatment team worked to hold the "long game" in tension with the microattention to daily fluctuations required by the insurance company. They were interested less in Caleigh's body weight than in her *willingness to get well* (epistemic authenticity)—not in some imagined future, but in the here and now.

Although the treatment team agreed with the insurance company that Caleigh was not thinking clearly in terms of her own health decisions, they relied on a different sort of anticipatory regime in imagining the future in relation to the present. That is, they anticipated that Caleigh would go through periods of struggle and even relapse on her way to recovery, but they believed that what was important was not whether she reverted to eating disorder behaviors but whether she developed an internal motivation to get well that would carry her through any trouble spots (recovery model). To this end, they talked about recovery not, like the insurance company, in terms of days meted out or "used up" in treatment (medical model), but in phases, loosely based on the model of motivational interviewing combined with mental health recovery discourse. They considered Caleigh to still be in the "stabilization" stage, where she had not yet even fully understood or accepted the seriousness of her problem (see chapter 7). Once she had done so, they maintained, she could begin the more concentrated work of recovery. But it was impossible to know when that might happen. They could provide psych-oeducation and therapeutic support to encourage it, but it couldn't be accomplished through direct intervention or by fiat. Caleigh, like all clients, would get there when she was ready.

COMPETING CHRONOGRAPHIES OF CARE

In Caleigh's case, we see two different chronographies of recovery, two different anticipatory regimes, and two different orientations to care. In the managed care chronography, "good care" meant setting clear expectations that mirrored "normal" functioning, surveilling Caleigh at all times, measuring her compliance to these regimes, and instituting negative consequences if she failed to comply. The task was to *rein in* Caleigh, to fit her into narrower and stricter parameters than she wished. In the recovery model chronography, "good care" was not about surveillance or monitoring or reining in; rather, it was about *opening up* Caleigh to the possibility of a different sort of future. To this end, clinicians were open, honest, accessible, and supportive with Caleigh while at the same time modeling recovery-oriented dispositions themselves. In this way, the managed care chronography and the recovery model chronography not only differently ordered how time was structured and utilized in day-to-day treatment but also differently framed how the client herself was viewed—as either an obstacle to or a potential ally in her own health process—and how relationships of care should be executed as a result.

One might suspect that such temporal frictions are common in all fields of behavioral health, where tensions inevitably exist between time-limited insurance coverage and longer-term visions of the recovery process. But I suggest something particular is going on in the field of eating disorders in this regard. Returning to the issue of chronicity, we will remember that chronicity in eating disorders is treated differently than chronicity in other conditions and that this has to do with perceptions of the patient's "willingness" to get well. How, then, does this issue of "willingness" show up in these two different chronographies, and with what effects?

In the medical model and managed care time, Caleigh's will is construed as diseased, starved, and evacuated of its rationality. There is even a name for this at the clinic: "ED head" (ED stands for eating disorder). ED head (sometimes called "hungry brain") is presumed to lead clients to seek disordered ends as long as they remain in a state of biomedical compromise. As a client reaches her discharge weight, however (usually somewhere around 90 percent of her ideal body weight), the assumption is that ED head will release its grip and the client will reorient toward a desire for health. The "will" of an eating disorder patient in the managed care chronography is therefore *by definition* always "sick" and capable only of seeking pathological ends. *The will becomes healthy only when the body becomes healthy.* (However, the patient is expected to work toward physical health in self-responsible ways, a clear double bind.) Because a change in practice is thought to produce a change in psychological orientation, the client's will is figured as an *obstacle to be overcome,* and care is structured around behavioral interventions and surveillance that can be generalized, routinized, and standardized. This situates the ideal patient as a passive passenger of interventions that alter the physical body, with the implication that the will eventually will follow suit. Any agency the patient may demonstrate in this process is seen as necessarily coming from ED head (especially if it appears to be at odds with the views of the treatment team in any way) and is therefore regarded as suspect.[43]

In the recovery model and the recovery chronography, the will is also problematized, but in a slightly different way. Like in the medical model chronography, the recovery model chronography reads the client's will as largely misdirected but not fundamentally diseased. In this view, many problems, including eating disorders, are thought to stem from a desire *to control;* to control people, circumstances, and experiences in ways that are unhealthy. The will is therefore part of the problem. However, this view also positions the will as a potential resource to be cultivated in the service of recovery. Yet it can be put in the service of recovery only when it is used to subvert itself— that is, through willing surrender and adapting a stance of receptivity.[44] In this model, change is dialectical, achieved through a tacking back and forth between willingness and surrender. Ultimately, while it has an element of "fake it 'til you make it" that resonates with the medical model's practice-based approach, the recovery model emphasizes that people will recover only when they are "ready" and not before; that is, psychological change comes first and behavioral change follows.

The medical model and the recovery model clearly figure the client's will differently in relation to recovery. In the medical model, physiological and practice-based changes come first and are believed to produce a change in psychological orientation. In the recovery model, a massive psychological shift must occur before lasting behavioral change will happen. In both cases, the client's "will" is rendered suspect. How, then, should client progress be assessed in treatment, and what effects does this assessment have on patients?

WILLFUL PATIENTS

As noted previously, the withdrawal of care in response to "chronicity" in eating disorders hinges on assumptions about a patient's supposed unwilling-ness to get better, an issue that sets eating disorders apart from other mental illnesses. If an individual suffering from schizophrenia, for example, doesn't want to take her medicine or adhere to treatment protocols, this is generally seen as an indication that she needs *more* care, not less. When it comes to eating disorders, however, such ambivalences about care are generally read as *willful choices* to remain ill, a rendering that, through the mediating con-struct of chronicity, becomes a justification for the removal of care. How the client's will is understood in relation to care is therefore a critical component of how chronicity in eating disorders is perceived and managed and, as a result, how the course of illness progresses in the presence or absence of needed care.

There are many historical and cultural reasons for why eating disorder patients are constituted as particular kinds of "willful subjects"[45] and why this is seen to justify the removal of care. As I've noted, in the clinical world, eating disorder clients are considered to be notoriously resistant, manipula-tive, and conniving. Their "will," in other words, is thought to be oriented toward remaining sick rather than getting well—they are seen as the quintes-sential noncompliant patients. While this is not wholly an artifact of dis-course (indeed, many eating disorder patients are highly ambivalent about getting well), in concluding this chapter I want to in examine how this notion of the patient's "will" is constituted through the process of the eating disor-ders treatment itself, impacting perceptions of chronicity and recovery.

Importantly, the convergence of the medical model's and the recovery model's different configurations of "will" means that configuring clients' wills as anything *other* than pathological becomes logically impossible (see chapter 10). Against this backdrop, the "truth" about a client's progress toward health is read through the biological markers of her body (in the form of weights, lab values, and vital signs), such that her body becomes situated at the center of anticipatory regimes and risk management strategies. This focus on the body at the expense of experiential or contextual factors dovetails with the symptoms of eating disorders themselves,[46] exacerbating client struggles and reinforcing clinicians' and insurance companies' perceptions that clients are resistant to getting well, thereby legitimating the removal of supports. While resistance to care and ambivalence about recovery can, indeed, be very real parts of an eating disorder (as well as other conditions), the specter of the "chronic" (and therefore "hopeless") eating disorder patient *is largely produced in and through the regimes of care that purport to treat these conditions and how these care practices configure the client's "willingness" to get well.* In other words, a deadly synergy among anticipatory projects, under-standings of patients' willingness to get better, and the delivery of care renders eating disorder clients unable to push back against these structures without being pathologized.

THE WILLING BODY? CALEIGH AND ANTICIPATORY COLLAPSE

Perhaps ironically—and certainly problematically, given the particulars of these conditions—the body comes to assume center stage in eating disorders treatment and is believed to "tell the truth" about a patient's willingness to get well in a way she herself is thought to be incapable of doing. Specifically, biological markers like lab results, weights, vital signs, and body changes are treated as bearers of truth and the locus of "willingness" to the extent that they come to elide the client herself and reinforce the notion that her body— sick and starving though it may be—is more authentic, more trustworthy, and more reliable than she is. This rendering of one anticipatory regime in the terms of another is what I call "anticipatory collapse."

This recruitment of biology in eating disorders is unique among mental illnesses. In no other psychiatric condition is a *biological* marker taken as a referendum on the *psychological* health of a client. While some blood tests can measure concentrations of antipsychotic medications in the body, if the person is hallucinating, he is hallucinating. He is not faulted or considered "resistant" or "attention-seeking" for hallucinating, even though his blood tests suggest he should have enough medication in his system to prevent hallucinations (though he may be seen as malingering).

This foregrounding of biology is, in fact, what happened in Caleigh's case. Everything changed in her fifth week of treatment: she got her period. This was a game-changing event. Caleigh hadn't menstruated in over three years, and the return of her period was both biologically and psychologically monumental. She was devastated, as it indicated to her that she had gotten "fat." The clinical team had mixed feelings about it. On the one hand, they were thrilled that Caleigh's body seemed to be repairing itself. On the other hand, they dreaded what the insurance company would say. And sure enough, despite the fact that Caleigh was at only 85 percent of her ideal body weight (still meeting the diagnostic criteria for anorexia), continued to hide food and exercise in secret, and was still highly ambivalent about recovery, her insurance company took the return of her period as evidence that she was ready for discharge. They stopped approving treatment (despite originally authorizing eight weeks), and two days later she was discharged.

Within two weeks, Caleigh was in full relapse. She called the clinic in tears, begging to come back to treatment. The clinic staff did what they could to obtain insurance approval, but after reviewing the case, the insurance company ruled that Caleigh had, in fact, "failed" her previous stay by relapsing after discharge, so she was denied coverage.

(UN)WILLINGNESS, FAILED PATIENTS, AND CHRONICITY

According to standard definitions, Caleigh had at this point developed a "chronic" eating disorder: she had been ill for over seven years and had now "failed" at several treatment attempts. Accordingly, based on the current best practices literature, one reasonable course of action would be to refer Caleigh to hospice and allow her to die.

But had she really failed treatment? If a relapse is precipitated by the removal of necessary treatment before it has had a chance to be effective, should it be considered failure? And if that removal of care is based on mutually undermining models of care and a turn to the (sick or relapsing) body for the verdict of "truth" about a patient's investment in recovery, we have to consider the ways in which our structures of care produce chronicity in some conditions more so than others. When those conditions are also uniquely identified as "hopeless" and its sufferers are referred to hospice rather than given more care, we have to ask what bigger issues are at stake that are producing this situation.

The reasons for this particular positioning of eating disorders are numerous and complex and are traced through the remainder of the book. What I wish to highlight here are the ways in which different chronographies become productive not only of illness conditions but of sufferers themselves as certain "kinds" of patients who merit (or do not merit) certain modes of intervention.

In the next section, we turn to the everyday life of the clinic and examine how these concerns about "truth," authenticity, subjectivity, and agency are enacted in daily practice and how clients themselves experience them.

Liquidated

NOVEMBER 1980

The thermos of chicken bouillon sits on Mrs. Brown's circular table in the guidance office, a few ounces of the still-warm liquid waiting in the top-turned-cup, staring at me. I can't really focus on what Mrs. Brown is saying to me, though I figure she is pleading with me to take a sip. Just a tiny sip. I am crying, tears streaming down my face.

"I can't," I weep. "I'm so sorry. But I just can't."

It's my second day without water.

Dynamics

In section 1, we looked at how eating disorders are constituted as objects of concern and as the target of specific kinds of intervention. In section 2, we encountered two distinct models of care that come together at Cedar Grove and the kinds of frictions that arise from their competing chronographies, different notions of the will, and divergent ethics of care. We saw in the case of Caleigh how these opposing ways of figuring the patient and the problem could lead to acts of "care" that look like—and feel like—harm and actually provoke the very conditions they are supposed to treat.

The process of recovery within Cedar Grove is meant to move clients out of a state of coagulated being or impasse and into one of growth and change, mobilizing them on a trajectory with both physical and emotional dimensions. In this regard, treatment is a distinctly *developmental* process in both scope and structure, as clients ideally transform from locally construed "sick" bodies and selves into imagined future "healthy" ones. A double movement of the anticipation of recovery on the one hand and the fear of chronicity on the other hand propels this process, even as it produces frictions, ambivalences, and contradictions that can become its undoing.

In this section, we look more closely at how clients move through the treatment process; how the tensions identified in the last section continually tug on, constrain, and morph this journey; and how clients come to bear the burdens of these (il)logics of care.

BETWIXT AND BETWEEN

Anthropologists have long been interested in how processes of change and transformation crystallize cultural values in profound and often dramatic ways. Anthropologist Victor Turner, best known for his studies of a particular genre of ritual practice that he termed "rites of passage" (building on the work of Arnold Van Gennep[1]), described three key phases to such transitions: separation (when people are removed from their prior social role either symbolically or, more often, by being physically sequestered from the larger community in a special space), liminality (the period of being "betwixt and between" two different roles), and reintegration (when individuals are reintroduced into society in their new role state).[2]

Turner was especially interested in liminality as the phase where ritual transformation occurs and where the work of culture is the most intense and potent. Liminality provides the occasion—and indeed the provocation—for a profound existential reflection on society and on one's position within it. When initiates have left one social role but have not yet attained another, they are challenged to relinquish their prior worldviews and trappings of identity and to begin to incorporate new ways of understanding the world and their own capacities and responsibilities within it. In the liminal stage, human potentiality is wrested loose from its prior moorings and carefully lead by skilled mentors toward a new tethering. This loosened potentiality, Turner argued, is highly charged, making it both sacred and dangerous— things could go right, or they could go horribly wrong. As such, the process of transitioning from one accepted social role to another is an awesome and monumental task, requiring the skillful attention and care of ritual experts who guide initiates and ensure that this potentiality is properly channeled.

Treatment at a clinic like Cedar Grove is a distinctly liminal phenomenon, in Turner's sense of the term. Clients have left their everyday lives and entered into a protected space within which they are learning to become new kinds of social beings: people "in recovery." They become entrained[3] in new bodily practices (e.g., healthy eating and sleeping patterns and other basic self-care activities) and learn new forms of knowledge and skills (e.g., how to articulate their feelings in words, how to navigate social relationships) that will prepare them to take on this new role.

But eating disorder patients are also liminal in another sense. Following a separate but related tradition of engagement with the notion of liminality— that of Mary Douglas—we can say that eating disorder patients are also liminal in that they don't fit cleanly into common biomedical categories that disambiguate the body from the mind.[4] A person with an eating disorder is therefore "matter out of place."[5] As such, she constitutes a form of "pollution" and is subject to targeted attempts to subsume her firmly within familiar and accepted paradigms.

Like other liminal processes, treatment at Cedar Grove is enervated with potentialities that are powerful as well as dangerous, and treatment is risky on a number of fronts.[6] It means at least temporarily leaving school or work, absenting oneself from family and friend relationships, and putting oneself at the mercy of a system one might reasonably suspect is motivated as much by economics as by health. Once in treatment, one must make oneself acutely vulnerable to strangers and be willing to uncover and access emotions and experiences that can be profoundly destabilizing and even traumatizing. When treatment ends, one must try to remain healthy after returning to daily life and relationships, which often haven't changed much. In addition to these risks, treatment is also fraught, as we will see, with challenges, interferences, and roadblocks that continually threaten its ideal(ized) trajectory, rendering the liminal process of treatment as fragile and precarious as it is critical and potent.

Despite these risks, such a radical removal from life-as-usual may be necessary to enable someone to redirect their energies and move forward. As we saw with Miranda stopping on the highway (described in chapter 6), people can become so entrenched in their behavioral, thought, and affective patterns that they cannot, of their own accord, wrest themselves free from them. It takes concentrated outside intervention and a great deal of structural and therapeutic action to disrupt these patterns and help people form new ones.

In the United States, this process happens in the context of significant material risk and precarity due to the insurance climate. This insecurity and instability has become folded into understandings of eating disorders themselves such that overcoming such obstacles and dangers can be considered to be part of the "achievement" of transformation and recovery. "How they [patients] handle the insurance situation tells us a lot about their progress," Zoë, a therapist, explained to me. "It [insurance] is largely out of their control. They have to practice their new skills of letting go and distress tolerance, and stay focused on recovery. It's not easy, but it gives us good information about where they are in their process." Eating disorders treatment, like the kinds of liminality Turner describes, is a time of radical unmooring, transformation, and retethering in ways that make acutely visible the cultural and social meanings and values that enable and constrain local ways of being.

Specifically, during the liminal period of treatment, key capacities having to do with regulating *affect*—its direction, amplitude, and saturation—are drawn out, foregrounded, and shaped in new ways. Notably, these modulations can be variously interpreted in the clinic either as healthy expressions of a "recovered" self *or* as pathological manifestations of a self that remains ill. Contradictions between the views of the recovery model and the medical model shape such interpretations, and when and how such distinctions are made has direct impacts on the course and outcome of treatment.

Treatment, in short, is a time of *gathering potentiality*, when all of a person's resources—emotional, physical, relational, and financial—are decoupled from their prior moorings, harnessed, and directed at the identified problem (the eating disorder), with the aim of restarting the client's life along a new trajectory. It is a time of dismantling, reconfiguring, and rebuilding, of radical dislocation from a world of illness, pathology, and misery and relocation (if all goes well) within a world of hope, growth, and health.

Far too often, however, things go terribly, terribly wrong.

DYNAMICS OF CHANGE

Like Turner and Douglas, I am interested in the concept of liminality. Specifically, I am concerned with the liminal dimensions of treatment at Cedar Grove—how the clinic conceptualizes and operationalizes the transition from "sick" to "recovered"—as a way of examining key cultural meanings and beliefs that shape local ways of being. Eating disorder patients disrupt and trouble existing categories of knowledge, even while, in other ways, treatment for eating disorders works to reinscribe them.

The chapters in this section conceptualize the treatment process as pivoting on three main "movements": unmooring, recalibration, and retethering.[7] While these movements in some ways resonate with Turner's stages of separation, liminality, and reintegration, I want to be clear that I am interested in what happens *within* treatment itself and in the clinic as a liminal space.[8] In other words, what I describe here are microprocesses *within* the liminal stage. At each of these junctures, we will see how understandings of what an eating disorder is and what kinds of care it requires are negotiated. We will see how key developmental tasks are put to the clients and how clients are scaffolded through them, and also how each is fraught with a series of ambivalences and contradictions that often place clients in untenable situations. Specifically, I direct our attention to the multiple and often contradictory messages and expectations that are communicated to clients at various stages of this process, disjunctures that then become sites of elaboration as clinicians and insurance companies try to make sense of why treatment isn't progressing as planned and clients try to figure out how to make it through one more day.

These tasks can be roughly mapped onto the two primary systems of measuring progress in the clinic—the "phase system" (loosely based on James O. Prochaska and Carlo C. DiClemente's stages of change model[9]) and the "treatment plan" (based on a biomedical model)—which share some overlap but are not isomorphic. The phase system is an older structure at the clinic and reflects the concerns and priorities of a recovery-based model. At the time of my research, Cedar Grove identified four phases—stabilization, initiation, recovery, and transition—each with its own parameters and attendant privileges and restrictions. Coexisting with the phase system, but more consistent with a medical model paradigm, the treatment plan is fine grained and problem oriented and breaks down the treatment approach according to the categories of nutrition, medical, therapeutic, and school/work functioning.

The tasks I discuss in this section resonate in different ways with both the phase system and the treatment plan modes of tracking progress. Like the phase system, these tasks sketch a developmental trajectory in that each requires and builds on the ones prior to it. Like the treatment plan, they entail specific indicators of "success" to which clients and clinicians alike appeal.

Rather than simply describe the phase system and treatment plan as separate technologies, then, I use the tasks identified above—unmooring, recalibrating, and retethering—as a way of considering how these different forms of reckoning illness and healing constitute eating disorders as different sorts of entities and examining the kinds of contradictions, paradoxes, and ambivalences this produces for clinicians and clients alike.

SEVEN

Loosening the Ties That Bind

UNMOORING

I just got here. But then I tell myself, or Ed [my eating disorder] tells me, I have to go back [home]. My kids need me. But I know I need to get better. But then the guilt steps in and the anxiety, because I've always had bad separation anxiety, which has been horrible for me. When I went to treatment the first time, I was in tears for the first week all the time. I mean, it was bad separation anxiety. I feel that in my chest being here. So I'm fighting that on top of everything else. And I've got horrible body image going on right now, and it's getting stronger.

—**AMBER**,
a thirty-three-year-old woman diagnosed with bulimia

Treatment for an eating disorder is, by design, radically disruptive. In the first part of treatment—the first one to two weeks—the client is systematically untethered from existing structures, practices, and relationships and reoriented toward new ways of being in and experiencing the world. While the client works through these processes, the clinic functions as a kind of living laboratory for a series of important tasks. As she habituates to life in the clinic, she (ideally) comes to see her previous life in a different light, understanding it as governed by pathology, and the clinic (supposedly) models new ways of healthy living. Then, as she begins to experience the world without the mediation of an eating disorder, she is mentored in understanding that what she previously thought of as control is actually its opposite and that by giving up control in treatment she is actually gaining more authentic control of her life. As she learns that what she thought was true about her self and her body was, in fact, distorted by the eating disorder, she learns to take her body and self as a new kind of object and to relinquish her claims of self-knowledge to expert others. And as the bonds of her old identity loosen, she comes to recognize her eating disorder as reflective of her interpersonal patterns and learns to relate to others from a new place of recovery. These tasks are accomplished through an *inversion of relationships of control,* a process that starts in this phase and is further elaborated as treatment progresses.

(DE)STABILIZATION: SAFETY AND PROVOCATION

REBECCA: What do you hope to get out of treatment? What are your goals for yourself, for your time here?

LILIA: I have to stop puking.

REBECCA: That's the part that's the hardest for you?

LILIA: Yeah. I wake up and my gut is killing me and my head is killing me and my tongue is stuck to the top of my mouth and I have chest pains when I run, which is scary. My bones are breaking. I want to continue running, but I want to be healthy. I'd like to make my fiftieth birthday. That's my goal.

• • •

KAREN: I feel like I'm in eating disorders camp right now.

REBECCA: What do you mean?

KAREN: I'm just learning a lot about what this disease is. It shapes you, and you learn more about yourself and about life.

Marly, a twenty-three-year-old woman diagnosed with bulimia, watched anxiously as Dee, a direct care staff member, emptied her belongings out of the suitcase and laid them out on Marly's bed in the residential house. Dee called out the items one by one as Armine, another direct care staff member, marked them down on a sheet of paper that would go into Marly's chart. Sweatshirts, leggings, underwear, shoes, belts, shampoo (which Dee opened and smelled to make sure it didn't contain alcohol or any other substance that could be used to induce vomiting), jewelry, makeup bag, razor—wait, that's not allowed. Dee put the razor to the side and continued. Underwear, lotion (opened and verified), socks, hairdryer, nail clippers (not allowed, put to the side), school books, journal, colored pens. Once the major items were sorted, Dee dumped out the makeup in the makeup bag and turned the bag inside out, running her fingers all around the seams. She shook out each piece of clothing and checked the pockets. She unbundled the socks and turned them inside out. She ran her hand around the insides of Marly's empty suitcase, checking all the pockets and seams. "What are you looking for?" asked Marly, mildly annoyed. "We have to check everything," Dee said somewhat apologetically. "People sometimes bring in laxatives or diuretics or things for cutting. We have to make sure none of that is tucked away somewhere. It's for your own safety," she explained.

Marly was in the middle of Cedar Grove's admissions process, a multihour sequence of getting settled into the residential house and oriented to the day suite, where the bulk of treatment took place. Paramount in this process is making sure that clients do not come in with anything that could be used to harm themselves or someone else, either directly (like razor blades) or by interfering with the process of recovery (like calorie lists or "thinspirational" images). Everything clients bring in with them is meticulously searched and catalogued, and clients are allowed access only to items deemed "safe."

Such paired dynamics of intrusion and protection are part of the self-consciously parental positioning of the clinic and are foundational to the developmental tasks set out in the process of recovery. "It's our job to make sure each client is safe and that the community as a whole is safe," Dr. Casey explained to me. "They are not in a position to know what is good for them right now. That's part of why they need twenty-four-hour care. It's up to us to be vigilant, even though they might not like it. In fact," she added, "if we're doing our job well, they *won't* like it. If they're comfortable, we're doing something wrong."

Not that Dr. Casey wanted things to be intentionally unpleasant for clients. On the contrary, the residential house is, as I noted in chapter 5, an actual house, and it is furnished and decorated with the explicit aim of being comforting and soothing. Dr. Casey was referring more to the fact that treatment takes people out of their comfort zone and puts them in a space of radical discontinuity with their lives outside. This is meant to be a productive disjuncture—like a grain of sand in an oyster—that provokes the development of greater intrapsychic, behavioral, and interpersonal capacities.

When clients first enter the clinic, they are considered to be in the most vulnerable of states and are accordingly assigned to what is called, in the clinic's phase system, the Stabilization Phase. Clients at this point are, by all measures, patently *unstable* both medically and emotionally and require the full press of institutional supports. All new clients start out in the Stabilization Phase and then work to progress through the other stages (the Transition Phase and Recovery Phase) as treatment proceeds.

During this early part of treatment, according to the Cedar Grove patient handbook, "clients may not recognize their eating disorder as a problem" and "may have no desire for recovery." Even if they do, "their commitment to the protocols of the program may waiver at times." Clients may also "require intensive medical monitoring and/or staff support in order to follow the basic program expectations." For example, a client might need continual reminders about not engaging in rituals at the table, extra encouragement to finish a meal, or frequent "check-ins" (brief conversations) with direct care staff to process difficult feelings. During this phase, the focus is on "medical stabilization, nourishment, and hydration, assessment of cognitive abilities, and assessment of capacity to participate in individual and group therapy." Due to the intensive nature of the staff supervision deemed necessary at this stage, clients are not initially eligible for passes, outings, physical activity groups, or daily walks.[1]

It is acutely ironic that this is called the Stabilization Phase, as most clients find it to be the single most *destabilizing* experience they have ever had. Indeed, the point of this first phase of treatment is to radically unsettle a client's current life situation and create *a seemingly paradoxical zone of both safety and provocation.*

On the one hand, clients in the clinic are held within a "biomedical embrace"[2] that seeks to ensure that they are made and kept medically stable and safe. Staff monitor and record their vitals several times a day. Nurses obtain and record their weights every morning. Activities are limited for clients deemed medically unstable. At the same time, however, clients are intentionally made to feel emotionally *unsafe* in very specific ways: they are prevented from "using their eating disorders" (restricting, bingeing, purging, exercising, and using food rituals) or engaging in other behaviors like self-harm or abusing substances to manage affect, and they are required to attend both individual therapy and group therapy sessions, where they are encouraged to explore how they are feeling and to listen attentively as others share. Clients are induced, in other words, to *feel their feelings* in ways that many experience as radically unfamiliar, intensely scary, and patently overwhelming. "The function of an eating disorder is to numb out," Edie, a twenty-eight-year-old woman diagnosed with anorexia, told me. "Here, we have to actually feel our feelings. It's really intense. I'm not sure I like it." Within the "holding environment"[3] of the clinic, clients begin—very tentatively—to experience the world without the protective filter of their eating disorders to help them modulate engagements.

When they come into treatment, then, clients are not only giving up all control over their bodies and their lives to strangers, they are also relinquishing their hold, at least to some significant extent, on their eating disorders, which are, as Amber described them, "like a security blanket." That is, they are being asked to simultaneously make themselves abjectly vulnerable to the power and control of others—intensely disquieting for most people, but even more so for someone with an eating disorder—and give up the one thing— the eating disorder—that makes them feel safe.

Despite the distress this generated, I found that clients generally recognized and largely appreciated the juxtaposition of safety and provocation, even if they didn't always enjoy it. As Bethany observed:

> It's really hard here. *Really* hard. I think they try to provide us with things to ease anxiety—plenty of art, the yoga, all that, the outings they take us on. To be candid, I think they really try hard to try to make things better. You can't really be happy in a place like this, but they try to make it better. And it's not perfect. There's things that go on, but so far I'm pretty impressed. And you know what? Nobody's going to be happy in a place like this. People come in at a variety of points in their lives with other things going on, and it's a weird circumstance to be in. You're thrown into a room with people you don't know, and doing a group therapy—helpful as it may be, it's not a natural thing for a lot of people to sit and talk about stuff. But as hard as it is, they do their best.

Karen's views echoed Bethany's: "The bathroom monitoring sucks. That was hard to get used to. But it's for our own safety, so I appreciate it, even if my eating disorder hates it."

The task in this portion of treatment can be characterized as a dual movement of *letting go* and *reaching toward*. That is, clients are asked to *let go* of "outside" behaviors, habits, and priorities, and they are assisted in doing so through programmatic structures and limits, like meal plans and set meal times, restrictions on exercise, and locked bathrooms. At the same time, they are encouraged to *reach toward* recovery by focusing on themselves and making their own health a priority, something that can be acutely uncomfortable for someone with an eating disorder, who feels unworthy of accepting even *basic nourishment* into her body, let alone putting her needs above those of others.

This challenge is heightened by the next task, (re)learning how to feel.

REAWAKENING: THE RUSH OF FEELING

Like the sensation of blood rushing back into a hand or foot that has fallen asleep, the flood of affect that many clients experience in the absence of eating disorder practices is intense, saturated, and often unwieldy. It is a profoundly and existentially destabilizing experience, as the following exchange with Edie, which took place about two weeks into her treatment, demonstrates:

> EDIE: I'm kind of in that helpless space. Where, like, I'm here and I don't really know my reasons for recovery or what's going to happen. And I'm so scared to death. I'm just kind of stuck, I guess.
>
> REBECCA: That's sounds like a very hard place to be. What do you do with those feelings of being stuck?
>
> EDIE: Well, I used to restrict [*laughs*]. And I actually used to do some self-harm. Otherwise, my anxiety just goes through the roof. I have to be busy all the time. I don't relax. That's what my husband says, "You don't know how to relax." And he's right, I don't. I think it's even harder here because I can't get out and walk. They won't even let me go on the walks. It's like a prison, you know? And I can't . . . I'm just sitting with a lot of that anxiety and stuff.

A conversation with Amber in which we were discussing her feelings of comfort when she's in her eating disorder also turned to this issue:

> REBECCA: You've used the word *comforting* a couple of times to talk about your eating disorder. For people who don't know much about eating disorders or have never had one, the idea that restricting can be comforting might sound weird. From the inside, can you tell me a little bit more about what that feeling of comfort is, that comfort of restricting?
>
> AMBER: It's like having a friend with you all the time that you'll have with you no matter what. Kind of like a security blanket, something that keeps you safe, keeps from you from feeling the pain of everyday life. Or having to deal with anything that goes on—problems with guys, or with friends, or family, or anything. It's just keeps you secure, safe. In some ways, it's like [how] some people turn to alcohol or cigarettes or compulsive shopping or gambling or whatever. I think everybody has something that they use as a coping mechanism, and that's what the eating disorder became for me. I think we all have a little weakness that we carry with us that could flare up, if we let it. I just think I couldn't control mine.
>
> REBECCA: So, what's it like being here and not being able to do that [act on your eating disorder]?
>
> AMBER: It's really hard. It's overwhelming. All these feelings and things that have been numbed out start coming back up, and then you're like, "Ugh, I have to deal with feeling all of this now." I can't sleep. My eating disorder thoughts are stronger, even though I can't actually do anything,

and I still have to eat my full meal plan or they might kick me out. So I have all the feelings *and* all the food. I'm just full of everything all the time. It's not fun. Not fun at all.

Without access to their eating disorders, clients in treatment often experience a resurgence of emotions, affects, and sensations, which they have few skills for managing and which can intensify the desire to return to the eating disorder.

One of the first and most intense of these affects to emerge in the absence of eating disorder behaviors is *pain,* which has both physiological and psychological dimensions in treatment. Pain is pervasive in the clinic. Clients' bodies are in pain: muscles and joints ache, stomachs bloat, GI tracts are dysregulated, heads hurt, NG tubes are uncomfortably inserted and removed, limbs swell. But the pain is more ubiquitous than this. The psychic pain in an eating disorders clinic is palpable and overwhelming. People are like walking exposed nerves, stripped of their usual protective defenses. Pain is everywhere; it can be seen in how people curl up in the foofs, how they cry in therapy, how they speak in groups, how they hold themselves, and how they force their way through meals and white-knuckle it through postmeal bathroom bans.

Clients readily described this welling up of emotional and psychological pain. As Marly recounted, "I just hurt. My whole body hurts. But it's more than that. My *being* hurts. I don't know how else to describe it. I'm in so much pain I don't know how I'm going to bear it from one minute to the next. I used to restrict or cut or purge, but I can't do any of that here. I just have to feel it, and it's excruciating." Jemma, a twenty-four-year-old woman diagnosed with anorexia, had a similar experience: "I just sit here now with all these feelings. And what comes to me most is the pain, the pain of all the things I've done. All the people I've hurt. All the ways I've failed. And I think of people I've lost in my life—my grandmother, for example. I was really close to her. And it hurts. It all just hurts so much."

Pain is not the only feeling that comes rushing forward. Clients also described anger, shame, grief, and sadness as among the most intense and unwelcome. "I didn't realize I was so angry," Amber noted. "I knew I had a lot of sadness, depression, and anxiety. All of that was pretty obvious. But the anger has surprised me. Things I've kept pushed down all these years. And now I have to find a way to deal with it constructively." Interestingly, hope was another troubling feeling for some, like Karen: "I think about the future now, and I want to get better. I want recovery. I want to get on with my career. But then again, I don't like that feeling. because I'm afraid it won't ever happen. I'd rather just not hope for it at all." The emergence of any emotion, sensation, or affect often caused distress for clients, who were habituated to the ambivalent anesthesia of their eating disorders.

Without their eating disorders or other behaviors to lean on, many clients reported feeling terrified, panicky, and lost, and they responded to this in a variety of ways. Some would cry uncontrollably, shake, curl up in a ball, rock back and forth, pace (until redirected by staff), wander aimlessly looking for something to do, or fidget (until redirected). Others would sit staring stonily at the wall or somehow manage to fall into the protection of sleep in the midst of all the noisy activity of the clinic. Others would engage more proactively, by journaling, talking to staff, or doing therapy assignments. A key aim of treatment is to help clients develop alternative, non-self-destructive strategies for managing their feelings, like using words, exercising distress tolerance, and employing constructive coping skills (e.g., journaling, grounding, and mindfulness practices). But such skills are built only over time and only through first feeling the rush of emotion that comes in the wake of having one's eating disorder blocked.

The tasks in this phase of treatment can be characterized as *affective affordance* (allowing affect to emerge or be experienced) and *distress tolerance*. That is, by not actively engaging in their eating disorder, self-harm, or other self-destructive behaviors, clients cultivate an opportunity for the reemergence of affects that may have been muted or blocked. And here I mean not just emotions but also physical sensations; often, the two are entwined. Without their eating disorders to rely on as mechanisms of regulation and presencing, clients struggle to exist from moment to moment.

I wish to be clear, though: it is not that people with active eating disorders don't feel any emotions, sensations, or affects. They absolutely do. It is just that these feelings are almost universally centered around and focused on things having to do with the eating disorder itself. As Edie described it, "When I was deep in my eating disorder, all I could focus on was how hungry I was, how much my stomach hurt. I was cold all the time, shivering, even in summer. My joints hurt. I was just miserable all the time, physically. So I guess while I was numbed out about some things emotionally, other physical things were heightened for me. That felt safer, though, because the physical is something you can deal with. Put on a sweater or whatever. It felt less overwhelming than the emotional feelings." We see here how an eating disorder functions as an affective strategy that enlists both the body and the mind in its project of altering one's state and quality of presence. In the clinic, without the eating disorder, the client can feel like everything is fragmenting and falling apart.

One way this sense of dissolution and being overwhelmed is attenuated is through the next set of tasks, which have to do with learning new techniques of self-scrutiny.

THE WEIGHT OF SCRUTINY AND
THE INVERSION OF EXPERTISE

It's really numbers focused here. I haven't been focused on numbers in a long time. My eating disorder took on a different form in this past year, and I really wasn't focused on my weight on a scale. So I'm trying, and I'm doing everything I can. I'm following the protocol. I'm not getting actually punished, but this [focus on numbers] is getting in the way of my recovery because I'm prevented from doing things because of my weight. Right now, it's such a numbers game, and that's the only thing that's keeping me back. That's just really frustrating.

—**KENNEDY**,
a twenty-seven-year-old woman diagnosed with anorexia

Each of the processes introduced above—encouraging clients to *let go* of old behaviors and patterns and *reach toward* recovery while also *making space* for feelings, which they must then learn *how to tolerate*—hinges on inducing clients to subject themselves to a new kind of gaze and new forms of monitoring and scrutiny.

Self-surveillance as a practice is intimately familiar to people with eating disorders; they are exquisitely habituated to practices of self-monitoring that are far above and beyond what most people can imagine or tolerate. They do things like create endless lists of what they will eat, what they did eat, what time they ate it, how long it took, how many calories they consumed, how many carbs, how much sugar, how much salt. They weigh and measure serving sizes down to each grain of rice or crumb of bread. They keep logs of miles run, elliptical steps accomplished, and calories burned. They ritually measure their hips, thighs, stomachs, and arms. They obsessively pinch their flesh and scrutinize the contours of their bodies in mirrors. They create spreadsheets of Fitbit readouts tracking how many hours they slept, how many steps they took, their respiration rate and heart rate, how many calories they expended. Eating disorders, in their daily practice, are largely about self-surveillance and constant evaluative scrutiny.

But subjecting oneself to the gaze of others is something completely different, and it is excruciatingly uncomfortable for someone with an eating disorder. Although the specifics are different for each person, At the root of any eating disorder is a toxic, necrotic, overpowering shame, a shame that can be managed—but never eradicated—by the technologies of surveillance and control of the eating disorder itself, which aim to shape the "disgusting" self, body, and affect into something passably acceptable, something others can tolerate.

Being in treatment turns the eating disorder inside out.

At the clinic, clients learn that their habituated forms of self-surveillance are pathological, part of their disease, and must be stopped. Yet at the same time they are asked to submit themselves to new regimes of scrutiny and critique. They are constantly watched, evaluated, counted, and quantified. They are weighed and measured, their blood siphoned and tested, their arms squeezed by blood pressure cuffs, the results noted in a logbook. Every crumb that enters their bodies, and every morsel of food or ounce of liquid that does not, is accounted for in a separate logbook. When they sleep, when they wake, when they cry, when they rage, when they are silent, when they pace, when they participate, when they refuse to participate, what they say, how they sit, whom they befriend—it is all recorded in their charts.[4]

In other words, treatment shifts the monitoring and management of the self and body from a private, intensely intimate and personal affair to something that is public and collective, on constant display, and a perpetual topic of conversation. It requires putting what feel like one's most shameful parts of the self and body—those parts that are needy, hungry, weak, and vulnerable—under the scrutiny and control of powerful strangers who not only see those shameful parts but also measure, document, and narrativize them to determine whether and how one is deserving of care.

The implementation of this regime of scrutiny and accounting requires an interdisciplinary team and a range of structures and technologies. On admission, as I noted in chapter 5, each client is assigned to one of several mini-teams, composed of a therapist, a dietician, a psychiatrist, and a physician and supported by nursing and direct care staff. These team members deploy stethoscopes, blood pressure cuffs, syringes, scales, feeding tubes, measuring cups, calorie charts, food plans, growth charts, medication logs, progress notes, group logs, and treatment plans to measure and track a client's changes over time. Privileges (passes, access to social media, permission to attend outings, the ability to exercise) are all tied to how a client's progress toward recovery is evaluated.

So what, exactly, are all these people and technologies looking for? As we have seen, there are two primary treatment models in tension at Cedar Grove (the recovery model and the medical model; see chapter 6) and three dimensions of being that are simultaneously targeted for intervention (medical/biological, cognitive/behavioral, and affective/psychological; see chapter 5). The data clinicians look for is therefore complex.

The targets of this monitoring in the clinic are threefold: (1) the body (the focus of medical interventions), which is measured through such things as weight, heart rate, temperature, blood pressure, and lab values and rendered in numerical terms; (2) behavior (the focus of behavioral interventions), measured through observation and reported both quantitatively (e.g., "Sarah was redirected from exercising three times today") and qualitatively (e.g., "Carly appeared skittish and fidgety waiting for the afternoon walk"); and (3) affect (the focus of psychological interventions), which is assessed through such things as reported emotions and cognitions and is articulated in terms of quality (e.g., positive, negative), frequency, and intensity. Each of these targets—the body, behavior, and affect—are important for different reasons in terms of measuring progress and "health," though there is an important disconnect here in terms of what is being measured and evaluated, how it is thought to relate to recovery, and what is prioritized by different stakeholders.

Insurance companies care primarily about a client's medical status. They want clients to become medically stable so they can be moved to a lower (less expensive) level of care (or out of care altogether). When a client is considered "medically stable," it means that she has reached a reasonable percentage of her ideal body weight (what counts as "reasonable" differs from insurance company to insurance company), her labs are within normal range, and she does not have any other indicators of instability, like bradycardia or orthostatic hypotension. Insurance companies expect underweight clients to gain on average two to three pounds per week in order to reach this state in what they deem to be a timely manner. Daily morning weigh-ins are meant to track this progress, and if a client does not gain the required amount of weight in a week (even if she has been fully compliant with her meal plans), her insurance company may refuse to certify further care, even if benefits are still available.

The clinical team at Cedar Grove cares about medical stabilization, too, and the clinic is nationally renowned for taking medical concerns seriously. But staff are just as interested in clients' affective lives and whether and how changes in troubling feelings, cognitions, and sensations are occurring. "It doesn't do much if they gain weight but are still deep in their eating disorder," Susan, a therapist, told me. "It's good that they're medically stable, but without that other piece they're going to relapse. It's only a matter of time." Such changes are more difficult to measure than lab values and weights, however, and are therefore assessed and communicated through chart notes and narratives rather than numerical values.

It is here that a focus on behavior can play something of a mediating role, as both the medical model and the recovery model look to behaviors as indexical of the issues they find most salient and important. For example, from the medical model perspective, behaviors like food rituals, continual subversion of program limits, and emotional outbursts can be read as characteristics of a "hungry brain" and a body and nervous system that need to be regulated. The same behaviors can be read, from the recovery model perspective, as indicating dysregulated affects like anxiety, which need psychotherapeutic attention to help clients manage them. But while both approaches look to outward behaviors as "evidence" of what they think is the core problem in an eating disorder, and both focus on regulation as an ideal and a goal, the underlying philosophy of the person and the epistemological framework of recovery in these two views are very different (recall the distinctions between procedural and epistemic authenticity). How, then, are these two kinds of assessment brought together in evaluating a client's location in relation to recovery? Often, as we will see in the coming chapters, this integration is messy and difficult, and it is not always successful.

During the early part of treatment, a key task for a new client is to turn over the intimate management of her body and mind to others, while retaining and even honing an acute attention to what that body and mind are *doing*—day-to-day, if not hour-to-hour or even minute-to-minute—and what this *means* in terms of her state of (physical and/or emotional) health. In other words, clients are led through a divestment of claims to knowledge about the (physical, emotional, and even behavioral) self but simultaneously encouraged to engage with a heightened curiosity about what that self is revealing about itself, although expert others are needed to interpret these messages. As Kendall noted, "I just have to wait to see what my labs say. I know I'm following my meal plan and not purging, but I'm always worried, you know, that something will show up as wrong. And that they'll think I was doing something I wasn't. Or that something is malfunctioning, like my kidneys or whatever. So I'm just waiting for them to tell me." Clients are induced to surrender their claims to knowledge of themselves to clinicians—and, even more so, to medical tests—who will determine the "truth" about where they are in recovery. "I think I'm doing pretty well," Bethany told me. "I'm still struggling with urges, but they're a lot less than they used to be. But we'll see what my weights are saying. They won't tell me what I weigh, so I have no idea. So I think it's going well, but who knows."

At the same time that clients are being guided to *relinquish* power and claims of legitimacy to biomedical authorities, however, they are being mentored to *reclaim* power and legitimacy from significant others in their lives.

RENEGOTIATING RELATIONSHIPS
AND BOUNDARIES

No one is sicker than the parent of a person with an eating disorder. I say that with all humility.

—ELEANOR,
mother of a daughter in treatment for anorexia

Once clients have adjusted (more or less) to everyday life in the clinic, begun to feel their feelings again, and subjected themselves to new techniques of surveillance, they begin the challenging process of refiguring intimacies, both inside and outside of the clinic. This task derives from longstanding beliefs about why people develop eating disorders that are rooted in psychoanalytic and psychodynamic theories about separation and individuation and are naturalized within contemporary approaches.

At Cedar Grove, food and eating are seen to both mirror the status quo of a client's affective and relational attachments and provide an avenue for her transformation. That is, how a client relates to food (Does she crave it, fear it, show ambivalence toward it, or seem disinterested in it?) is thought to express how she experiences and enacts human attachments. Does she "binge" on relationships to the point of exhausting other people's emotional resources? Does she avoid others, allowing herself only tiny "crumbs" of connection at a time? Does she have no interest in attachments at all? Do they make her anxious, nauseous, or "hungry" for more? "In general, people in the throes of anorexia tend to be more reserved in their relationships, whereas people actively struggling with bulimia tend to be more erratic," Joan, Cedar Grove's assistant director, told staff during a clinical training meeting. These relational patterns are thought to precede the eating disorder rather than to arise from it (though they may be exacerbated by the illness). We can see here an underlying premise that food behaviors are expressive of psychodynamic issues and become a way of articulating and possibly trying to navigate interpersonal dynamics. Critical to the practice of recovery at Cedar Grove, then, is the shifting of patterns of interpersonal relating.

This understanding of eating disorders, what we might call the classic view, positions the child's struggle for autonomy, usually from an overinvolved mother, as the core conflict of these illnesses. It is believed that as a result of this enmeshment, the eating-disordered girl has not formed a sufficiently solid sense of self as separate from others. As she moves into adolescence, this is thought to lead to a host of other difficulties, including the need for validation, to feel seen—by becoming the "perfect" daughter or student, the most popular girl in school, or a star athlete, for example. In this context, food is understood to be the one area over which the eating-disordered girl feels she has sole control. Acting out against her own developing female body is understood as a rejection of adult womanhood (which is associated with the mother) and a desire either to remain childlike or to attain a more androgynous (or even masculine) appearance.[5]

Although the assumptions of this classic view might translate into very different types of therapeutic action (e.g., a psychodynamic therapist might focus on ego functions, whereas a cognitive-behavioral therapist would target problem thoughts and behaviors), this core developmental tale has structured most eating disorder theories and therapies since at least the 1920s, including those at Cedar Grove, even in the face of a push toward more biomedical models. Such approaches share the core belief that the cause of eating disorders, and the enduring problem keeping a client in distress, is a lack of an adequately and properly individuated self.

Given this focus on separation and individuation, the classic view considers boundaries to be paramount in the process of eating disorders treatment, and Cedar Grove places significant emphasis on them as well. In this context, "boundaries" refers to the psychological, emotional, and affective differentiations between the self and the other but also to limits in a broader sense, such as limits on time, attention, and resources. "Teaching clients to recognize and respect boundaries is key to what we do," Dr. Casey emphasized during a training session for Cedar Grove therapists. "Often, the family environment is such that they haven't learned good boundaries, either interpersonal boundaries or limits more generally. That's why it's so important that we have clear limits here and that we hold those limits. And why therapeutic boundaries are so critical." (See chapter 10 for more on how clinicians cultivate and understand their therapeutic relationships with clients.) Dr. Casey's observations highlight the clinic's emphasis on resocializing clients and remobilizing "healthy" developmental processes, which, in this context, means a certain kind of individuation that privileges autonomy, boundedness, and emotional containment. In this way, the clinic is positioned as a sort of "do-over" for the family environment that produced the eating disorder.

Before going on, I want to pause here to offer a few words about families. The "typical" family that produces a child with an eating disorder, according to the classic eating disorder literature, involves an overbearing and critical mother, a largely absent or "weak" father, a child who wishes to regress to prepubescence as a way of managing overwhelming affects of different sorts, and unclear emotional boundaries all around.[6] "Anorexic" families are thought to be rife with double messages about nurturant affection and neglect, while "bulimic" families are thought to be characterized by hostile enmeshment.[7] (The fact that most people with an eating disorder will move back and forth between diagnoses does not seem to trouble such theories.)

While I did occasionally observe such family patterns at Cedar Grove, they were decidedly not the norm. And in those cases where they did appear, I found myself wondering whether they were the *cause* of the eating disorder or a *result* of it. Likely, they were both. It is difficult and problematic to assess the nature of intimate relationships when observed in times of crisis. It is not surprising, for example, that one or both parents may become extremely involved and even "enmeshed" with a child whose very life hangs the balance, or that a family in crisis may appear to be chaotic and fraying at the seams.

Generally speaking, from what I observed, fathers seemed to have more difficulty than mothers wrapping their heads around what an eating disorder is (and isn't) and would sometimes, as a result, step back, lending their support primarily through financial means rather than by being involved in the day-to-day work of recovery. This would leave mothers, step-mothers, or other female partners (all parental couples I observed were heterosexual pairings) to pick up the slack, and the women would generally step in to do the more hands-on work of, for example, getting their daughter to outside doctors' appointments, making sure she was following her meal plan when at home on pass, and intervening when problems arose. Such arrangements could, in practice, look very much like the overinvolved mother/distant father dynamic identified in the literature. Whether this sort of configuration reflected longstanding familial dynamics that were simply intensified during the crisis of an eating disorder or whether these dynamics emerged within the context of the eating disorder crisis itself differed from family to family. Notably, however, the literature naturalizes such dynamics as endemic to the family system and tends to blame mothers for being too controlling and invasive rather than, for example, faulting fathers for being largely absent and leaving the work of daily crisis management to their female counterparts. I mention this not to place the blame on fathers but to point out how gendered patterns of engagement are tied to much bigger and broader structures than family systems or individual psychological proclivities, and how these gendered structures have been folded into theories of cause and cure.

What I saw more than any sort of typical gender arrangement in terms of enmeshment and distance, however, was something more fundamental: a combination, often enacted by *both* parents, of heightened scrutiny and control of their daughter coupled with significant difficulty in genuinely seeing and empathizing with their daughter's emotional needs. For example, parents might be deeply involved in monitoring and managing their daughter's academic or sports performance—attending every event, supporting every success, celebrating every accomplishment—while at the same time having little capacity to recognize their child's emotional needs, or even if they do recognize them, to validate those needs. Now, this in and of itself would not cause an eating disorder. But such dynamics of intrusion and control combined with elision and erasure can be emblematic of broader patterns of relating that, over time and in conjunction with temperamental and situational factors, lay the groundwork for an eating disorder to emerge as a strategy of affective regulation and *presencing*. In Dorothée Legrand and Frédéric Briend's terms (see the introduction), we might say that such parents are adept—or even brilliant—at providing *answers* (being, for all intents and purposes, supportive parents in a procedural sense) but less so at providing *responses* (actually being attuned to and responsive to their daughter's needs in a more epistemic sense). In my terms, we would call this a misattunement in terms of *presencing*—either clients were not adept at presencing so they could be adequately seen, parents were not adept at seeing what clients were presencing, or (more often) both.

I want to emphasize that this hypervigilance/misattunement dynamic did not, as far as I could tell, reflect a lack of love or concern on the part of most parents. And it was certainly compounded by clients' difficulties in recognizing and articulating their own needs (though one could argue that this could be, at least to some degree, a consequence of parental modeling). My point here is that I am not interested in assigning blame. We can acknowledge this misattunement without specifying its origin, which is, in any case, probably due to a combination of historical, psychological, biological, temperamental, and situational factors as well as interpersonal ones.

Regardless of the cause, a marked degree of parental hypersurveillance and hypercontrol coupled with a misalignment of emotional and temperamental inclinations characterized almost all of the families I engaged with at Cedar Grove, and from talking with both parents and clients, it seemed that such misattunement had a history that began long before the emergence of the eating disorder itself. This could be significant not only for understanding how and why some people develop eating disorders (an eating disorder, after all, is animated by invasive self-control and self-surveillance paired with a deliberate ignoring of one's actual physiological and emotional needs, thereby mirroring relational dynamics) but also in thinking about the ways that managed care replicates the conditions under which eating disorders emerge and thrive. I will return to this issue in subsequent chapters.

Living under such conditions of hypervigilance and control combined with a lack of empathic attunement, people learn to form and engage in relationships in particular ways. Among other things, they devise strategies and workarounds for getting their needs met that are not always direct. This can look (or actually be) quite "manipulative," which can further exacerbate interpersonal tensions.[8] Overtly ignoring or silencing one's own needs while simultaneously using back channels to get them met (often unaware that that is what one is doing) is one of the key interpersonal strategies targeted for change during eating disorders treatment, although the conditions themselves that give rise to the need for such strategies persist in the clinic and can even become intensified, making the unlearning of such mechanisms not only challenging but also highly unlikely (see chapter 10).

Returning to the issue of boundaries: The work of recovery at Cedar Grove, as I noted, is conceptualized as developmental, in the sense that it helps clients achieve independence and autonomy. To this end, clinics like Cedar Grove often configure themselves as a sort of substitute family system whose job is to reparent the client, facilitating the development of a more solid sense of self. The task is to help clients develop and maintain "healthy" boundaries between themselves and others and to learn to know and trust themselves.

But we will also remember that eating disorder clients are considered to be notoriously "difficult," "controlling," "manipulative," and "resistant." This poses something of a conundrum. Being a "good" patient means accepting the direction and authority of the treatment team, even when (or perhaps especially when) it goes against one's own instincts. Yet to individuate, one must assert one's own will and follow one's own priorities even in the face of the influence of powerful others. What, then, do individuation and "healthy boundaries" look like in such a system? And how does this inform relationships of care?

DOUBLE BINDS

Unlearning longstanding interpersonal strategies and learning new ones is a tricky and multidimensional task, particularly when structural dynamics mirror and reproduce relational ones. Critical to this process in the clinic is the foregrounding of both dependence and independence in ways that can sometimes be confusing and contradictory. For example, by coming into residential treatment, clients make themselves completely dependent on the treatment team not only pragmatically (they depend on the team for food and housing, and must ask permission to engage in basic functions like using the bathroom, sleeping, or stepping outside) but also dispositionally, as they are induced to "give up control" and "allow the team to take the lead." At the same time, clients are constantly reminded that it is up to them—and *only* them—to take charge of their recovery, and they are chastised and even shamed if they seem to find comfort or relief in being cared for in the clinic (recall Dr. Arnold's comments about Felicia in chapter 4). Similarly, clients are mentored to be able to separate themselves from purportedly destructive family dynamics and encouraged to institute new forms of independence, but many of them rely on family members to provide financial, structural, and oversight support during the process of recovery. Amber felt this tension acutely:

> I know it's not a prison. Whenever I want to leave, nobody can hold me here because I'm an adult. I mean, unless I'm underweight. I'm low weight, but I'm not medically unstable. I just don't want to have to go out there and do it alone. I don't want to have to just do what everyone else wants, because that's not going to work. But I also don't want to have to do it alone. It's like I have to make a choice between getting support and doing what I think is right for me. I have to pick one or the other. And that's not a very nice choice to make.

The following transcript of a phone call between Sheila and her mother further demonstrates some of these dynamics. At the time of this call, Sheila, age twenty-three, was in the day treatment program at Cedar Grove for the second time (this was her third treatment overall, not counting ongoing out-patient therapy). She struggled with bulimia and self-harm and had made two serious suicide attempts. I was working as Sheila's therapist at the clinic—hence my inclusion in the conversation. A few nights before the call, Sheila had tried to talk to her mother (who lived out of state) about her desire for additional support but had felt the conversation "went nowhere," so she asked to call her mother again during our session. Here's how the conversation went:

SHEILA: Hi, Mom

MOTHER: Hi, Sheila. [*Pause.*]

SHEILA: Yeah. Well, I wanted to call you back with Rebecca here.

MOTHER: Hi, Rebecca

REBECCA: Hello.

SHEILA: Um, because I think things really ended badly the other night.

MOTHER: Yeah, they did. I was a complete mess the rest of the night. I really didn't sleep much.

SHEILA: Um, yeah. So I thought maybe we could try again to talk about things.

MOTHER: OK. I think that would be good.

SHEILA: So um, yeah. So as I told you the other night, I'm really struggling right now with behaviors.

MOTHER: Yes.

SHEILA: And I'm really having trouble.

MOTHER: Yes. So what are you asking me for? Because I know that when you start to talk like this you want us to do something.

SHEILA: Well, actually, I just want to talk to you about my options and what you guys are open to.

MOTHER: What do you mean?

SHEILA: Well, I mean that I think I really need more support right now.

MOTHER: And what does *that* mean? More treatment?

SHEILA: Well, I think I might need to step up my days a bit, maybe from three to five.

MOTHER: Because you know how your father and I feel about that. We don't want to pay for more treatment unless you can tell us what will be different this time. We've been down this road already several times, Sheila.

SHEILA: I know. I'm not sure how to tell you for sure what will be different this time.

MOTHER: So that's the problem, you see? Why should we go through this again if nothing's going to be different? You need to take charge of your recovery. Nothing is going to change until there's an internal shift. Otherwise, it's just going through the motions.

SHEILA: Well, yeah. OK. So I'm trying to think about what my options are.

MOTHER: And what have you come up with?

SHEILA: Well, one idea—I don't know if this is possible—but one idea would be for either you or Dad to come out here for a while and help me break the cycle of behaviors. You know, just be here.

MOTHER: What do you mean by "a while"?

SHEILA: Maybe two weeks?

MOTHER: Sheila, we can't possibly do that. Your dad can't take a leave from work, and you know I'm starting up a new job. We have lives, too! You can't just expect us to drop everything and come out and rescue you! You're a twenty-three-year-old woman now. You are an adult, and you are in charge of your choices. You have total autonomy here. We're not in charge of your choices

SHEILA: Um, OK.

MOTHER: We have made sacrifices for you for years, Sheila, and it's time we take care of ourselves and the rest of the family. We can't always just think about "What's best for Sheila?" and put everyone else last.

SHEILA: [*Pause.*] OK. So what should I do?

MOTHER: That's just it, Sheila. These are your choices, and you need to make them. You need to be responsible for yourself. You need to be in charge of your own recovery

SHEILA: Well, I think I need to increase my days at the clinic.

MOTHER: We are just not going to support that when we think it's a dead end.

SHEILA: So what am I supposed to do, then?

MOTHER: It's not my job to figure that out for you, Sheila.

We can see the dilemma Sheila is put in. She is told repeatedly that it is up to her to "take charge of her recovery," but every time she tries to do that, to assert what she needs, she is shot down and told, effectively, that she is expecting too much of others. She is depleted in that she is clearly ill and needs help and support, but in trying to address those needs she is constituted as depleting those around her. These are the kinds of double binds that suffuse not only the families of people with eating disorders but also the structures and practices of treatment itself.

At the same time, I want to be careful not to demonize Sheila's mother. She is clearly frustrated in this conversation. And while she may come across somewhat harshly, we have to remember that she and her husband had spent the past nine years of their lives and many, many tens of thousands of dollars trying to help Sheila, only to watch her relapse again and again and again. It is understandable that she would be skeptical of Sheila's motivation to get well and would want assurances and even evidence that "things will be different this time" before agreeing to commit additional time and resources to Sheila's care.

If we can understand this perspective from a parent, certainly we could understand that an insurance company would take a similar position. My point is that Sheila's double bind is emblematic of the kinds of struggles around choice, agency, and responsibility that characterize this part of treatment. And, like with Sheila's mother, the insistence on personal and individual autonomy and "choice" creates a situation where clients are caught within webs of expectations from which it is almost impossible to disentangle.

A discussion about Jenna, a nineteen-year-old woman diagnosed with anorexia, at a treatment team meeting reveals both the double binds within relationships that ensnare clients and the ways these kinds of double binds can be recapitulated clinically. Jenna had complained to her therapist, Susan, that her mother was not reminding her to eat her snacks when she was home on pass. As a result, Jenna admitted, she regularly threw out half of her snack. Her mother was not reminding her to eat her desserts either, so she was skipping them. Here's how the team conversation went:

SUSAN: I told her [Jenna] that she's nineteen and she's responsible for making sure she's doing what she's supposed to.

NADIA [JENNA'S DIETICIAN]: Yes, but she also needs that support and oversight right now. Mom said she would provide that.

SUSAN: The thing is, Mom is lying to me. She says, "Sure, Jenna is eating her snacks and desserts." I also think Jenna may be manipulating because she wants to go live with her father.

DR. CASEY: OK. Is Mom still having her boyfriend spend the night every night?

SUSAN: Yeah. It's the same guy she had the affair with.

DR. CASEY: You need to confront her about this. Tell her we want her to do a two-week trial of focusing solely on Jenna.

NADIA: I don't have the confidence that she'll do that. She'll probably lie, whereas Jenna will say he's spending the night. So how will we know what's happening?

SUSAN: Yeah, Jenna says to me, "Why didn't she just give me dessert?"

NADIA: OK, but she needs to take responsibility.

SUSAN: I told her that. She said, "But I'm the one who's sick with an eating disorder. Why doesn't she [Mom] pay attention to it?"

NADIA: Mom and Dad both think she's purging. She denies it.

DR. CASEY: Her labs don't indicate purging.

SUSAN: Should we take her off bathroom monitoring?

DR. CASEY: We can try and then wait to see what the labs say next week. There's lots of lying going on.

SUSAN: This sounds awful, but she's actually kind of a brat. She kicks her mom when she gets angry.

DR. CASEY: Yeah, I think it's a family issue. Mom also hates being alone. They really need family therapy.

There are a lot of things are going on here. Clearly, the clinical team doesn't trust Jenna. Nor do they trust her mother. Despite some harsh language, though, the tone of this meeting was not one of anger or frustration—these are the kinds of cases and situations these clinicians deal with all the time. Their intent, rather, was to figure out how to help Jenna get well within a family context that was at best unsupportive and at worst actively harmful. The team vacillates between placing responsibility on Jenna's mother (to not have her boyfriend spend the night, to focus on Jenna for two weeks) and placing it on Jenna, even though (as Jenna herself notes) she's the one who is sick and needs the additional support. Although Jenna's parents think she's purging, the team relies on her labs to render the "truth" about this and, despite the parents' suspicions, decide to take her off bathroom monitoring. The decision to "wait to see what her labs say next week" suggests that the medical tests will give the treatment team the knowledge they need to cut through all the lying and determine what is really going on.

The double binds here are subtle but profound. Jenna is constituted both as a child who needs care and as an adult who should be responsible for herself; both as a patient who needs extra support and as a liar who games the system; both as vulnerable and deserving of attention and as malignant (she manipulates, she kicks her mother, she's a "brat"). Importantly, however, the team does not blame Jenna for the entirety of the dysfunctional system—they clearly see Jenna's mother as a key part of the problem. Yet they seem to place the responsibility for rehabilitating the family system primarily on Jenna. Although they do want Jenna's mother to change her behavior for two weeks, recovery is ultimately seen to be up to Jenna, regardless of what her mother is doing or not doing.

· · ·

These processes during the early stages of treatment—destabilizing old patterns, reawakening feelings, withstanding the weight of scrutiny, and loosening the ties that bind—unfold in overlapping and complex ways. To look at them a bit more organically, I turn now to the case of Carly, which is illustrative of these dynamics and the kinds of challenges they produce for clients and clinicians alike.

CARLY

Carly was nineteen years old the summer I met her. At five-foot-two, she was petite, and she had long, dark brown hair, bright blue eyes, and a pronounced Southern accent. She had come to Cedar Grove from a small Southern town, where she had moved back home to live with her mother and maternal grandparents after having dropped out of college because of her illness. Carly became a therapy client of mine, and as we worked together over the next year and a half, I watched her variously struggle, improve, relapse, and try again.

Carly traced the origins of her eating disorder to conflicts with girlfriends during her senior year in high school. She had been friends with the same circle of girls since preschool, but she said that when she began earning awards and scholarships and serving as student council president, they had "turned against her" and wanted to "bring her down." As is common in relationships between American adolescent girls, this tectonic shift in allegiances was veiled by a veneer of civility and niceness that added layers of complexity to every interaction. In keeping up the appearance of friendship, Carly ate lunch with this group of girls every day and endured (as she represented it) a mounting litany of subtle barbs, backhanded compliments, and jokes at her expense. She began to find it physically hard to eat. "I would just sit there with my lunch, and I would stare at it," she told me. "I had this horrible gnawing feeling in my stomach, like an animal was eating me from the inside. It was awful. And I just couldn't eat. I literally couldn't." Carly began to lose weight. She dropped about fifteen pounds in two months, which was especially dramatic on her petite frame. But she loved the way this changed her body and began to consciously restrict her intake to lose more weight. Teachers, coaches, and parents of friends began to express concern. Carly's mother took her to see a gastroenterologist. They couldn't find anything wrong with her.

The following fall, significantly underweight, Carly went off to college at a large Southern state school. She participated in sorority rush and was invited to join the most prestigious sorority on campus. She relished the sorority girl persona, and even while in residential treatment at Cedar Grove, she continued to wear t-shirts, shorts, and flip-flops sporting her sorority letters and would doodle her sorority insignia during group therapy sessions.

At college, Carly's weight kept dropping, and her energy and motivation plummeted. She started having trouble getting to classes. She barely finished the fall semester before dropping out of school and moving back home. She continued to lose weight. Five pounds more. Seven pounds more. Ten pounds more. By the spring, Carly's mother had taken her to every doctor and every specialist within a two hundred mile radius. Doctors began using words like "anorexia" and "psychosomatic." Finally, Carly's mother became alarmed enough to seek out eating disorders treatment. "Nothing else had worked," she told me, "and I was just at the end of my rope. I hoped that maybe y'all could fix her." By the time she arrived at Cedar Grove, Carly weighed just sixty-four pounds and easily met the criteria for anorexia nervosa.

Carly's treatment was complicated in unexpected ways. Carly and her mother engaged in something like a shared hypochondriasis or an attenuated form of Munchausen syndrome. Beginning when Carly was a baby, and continuing through the time I met her, her mom took her to doctors and specialists regularly—sometimes as often as four or five times per week—for a variety of concerns, including muscle pain, constipation, headaches, and vague malaise. Although there was never any indication that Carly or her mother induced these medical conditions (as is the case in Munchausen's and Munchausen's by proxy), Carly had undergone dozens of tests, examinations, and procedures in her lifetime without anything serious ever turning up. By the time she arrived at Cedar Grove, Carly had become proficient at medicalizing any sort of distress and reported feeling comforted and cared for in hospital and clinic settings. Her engagement with treatment, therefore, was multilayered.

It is not uncommon for people with eating disorders to have a great deal of bodily discomfort related to eating and digesting food. As noted in chapter 5, slow gastric emptying and other such difficulties can cause significant pain. This was true for Carly as well. "My stomach just hurts all the time," she told me about a week into her treatment. "I mean *really* hurts. I'm trying to eat my full meal plan, but I tell you, I don't see how it's therapeutic to keep shoving food down my throat when I'm literally stuffed to the gills and in pain. It's not making me feel any better about eating outside of here, I can tell you that." At this point in her treatment, Carly still insisted that her massive weight loss was not due to any intention on her part or a desire to be thin but was purely the result of emotional and medical issues that made it difficult to eat. "I have always been small," she said. "I wasn't really trying to lose weight. I just felt that animal gnawing at my stomach because of the social things and stress, and it hurt to eat. I don't even think I have an eating disorder, to be honest."

I want to pause here for just a moment and take a brief detour. In clinical terms, Carly at this point was considered at best to be in denial about her eating disorder and at worst to be purposefully lying and manipulating by saying she didn't even have an eating disorder and wasn't trying to lose weight. I am ambivalent about this issue. Carly did eventually (many months later, and after being subsequently discharged from and readmitted to the clinic) acknowledge that she had an eating disorder and that she had indeed been intentionally trying to lose weight both prior to her first admission to Cedar Grove and after her various discharges. But what does this really tell us? Does this mean that Carly was in denial or lying early on, that she had really had an eating disorder centered on thinness and distorted body image all along? That she was (intentionally or not) "somatizing" her eating disorder in the early stages as a strategy of denial, manipulation, or both? Or is it possible, instead, that she learned to "psychologize" her distress in the process of treatment so that it came to look more like something the clinicians and managed care companies could understand? And what difference does it make knowing which of these was true? It actually makes a great deal of difference because these two accounts position Carly very differently as a subject who is variously deserving or not deserving of care. I will revisit this in more detail later.

Let's return to the issues that complicated Carly's treatment. In addition to having difficulties with food and eating, Carly was palpably enmeshed with her mother, even more so than is thought to be common among eating disorder clients.[9] Most notably, they both used the plural *we* when referring to themselves, even when alone. For example, Carly might say something like, "We think I should make an appointment with Dr. Davis for tomorrow," meaning that her mother wanted to see the doctor; and her mother might say something like, "We had a hard time sleeping last night," meaning that Carly had had a rough night. Carly had great difficulty thinking or acting outside of reference to her mother.

Through intensive therapy, Carly was gradually able to understand that her anorexia was, at least in part, keeping her dependent on her mother by taking adulthood off the table. Interestingly, though, Carly did not simply want to remain a child—she was very bright and had clear ambitions for her education and career. She tried to resolve this dilemma, she discovered, through a fairly ingenious process of essentially becoming geriatric at age nineteen. Due to her anorexia, she had full osteoporosis. She had digestive problems that required daily medications. She had difficulties with her joints. Her hair was falling out. In short, she had the body of a seventy-year-old woman. Carly was not using her illness to stop developing all together, she just wanted to leapfrog over the adult stage, which, based on what she saw with her mother, entailed endless caretaking and self-sacrifice in the service of others.

Carly was torn in terms of self-actualization. On the one hand, being different from others was dangerous; it brought rejection from her peers and threatened her intimacy with her mother. On the other hand, being "special," at least in terms of being sick, kept others close to her and concerned for her well-being. The question of how to forge an independent identity outside of the sick role, however, completely confounded Carly.

If we look at Carly's case, we can see how the markers of an eating disorder that are scrutinized by most managed mental health plans (including Carly's)—things like labs and vitals, weight gain, compliance with treatment, and discharge planning—would give a very limited picture of her situation. As it turned out, despite being on a very high-calorie meal plan (over four thousand calories per day), Carly gained weight extremely slowly, putting on only one half or one pound per week rather than the two to three pounds required by her insurance. Her blood work and vitals were fairly stable, which was actually a bad thing in terms of treatment because it meant that her insurance would be more likely to discharge her sooner. Carly appeared very engaged in treatment and discharge planning, although she rarely followed through on her commitments outside of the clinic context. In other words, from the point of view of her insurance company, Carly was "failing" treatment.

But her treatment team—which consisted of myself (as therapist), a psychiatrist, an adolescent medicine specialist, and a dietician, with input from nursing and direct care staff—saw real recovery for Carly as entailing more than just weight gain and compliance. For us, it also involved a process of identity clarification. We followed her weight, vitals, and labs closely but were also attuned to the subtle changes we saw occurring in Carly's relationship with her mother. Was Carly able to state her needs directly to her mother in family therapy sessions? Would Carly allow herself to become frustrated with her mother? Was her mother getting better at setting clear limits and upholding them? How well did Carly manage her anxiety while her mother was away? We viewed changes in these areas, no matter how small, as Carly's attempts to launch—to separate from her natal family and begin to build her own life. They had been aborted attempts to date, but they were seen as attempts at healthy behaviors nonetheless.

BLACK FINGERNAIL POLISH

Then, one day, something happened. In therapy, Carly had been working on recognizing how narrow a scope of experience she allowed herself and how she tried to contort herself in infinite ways to fit others' expectations of her: sorority girl, dutiful daughter, good Christian, Southern belle. Carly had absolutely no idea what she really wanted for herself, but she knew how to follow the rules of these roles so that she could feel safe.

Imagine my surprise, then, when Carly—sorority girl, pastel-wearing, ribbon-tied-around-her-ponytail Carly—came into session one day sporting *black fingernail polish*. I noticed it right away but didn't remark on it. She brought it up. "Rebecca, I don't know what got into me!" she said with her eyes wide, holding out her hands for me to see:

> I stopped at Walgreens yesterday [on pass], and all I could think about was black fingernail polish! Oh my gosh! I walked up and down that aisle like five times, trying to decide if I should buy it. I even made myself go over to the other side of the store and pick up the other things I needed. I planned to head straight for the check out, but before I knew it, there I was again! Back

in front of that nail polish! So I grabbed one and quickly paid for it. When I got back, I set it on the bedside table and just stared at it for about an hour. Should I? Shouldn't I? Finally, I decided to just do it. It felt so good! I really like it! When I talked to my mom on the phone that night I told her about it, and she *freaked!* "Carly!" she said. "What's gotten into you?!?" "I don't know, Mom!" I told her, but I said I liked it and was leaving it on. I'll probably have to take it off before she comes back here next week. But oh well. I can enjoy it until then!

I observed to Carly that it was great that she was exploring new ways of expressing herself. "Well," she said with a hint of a smile. "Not *completely* new. I *did* get the kind with sparkles in it."

This seemingly minor incident was the single most encouraging thing I had seen from Carly in the time I had known her. This was a young woman who, just months earlier, could not even conceive of a life or a worldview outside of the one she and her mother had crafted. She was so welded to the Southern sorority girl identity that she would not even let herself test other waters. Yet here she was, wearing black fingernail polish and enjoying it. To me, and to the other clinicians at Cedar Grove, this indicated that something, indeed, was shifting for Carly and that she was taking small steps toward discovering her own sense of self.

This is not, however, the kind of information insurance companies tend to find particularly relevant. "It's not enough," the insurance case manager told me when I tried to advocate for further coverage by sharing the black fingernail polish story. "It doesn't mean anything if she's not gaining weight." Overall, the insurance company felt Carly was not using treatment effectively, and it denied further coverage.

In my experience, these kinds of things happen regularly with clients in treatment. Clients make apparently small changes—like being more engaged in group therapy sessions, socializing with the other clients, asking staff for something they need when before they would have just gone without it—that suggest deeper shifts. Yet there is no way to effectively translate these kinds of everyday victories into the language the insurance companies find relevant. Although insurance case managers might be personally heartened by such things, their decisions are ultimately constrained by numbers, diagnostic codes, and quantitative thresholds. How does one code for black fingernail polish?

Carly's case demonstrates how the early phases of treatment set the tone for a client's "addiction trajectory."[10] When she entered the clinic, Carly had to become habituated to eating "normal" amounts of food at regular intervals and to working, playing, sleeping, and engaging according to the clinic's schedule. These changes (especially regarding food) brought up overwhelming anxiety for her, which she had to learn how to navigate without resorting to restricting or overexercising. Carly was quite invested in the notion that biomedicine had answers to which she was not privy, so relinquishing control and claims to knowledge to the treatment team and to medical tests was familiar and comfortable for her, though she definitely did not like certain forms of knowledge (like weight) being withheld from her. The most challenging part of treatment for her was beginning to separate from her mother and forging a sense of herself outside of her family nexus. But she made tentative steps in this direction. Unfortunately, it was not enough. From the perspective of the insurance company, she was getting worse, not better.

As we can see in Carly's case, what counts as the object of concern and the target of intervention is not a stable entity, and it is constituted differently in different contexts and through different relationships. Significantly, strategies of care must be nimble enough for clinicians to be able to accommodate these shifting iterations of the "problem" as well as to preserve their own sense of doing ethical work in the face of challenging conditions. This is all good and well, but clients are not afforded the same luxury. They are the ones who ultimately pay the price of a broken system.

REFLECTIONS

The initial part of treatment is focused on unmooring the client from external behavioral and affective routines, habituating her to new rhythms of engagement, and establishing new regimes of dependence and independence, while also inverting her claims to expertise about her own experience. In the following phase of treatment, clients begin to turn these processes inward. At this point, however, the focus is on setting the stage for this internal shift. To do this, clients must come to experience themselves, their bodies, and their relationships in new ways.

Importantly, as we've seen, during this stage clients learn to draw connections between their disordered eating behaviors, affective attachments, and modes of relating to others. For example, as clients are learning to renegotiate boundaries with others (where one ends and the other begins), they are also learning to recognize their own affective and sensational boundaries of hunger and fullness. In other words, the work clients are doing emotionally and in terms of interpersonal relationships mirrors what they are learning to do with food and eating, and vice versa. This is in keeping with the clinic's understanding that food behaviors associated with eating disorders parallel relational and attachment strategies. Because of this, the setting of healthy boundaries and limits for clients in the clinic (being told how much they will eat and when, having specific times designated for activity and rest, enforcing rules regarding program times and client responsibilities) is seen to be crucial in modeling for clients healthy experiences of need and satisfaction and showing that neither need be scary or overwhelming, that these feelings are part of the everyday flow of life, and that clients themselves have the resources necessary to get their needs adequately met without depending on others to do so for them.

Critically, however, such work proceeds within the broader context of American managed care, which operates with a very different set of logics. In treatment, clients learn to moderate "need" and "satisfaction," striving toward balance. But the managed care system operates through extremes— one must be radically medically unstable to obtain treatment, and as soon as medical stability is achieved, treatment is withdrawn. In other words, treatment encourages clients to modulate and fine-tune their needs, akin to using a dimmer switch on a light, but the managed care framework operates with a binary on-off logics.

Importantly, we can see how the issue of *control* plays a central role here, becoming a site of significant friction and disconnect. As we saw in chapter 6, both the medical model and the recovery model identify the client's *desire to control*—to control her food intake, her affects, her relationships, her body shape and size, the ways others perceive her—as emblematic of eating disorder pathology at its most fundamental level, and as a key target of intervention. I want to elaborate on this here. Both models endorse the perspective that what clients think of as control is, in fact, indicative of a life lived *out of* control. But it is here that they diverge. The message of the recovery model is that attempts to control are *themselves,* by nature, unhealthy, and that recovery depends on learning how to *let go* of the desire for control. The medical model, however, takes a different stance. It maintains that attempts to control are not problematic in and of themselves and that control is, in fact, a *good* thing; it is simply that, in an eating disorder, such efforts at control have become misdirected. That is, "good" control is oriented toward "health" and is bolstered by the expertise and oversight of experts, and clients should be encouraged toward this sort of orientation. In other words, in the recovery model, health is accomplished by *letting go* of the need to control oneself, whereas in the medical model, it is accomplished by *intensifying* control and controlling oneself more effectively. I will return to this issue again in the following chapters.

In the clinic, under the pressures of managed care and against this backdrop where control is considered both healthy and pathological, clients have to learn to develop and remake attachments and affects within a logics of excess and deprivation. This attachment work is predicated on the notion that the client *is responsible for herself* while at the same time *is alienated from her self and cloaked from authentic subjectivity by layers of denial and not knowing*. These dual imperatives—to know the self and simultaneously recognize the impossibility of that knowledge—characterize this phase of treatment and put clients in a series of double binds within which they remain suspended. The "good" client is one who does not know her own motivations or intentions (which makes her "ripe" for therapeutic engagement), yet she must not be in denial (which makes therapy and other interventions difficult). These politics and logics of not knowing produce knots for clients that they cannot easily escape. In the next chapter, we turn to how these knots affect internal processes of regulation and reshaping.

Mortifications

JANUARY 1981

My friend Katie came to see me in the hospital today. I'm in the adult psych unit because there's no child or adolescent unit within two hundred miles of where I live, so my parents chose to put me here rather than send me away.

When Katie walks up to the door, I can tell she is scared to be here. I don't blame her. I'm scared here every day, though I'm mostly used to it now, I guess. The nurses let me leave the unit to talk with her so she doesn't have to come in. "It's not really an appropriate place for a child," they say. Ha, I think. That's funny.

I know it's mortifying for my dad that I'm here. Some of the nurses are his patients, but there's nothing I can do about that.

I won't sit down. Not unless I absolutely have to for some reason. I read somewhere that standing burns more calories than sitting. So I stand all the time. It makes people uncomfortable, especially during meals. I don't know why they care so much, and I'm not doing it to bother anyone. Sitting feels lazy and wasteful, and I just can't do it. Even when my hips and back start to throb.

The Jesus lady came again today. She says I'm sick because we're Jewish, and if I accept Jesus as my personal lord and savior I'll get better. If only it were that simple.

My hands are raw. I wash them every half hour to make sure there are no calories on them. I'll do an extra hundred jumping jacks in the mornings, just in case.

EIGHT

Me, Myself, and Ed

RECALIBRATING

By the end of the first few weeks of treatment, a client should, in theory, be able to follow the basic rules of the program and be inching toward a proactive engagement in the therapeutics of Cedar Grove. She is expected not only to attend groups and accept medical interventions but also to demonstrate a consistent ability to follow guidelines without constant encouragement and surveillance. The emphasis, then, moves from containment—the focus of the early part of treatment—to *cultivating a desire to meet the expectations of the clinic.* At the same time, the client is afforded additional strategies for individuation and is encouraged to further evaluate and renegotiate her interpersonal relationships.[1] The double movement of pressures toward both compliance and independence primes the client for the next phase in the process: an engagement with *agency,* or the capacity to act and make choices independent of their eating disorders.

While the early part of treatment is concerned with helping the client disrupt old behavior patterns, affective strategies, ways of inhabiting the body, and relationships of dependency, the next set of tasks is focused on *recalibrating the experience of the self.* This is a radical process that leads to a jarring experience of suspension and dislocation. It is also at this juncture that insurance approval for treatment is most likely to be withdrawn.

WHO AM I (NOT), ANYWAY?

Nobody's listening to me. They say it's my eating disorder talking. It feels like every time I try to claim my voice and make my own decisions, people just kind of shoot me down or doubt me or tell me that I'm malnourished. And I know I'm malnourished. But I'm still a person, and these are still my feelings.

— JULIE,
a twenty-four-year-old woman diagnosed with bulimia

Once a client has become habituated to new regimes of behavior, affective practice, and surveillance and has begun to renegotiate her boundaries and relationships with others, she learns to turn this process inward.

The clinic, drawing on an American therapeutic modality called Internal Family Systems Therapy (IFS), various recovery traditions (e.g., Alcoholics Anonymous), and the perspective articulated in the book *Life Without Ed*,[2] encourages clients to come to think of their eating disorders as separate from their real selves, as a sort of subpersonality that coexists with other parts of who they are but has taken over the internal "self-system." This phase of treatment (lasting from approximately weeks two through eight) involves progressively separating out the eating disorder from the rest of a client's sense of self and reconfiguring the client's agency—or capacity to act—vis-à-vis her illness. I will spend a good deal of time describing this dimension of treatment, as it is in many ways the crux of the treatment process.

I want to be clear, at the outset, that while I spotlight IFS here, it is only one of many therapeutic modalities used at Cedar Grove. The clinic is by no means IFS-centric, although many of the basic principles of IFS infuse the program, even if the full therapeutic techniques are rarely used. Nevertheless, I have chosen to focus on IFS in this chapter about recalibration for four reasons: (1) IFS crystalizes and operationalizes two core propositions of the Cedar Grove program—namely, (a) clients are *not* their eating disorders and (b) separating out the client from her eating disorder and helping her forge a new relationship with it is a key to recovery. (2) IFS foregrounds the belief that an eating disorder performs a necessary function for the sufferer and will not fully remit until and unless the individual has other ways of getting those needs met, and this is central to the clinic's philosophy. (3) IFS gives us a language for describing certain micropractices involved in this recalibration that are central to the Cedar Grove program more broadly and are common to other modalities as well, albeit in less explicit ways; these micropractices help clients cultivate what I call a "dialogic interiority." And (4) IFS, in proposing an alternative model of how our internal lives function and should ideally be organized, opens up a place for productive discussions about how psychotherapies intersect with political and economic systems. Accordingly, while IFS is not the only modality used at Cedar Grove, it is a useful site for exploring the clinic's understanding of how people change as well as the practical constraints that shape these processes.

I am intimately acquainted with IFS therapy. In 2011–12, after learning about IFS at Cedar Grove, I attended a Level 1 training program in IFS, a ten-month professional course for licensed clinicians wishing to become IFS therapists. Additional levels of training are needed to become fully certified in the model and be able to train others (see chapter 11 for more on these kinds of certification programs for therapists), but Level 1 training is sufficient to present oneself as an IFS therapist. The training was multidimensional and included didactics, engaged learning activities, supervised role-playing (as both client and therapist), group work, and individual consultation with trainers. Several of the training sessions were led by Richard Schwartz, the model's creator.

IFS: MULTIPLE SELVES, SYSTEMS THEORIES, AND THE SOCIETY OF THE MIND

Internal family systems theory, developed in the 1980s by marriage and family therapist Dr. Richard Schwartz, explodes the conventional Western understanding of the self by viewing the mind not as a singular entity but as a system of different subpersonalities, each with its own history, emotions, cognitions, and ways of interacting with the world. IFS calls these subpersonalities *parts,* "inner people of different ages, temperaments, talents, and desires, who together form an internal family or tribe" that organizes itself in the same ways other human systems do and "reflects the organization of the systems around them."[3] IFS holds that we each have an indeterminable number of these parts, which have developed out of our idiosyncratic life experiences to help us adjust to and cope with different circumstances and events, and which remain in our self-systems as functional clusters of thoughts, behaviors, affects, and abilities. Each person's specific parts are different, entirely unique to them and their experiences. The self, according to IFS, is not singular but multiple.

This view of multiplicity, Schwartz says, "transports us from the conception of the human mind as a single unit to seeing it as a system of interacting minds."[4] Once we make this shift, he argues, "the mind ... becomes just a human system at one level, embedded within the human systems at many other levels. It can be understood with the same systemic principles and changed with the same systemic techniques."[5] The task then becomes how to understand this inner society of mind as such a human system.

Here, Schwartz (who initially trained as a marriage and family therapist) turns to the insights of family systems theory to understand the internal workings of experience. Family systems theory, broadly described, holds that families are constituted by differently positioned actors who work together in mechanical solidarity, with the system as a whole continuously striving toward balance or homeostasis. In response to internal or external pressures, members within a family assume different roles or functions. When polarized (the family "hero" versus the family "scapegoat," for example), members of the family system maintain their roles to avoid system fragmentation. But if one family member moves out of his or her role (through recovery, for example), the system's balance is disrupted. This exerts pressure on others in the system to modify their own roles to regain homeostasis, or to persuade the errant family member to resume her previous position. For the system to remain intact, parts of the system must continuously (re)calibrate to the other parts of the system to ensure that balance is maintained.[6]

Building on family systems perspectives, Schwartz argues that the mind is like an internal family, composed of multiple parts that play different roles, continually responding to one another and to the outside environment and seeking homeostasis. To keep the system functioning, these parts configure themselves in continually shifting patterns of collaboration, competition, strategic alliance, polarization, and coalitions as the person navigates his or her daily life. Just like in a family, the parts can collude with one another or be diametrically opposed. They can triangulate. They can be deeply hidden or easily activated. A person's parts are in constant dialogue with one another as well as with other people's parts, extending the possible network of the self-system beyond the boundaries of the individual body. The self, then, according to IFS, is always relational and social, even its most interior.[7]

IFS identifies three main components of the self-system: Managers, Exiles, and Firefighters. Managers are the parts that help us handle the frustrations and difficulties of daily life by maintaining control over inner and outer environments. They do this by making sure we don't get too close to people if we fear becoming too dependent, for example, or by rationalizing away our anger in circumstances where we fear it would be inappropriate. Exiles are the parts that develop if we have been repeatedly hurt, humiliated, frightened, or shamed. Managers work to keep these scared, vulnerable parts sequestered away, out of everyday awareness. But when an Exile becomes too upset and floods us with emotion or puts us at risk of being hurt again, the third category of parts is mobilized: Firefighters. Firefighters come in and douse the flames of overwhelm, shame, or vulnerability brought by the exposed Exile. They do this in extreme ways, generally by pushing for stimulation or dissociation that will override the Exile's feelings. Bingeing and purging, restricting, drug use, cutting, and overwork are examples of common Firefighter activities.

IFS acknowledges that most people do not experience themselves as systems of moving parts but instead (at least in the postindustrial West) as mostly integrated, most of the time. This sense of integration—what is often called "the self"—is an illusion, according to IFS. It is a functional fantasy. It enables us to move through the world with some degree of coherence and organization, but it belies the fact that agency, moral responsibility, and interpersonal positioning are continuously shifting among our inner parts rather than resting in any one place.

MY PARTS MADE ME DO IT: LOCATING AGENCY AND MORAL RESPONSIBILITY

If IFS understands the self to be a system of multiple, relatively differentiated parts, where does the model locate agency, or moral responsibility for one's actions? If "the self" is a distributed network, who's in charge?

These questions resonate with philosopher Harry Frankfurt's discussion of the "willing addict" and philosopher Marina Oshana's distinctions between procedural and epistemic authenticity.[8] I will go into some degree of detail here, as the nuances of these concepts are critical for understanding the IFS model and its function in the clinic. Although some of the terminology is opaque, the ideas are actually quite straightforward, and I will unpack them as we go.

Regarding the basic proposition of human agency—for example, A wants to do X—Frankfurt argues that there are a number of possible conditions that are obscured unless this assertion is further unpacked. He teases out what he calls first-order desires and second-order desires. An example of a first-order desire is "I want to go for a run." In this scenario, if I go for a run it is because my desire to run motivated me to do so. A second-order desire would be wanting a first-order desire be our will. For example, an affirmative second-order desire would be "I *want to* want to go for a run." Second-order desires do not presume any particular first-order desire orientation, nor do they presume that the second-order desire will motivate any particular action. If I want to want to go for a run (second-order) *and* actually desire to do so (first-order), my going for a run reflects an agreement of both levels. But first- and second-order desires can also be in conflict. If I want to want to go for a run but actually hate running and want to take a nap, the act of running *is not the same action* as running because I actually desire it and embrace that desire. What Frankfurt is emphasizing is that simply observing someone doing an action doesn't tell us anything about whether or not they wanted to do it, and that two people doing the same *action* may actually be exhibiting very different *behavior*.

Frankfurt's approach to agency is similar in some ways to Oshana's discussions of procedural and epistemic authenticity, introduced in chapter 6.[9] In Oshana's framework, we will recall, procedural authenticity refers to an assumed synergy of action and intention, so that a person performing a certain action is presumed to be demonstrating a desire to engage in that action (which Frankfurt says is a mistake). Epistemic authenticity, by contrast, holds that an action is only "authentic" inasmuch as it actually reflects a person's subjective intention or desire.

For example, consider the following scenario: Julia, in treatment for anorexia, begins to eat all of her meals without protest and is advancing toward her weight goals. From a perspective of procedural authenticity, Julia is performing the acts of recovery and is therefore authentically progressing in her treatment. But let us add this additional information: Julia and Colleen, another patient diagnosed with anorexia, have made a pact to get out of treatment as quickly as possible, move into an apartment together, and jointly resume their eating disorders with a vengeance. How, then, should we understand Julia's apparent "compliance"? Is it still a step toward recovery? This goes to the heart of epistemic authenticity: Is a person engaging in behaviors that signal "authenticity" for the reasons assumed to be conditions for that behavior? In this case, Julia was exhibiting procedural but not epistemic authenticity.

So why does this discussion of desires and authenticity matter? It matters because perceptions of patients' desires and intentions are critically important in decisions about how *deserving* they are of care, made by both clinicians and insurance companies, as well as by families (as we saw in the case of Sheila in chapter 7). It is a client's *desires* that make her a "good" (or "bad") patient according to managed care algorithms. But how do clinicians and insurance companies actually know what these desires are, especially when clients are constituted as always already manipulative, deceitful, and resistant?

To "get around the patient," such decisions in eating disorders treatment generally rest on first-order (procedural) evidence (e.g., weight, lab results, number of calories consumed), and then infer from this a client's second-order (epistemic) intentions (as we saw with Carly and Caleigh). But, as both Oshana and Frankfurt emphasize, this is a highly risky and flawed way of doing things. And in the case of eating disorders, it can be deadly. Care is rendered at the level of procedural authenticity (healthy is as healthy does), while *deservingness* for care is assessed at the level of epistemic authenticity (healthy is as healthy intends), and there is no agreed-on mechanism, philosophy, or structure for translating between the two. This requires clinicians to generate ad hoc philosophies of intention and action and to convince insurance companies of them on a case-by-case basis. Quite a hefty job.

With Oshana's views on authenticity in mind, we can now take up another concept from Frankfurt's work—his distinction between what he calls the "willing" and "unwilling" addict. In Frankfurt's terms, both willing and unwilling addicts have a first-order desire to use a drug, say heroin. The willing addict, Frankfurt says, knows she wants to use heroin, and she *wants* to want to use it—that is, she embraces her desire for the drug. The unwilling addict wants to use heroin but does *not* want to want to use it. She feels compelled to use heroin due to whatever physiological, psychological, or social reasons fuel her addiction, but she does *not want* to have this desire. She wants to be free of it. We have, then, two people engaging in the same behavior (using heroin) but with two very different orientations to that behavior.

In terms of eating disorders, Frankfurt would make a clear distinction between a person who restricts (or binges and/or purges), and *wants to* want to do so (in the clinic, they would say this person is "in" her eating disorder) and one who engages in these behaviors but *does not* want to want to do so (in clinic terms, this person would be "struggling" or "in recovery"). And Oshana would make a clear distinction between a person who is enacting recovery behaviors in a performative way but is not necessarily invested in them (procedural authenticity) and a person whose health-oriented behaviors are consistent with an actual personal investment in recovery (epistemic authenticity). Both Frankfurt and Oshana, therefore, caution us to be wary of attributions of moral responsibility based on exhibited behavior and call, instead, for a focus on *how someone experiences herself in relation to* that behavior.

Why does this matter? This more nuanced understanding of intention, behavior, and moral responsibility is critical when thinking about behaviors associated with psychiatric conditions, such as eating disorders. But the situation is even more complex than what Frankfurt and Oshana suggest. Both models assume a subject whose relationship to her behavior is relatively consistent. According to them, if I do not want my eating disorder now, I won't want it an hour from now. And if I eat my 10:00 a.m. snack because I am authentically invested in recovery, then eating my lunch indicates a similar investment. But intentions and orientations to behavior are not always consistent, particularly for someone recovering from an eating disorder. First- and second-order desires can align, diverge, and realign multiple times per day (or even per hour) as the person struggles through complex issues of being-in-the-world.

It is here that IFS can be helpful. Clinicians working in the field of eating disorders must be agile enough to continuously reassess and respond to these fluctuating orientations. At Cedar Grove, this happens in the stream of everyday life in the clinic and is often implicit and emergent within dense thickets of interpersonal and social interactions and assumptions. Yet the stakes are very high: how clinicians understand and represent a patient's motivations is critical, because it often directly affects whether or not she will get continued care. Clients, too, must learn how to understand and manage these fluctuations as they move toward recovery.

IFS offers both clinicians and clients a shorthand for thinking about and representing complex issues of agency within the flattened agentic space of the managed care system. It provides a way of talking about shifting relationships between desires and actions while also rendering these dynamics intelligible within the priorities of managed care. It does so by introducing what we might call a third-order desire, a desire that seeps in around experiences of wanting, and wanting (or not wanting) to want, motivating them with its own intentionality.[10] And in IFS, this third-order desire is believed to be always already oriented toward optimizing health and minimizing harm.

THIRD-ORDER DESIRES: SELF VERSUS SELF

Instead of having "a self," IFS says, we have "Self" (capitalized, and without the definite article), which is quite different from standard Western understandings of the term. Rather than standing as the core of one's unique individual identity, Self in IFS is characterized precisely by a loss of boundaries and self-identification. Self in this view is actually more akin to the Buddhist concept of *anatta,* or "nonself." It is a state of mindful compassion; it is the place through which we experience our connectedness with others and with the universe. Schwartz describes Self as "both an individual and a state of consciousness, in the same way that quantum physics has demonstrated that light is both a particle and a wave. . . . It is the same Self, but in different states."[11] When in the wave state, Schwartz says, "our waves can overlap with other people's waves creating a sense of ultimate commonality and compassion."[12] In IFS training, we were told that we would know if we were "in Self" because it would feel like the experience of flow described by Mihaly Csikszentmihalyi.[13]

As desirable as it is to "be in Self" or "act from Self," the goal of IFS therapy is to *not* subsume all of the parts into Self or always be "in Self" rather than "in parts." This is thought to be impossible and also psychologically and socially crippling; we need our parts to function in the world because they help us adjust and adapt to changing circumstances.

What distinguishes a healthy self-system from a less healthy one, according to IFS, is not getting rid of one's parts and only having Self but becoming what is called "Self-led." "Self-leadership" means that Self can productively harness the energies of a person's parts and strategically invoke them in everyday life. In this view, Self functions similarly to the conductor of an orchestra, with the parts as the instrumental sections. In any given situation, Self might call on more strings, or more brass, or more drums, depending on what is needed. Or Self might quiet down one section so another can be heard. Self can regulate tempo and tone and make sure that the orchestral performance—the lived experience of the self—is collaborative, intelligible, and effective.

For most of us, IFS says, becoming Self-led requires a lot of time and effort to get our parts to "step back" and let Self be in charge. This is because the ultimate goal of any self-system is to protect Self. In situations of perceived danger, parts "come forward" (that is, they take over, orchestrating thoughts, affects, sensations, and interpersonal patterns) to manage the system, sometimes assuming extreme or overdeveloped roles. Schwartz provides the following analogy:

> It may be useful to compare a person's Self and parts to the functioning of a country. As another country threatens to attack, the president [Self] is moved to a special place of safety (in the United States, he or she is in a jet flying above the fray), civilians [Exiles] are sent to shelters, and the military [Firefighters] takes over. If through the crisis the president stays calm, and provides the strength and comfort that leads to a satisfactory resolution of the crisis, then the trauma may increase the people's trust in their leader. If,

however, the president cannot prevent the devastation of the country, the president loses credibility, and military leaders are likely to remain in power to protect and manage the country.[14]

Inner systems function in a similar way, according to IFS. Depending on the perceived severity of external threats to Self, inner systems will organize so that those parts that can effectively deal with the danger are in charge, and they will remain in these roles as long as the perceived danger exists. This threat response can produce all sorts of conditions that we call psychiatric illnesses, including eating disorders.

As Self is strengthened and resumes its rightful place at the center of one's experience, the client can work on getting the eating disorder to "step back"—to return to its role as a *part* of Self rather than running the show.

With this in mind, we can now return to Cedar Grove to examine how the IFS model informs treatment at the clinic.

MEETING ED AT CEDAR GROVE

I don't know what to say about Ed. I don't even know if there is an "Ed" per se. Ed is me. I can't really distinguish between the two, and it feels weird to talk about it that way.

—BETHANY,
one week into treatment

. . .

Ed wants to kill me.

—BETHANY,
six weeks into treatment

At Cedar Grove, clients learn to identify their eating disorder as one of these parts of self, or rather, as an identifiable subsystem of other parts that hang together in something called an eating disorder. As a way of helping clients conceptualize this subsystem, clinicians personify it and give it a name: Ed (for eating disorder). Ed—gendered male[15]—is himself composed of many parts. These may be self-critical parts, competitive parts, or parts that need approval or acceptance. Ed might have restricting, bingeing, exercising, purging, or self-destructive parts. Ed can work to maintain homeostasis in the system by helping to regulate strong affect, and this is thought to be one of the main reasons Ed is able to take over leadership of a system in crisis.

But Ed increasingly becomes complicit in generating that affective dysregulation as well as alleviating it, thereby gaining more and more power. Clients learn to think of Ed like a partner in an abusive relationship. He is controlling and possessive. He wants to dictate your every action and thought. He feeds you a constant string of lies to keep you dependent on him. He tells you that you are ugly and worthless and that you cannot possibly exist without him, wearing you down so you cling ever more desperately to him. He punishes you if you stray, barraging you with abusive messages about how bad, disgusting, and horrible you are. Above all, Ed is powerful, resilient, and entrenched. And he expects to be obeyed. In return, he promises acceptance, love, and above all, safety.

This framing of Ed as a part (with his own parts) within clients' larger self-systems complicates understandings of agency and moral responsibility for disordered eating behaviors such as bingeing, purging, compulsive exercise, or calorie restriction. Cedar Grove's adaptation of IFS stresses that it is not really the client herself who does these things; it is her eating disorder *part* of her that does them. Ed drives clients to yell or sulk or lie or say they wish they could die. Clients learn that Ed is the one who has causes them to isolate from friends, obsessively calculate calories, and cruise pro-anorexia websites. He's the one who pushes them to obsessively check their bodies in the mirror every morning for any sign of weight gain, to cut up their food into miniscule bites and eat them at precise four-minute intervals, to run for ten miles every morning before hitting the gym for two hours. He is the one who lures them to the scale, sometimes a dozen times a day, for a verdict on their worth. Within treatment, Ed pushes clients to hide food, purge in secret, or do jumping jacks in the bathroom to burn extra calories. Ed makes them mistrust the dietician, keep secrets from their therapists, and feel jealous of the new patient who is so thin and weak she needs a wheelchair. Ed tells them to leave treatment because he misses them and loves them and is waiting for them with open arms.

In recovery, clients are mentored in how to distinguish Ed's desires from their own. They practice convincing him to relinquish power and to step back so Self can assume its role as rightful leader. This cannot be achieved by a coup. Clients learn they must persuade Ed to willingly release his hold on the system. In other words, they have to cultivate a new inner relationship with Ed that reverses the dynamics of power in the system and hopefully leads them toward health.

To illustrate one way clients at Cedar Grove are mentored in how to experience Ed as a separate, yet still internal, locus of agency, I turn now to a group therapy session at Cedar Grove.

SCULPTING ED IN A GROUP THERAPY SESSION

The group session I describe here is typical of many I attended at Cedar Grove over the course of my seven years there. I did not take notes or use a voice recorder during groups but would generally write up my recollections as close to verbatim as possible as soon as I could after the event. In more extended write-ups, like the one presented here, I asked participants to review my rendering of the group and to make any corrections or edits they saw fit to ensure accuracy.

The session I describe here combines a therapeutic technique adapted from family systems therapy known as "sculpting" with the principles of IFS. Sculpting is aimed at helping clients conceptualize their inner and outer systems by enacting them visually. During the exercise, one client asks others in the group to act as stand-ins for various important people (father, mother, siblings, etc.) as well as for key parts (various managers, exiles or firefighters) and emotions such as anger, sadness, or loneliness. The group facilitator assists the client in talking to these different characters and exploring her relationships with them. In this way, clients learn to observe and interact with their internal psychological processes and their various parts as if they were interlocutors who are just as real (and complex) as the actual people in their lives.

On the day of the group in question, Trudy, the group therapist, gathered everyone into a large circle in the center of the room and reviewed the purpose and the structure of the session. She then asked for volunteers for the sculpting activity. After a few moments of awkward silence, Jill, a twenty-one-year-old woman diagnosed with bulimia, raised her hand. "I'll do it," she said, moving forward into the center of the circle. "Great!" said Trudy. "Thank you, Jill. Now, let's have everyone back up, and Jill, let's start identifying your parts."

Picking up a stack of three-by-five-inch cards, a roll of tape, and a black Sharpie marker that she had brought with her, Trudy turned to Jill. "OK. We're going to sculpt your inner system. What we want to do is to get as accurate a representation as possible of what it *feels* like to be you, what your *experience* is. OK? There's no 'right' or 'wrong' here. *You* are going to tell *us* what it should look like. Now, where do you want to start?"

This last question was slightly disingenuous; Trudy had premade a card that said "ED" in bold black marker, and it was right on top of the pile. "I guess I'll start with Ed?" Jill said somewhat tentatively. "OK," said Trudy. "Who would you like to play Ed?" Jill looked around the group, brow furrowed in thought. "Ummm ... I think maybe Molly?" Molly moved into the center of the circle with Jill and Trudy. Trudy taped the card labeled "ED" to Molly's chest.

"OK, Jill," said Trudy, "where do you want to put Ed?" "Where do I *want* to put him?" asked Jill, perplexed. "I mean, where is he right now in your experience," Trudy clarified. "Does it feel like he's right up next to you, or maybe a few steps away? Is he in front of you facing you, or maybe behind you? It's really up to you. Again, there's no right or wrong, it's just how it best represents what it feels like inside."

"He would be right in front of me," said Jill. "Facing me. "OK," said Trudy. "Ed ... and let me pause here to tell the new people that this is not Molly anymore. This is Ed. For the purposes of this group, she is going to be Ed in the way that Jill experiences Ed, OK? So, Ed, you come here and stand right in front of Jill. That's right. As close as the two of you feel comfortable." Ed sidestepped over to stand about a foot away from Jill and looked directly at her. Jill appeared nervous and uncomfortable and avoided eye contact.

"Now, what kinds of things does Ed say to you?" Trudy asked Jill. "Um ... well ... ," Jill began haltingly and then stopped. "Does he tell you things about how you look? Or what you should or shouldn't do?" Trudy offered. "Yeah," said Jill. "He tells me I'm ugly and fat and disgusting. He tells me I'm selfish and lazy." "Anything else?" asked Trudy. "He says no one would ever love me," Jill responded. "Why would they? But if I'm thin, at least people won't be totally grossed out by me."

"Ed, now I want you to say those things to Jill. And remember, you're not you, you're Ed. So say them as if you're Ed. We know this is not *you* saying them. Go on."

"You're ugly and fat and disgusting!" Ed snarled. "You're selfish, and you're lazy. No one is *ever* going to love you—why would they? At least if you're thin, people won't be totally grossed out by you."

Jill visibly shuddered and looked pleadingly at Trudy. "Did that sound about right?" Trudy asked. "Oh yeah," said Jill.

"OK," said Trudy. "Who else is in this system? Who else should we put in here today?"

Jill identified her parents, who were pressuring her to leave treatment and go back to college, as well as a "Good Girl" part and a "Hopelessness" part. Jill chose other clients to role-play these parts and configured them around her. She identified lines for each of them to say based on her own inner narratives and experiences.

Once everyone was in place, Trudy asked Jill to take a moment and sense if the sculpture felt right, if it mapped on well to her internal experience. She nodded that it did. "OK," said Trudy. "Let's try putting the sculpture in motion, and you can always make changes as we go, OK?" Jill nodded. "So when I say 'go,' I want each of you to speak the lines of your part and to move and act just as Jill told you to. Got it? OK. Go."

Jill's sculpture came alive. Her parents, Ed, Good Girl, and Hopelessness began speaking their lines, all at the same time. Hopelessness and Good Girl slowly moved around as they spoke, just as Jill described. For about sixty seconds, we all experienced part of Jill's inner world along with her. It was clamorous and confusing, and the negative messages seemed to hammer Jill from all sides. During the enactment, Jill went from turning her attention from part to part to closing her eyes and sobbing softly. Clients observing the activity were riveted. Many had tears in their eyes.

Trudy called a stop to the enactment. She asked all of Jill's parts except Ed to step way back, to the edge of the circle. Facing each other, Jill and Ed still avoided eye contact. "So now we're going to give you a chance to say something back, Jill," said Trudy. "Before, we were looking at how parts of your system communicate with *you* and how they relate to *each other*. But now *you're* going to get a chance to say something back to Ed. OK?"

The facilitator asked Ed to move in even closer to Jill, to encroach on her personal space in a menacing way, and to repeat again the words Jill herself identified: "You're ugly and fat and disgusting! You're selfish and you're lazy! No one is *ever* going to love you! Why would they? At least if you're thin, people won't be totally grossed out by you." As Ed spoke these words to her, Jill's eyes dropped and her head bowed. She curved in her shoulders. Trudy asked Jill how she felt. The exchange went as follows:

JILL: Hopeless.

TRUDY: Right, we know about Hopelessness. What else?

JILL: I feel like maybe he's right, like I need to do those things.

TRUDY: Yes, that's Good Girl, the one who wants to do things right and be accepted. What else?

JILL: Like I'm not worth anything.

TRUDY: What else?

JILL: I don't know.

TRUDY: Yes you do. What else?

JILL: I don't *know!* [She was becoming more on edge.]

TRUDY: You *do* know! How do you feel that Ed has made you feel so worthless? How do you feel that he has taken you away from your friends and made you drop out of school? How do you feel that he's telling you you're ugly and disgusting?

JILL: [*Mumbling*] I hate it.

TRUDY: Say more.

JILL: Well, I mean, I *hate* it. I *hate* feeling so bad about myself all the time, like I'm not worth anything, like I'm gross and disgusting and unlovable. I hate feeling like I have to work so hard just to not be repulsive to people, just to be *normal.* It's exhausting, and I hate it. Why do I do that?

TRUDY: Because Ed tells you to.

JILL: But that's so stupid! It sounds crazy when I say it out loud like that. Why do I let him control me like that? Why do I listen to him?

TRUDY: Because he's powerful.

JILL: Yeah, but I don't like what he's doing to me, what he's done to my life.

TRUDY: That's right! [She stepped a bit closer to Jill so she was just behind her left shoulder, facing Ed with her.] Ed, tell Jill again what you said before, that she's ugly and disgusting.

ED: You're ugly and disgusting!

TRUDY: Jill, what do you have to say to that? What do you want to say to Ed?

JILL: [*Silence.*]

TRUDY, TO ED: Say it again.

ED: You're ugly and disgusting!

JILL: [She paused for a second and then looked right into Ed's eyes.] I HATE YOU.

We can see that the focus of this group was to help Jill identify Ed as separate from her Self, as a force that wants to control, abuse, and manipulate her. This is an early stage in the IFS process called "unblending," aimed at helping Jill accept the idea of the multiplicity of the self and to identify her parts and their functions, particularly those parts that have self-destructive components. In Frankfurt's terms, unblending is meant to help Jill become an *unwilling* addict, to make her aware that although she still has an eating disorder, she can reorient her view of the behaviors as something she *does not* want to want to do. Ed *does* want her to want to engage in those behaviors, but she does not.

A useful mechanism for unblending from Ed, as we see in this group session, is for a client to get really, really angry at her eating disorder. But the ultimate goal for clients like Jill is to eventually move from this antagonistic relationship with Ed to one of understanding and compassion—that is, to relate to Ed from Self. This is incredibly difficult. As Jill told me in a conversation a few days after this group therapy session, "Ed's an asshole. He made me trust him, then took everything from me and tried to kill me. How can I possibly feel compassion for *that?*" But IFS holds that as long as a part is unreconciled with Self, it retains its power. The more a client hates Ed, the more he remains a threat to her system. Clients are taught that they must instead learn how to relate with compassion to Ed so they can understand what, although his methods are destructive, he has been trying to do for them, for the self-system. Only then can they gradually ask him to move out of the driver's seat and head to the back of the bus.

As I learned more about IFS, I began to see the subtle ways in which this refashioning of the self as a system of interacting parts was not just employed in therapy sessions but integrated into everyday interactions in the clinic. For example, one day when Carly argued with the dietician about a meal plan increase, she was told, "That's not you but your eating disorder talking." The stronger Carly would insist that, no, she was legitimately upset about the meal change (which she said went against the agreed-on treatment plan in her chart), the more adamant staff would become that it was clearly her eating disorder that was in control. Similarly, when Bethany became panicky because the timing of the afternoon walk was changed, she was told that it was her eating disorder—not really *her*—that was being thrown into such states of anxiety and that *she* could be flexible, even if her eating disorder could not. At other times, therapies and everyday interactions focused on what Ed did *for* a client, what functions Ed served in their everyday lives. When a client's "eating disorder was talking," she was encouraged to look at what constructive purpose it was serving, even though it was also making her life more difficult. Was she trying to avoid conflict? Manage difficult emotions? Communicate something? The therapeutic task was to help the client find other ways of dealing with the issues Ed had taken on as his job so that Ed could "step back" and let Self take the lead.

THE DIALOGIC SELF AND MANAGED CARE

Building on the "dialogical self theory" of Hubert J. M. Hermans and Giancarlo Dimaggio, I call this internal diversification and restructuring "dialogic interiority"—a rendering of one's "self" as constituted in and through ongoing (and shifting) dialogues between two or more internally experienced aspects of the subject.[16] This reorientation of inner experience proposes (and also generates) an epiphenomenal or holographic "self" that arises from a buzzing, dynamic *network of internal relationships* rather than from any sort of identifiable, stable, or even especially predictable state of being. In this sense, developing dialogic interiority shifts the client's understanding not only of the *structure* of self (multiple versus singular) but also, more fundamentally, of what self *is,* so that "self" becomes an action rather than a noun. Interior experience is reconceptualized as always already diversified and intrarelational. In other words, the clinic deploys specific techniques not only for observing or articulating internal dialogue but also for actually *restructuring* it, thereby reconfiguring the relationships within one's internal system.[17] This is critically important for understanding how broader cultural values about power, governance, and moral responsibility become entangled with psychotherapeutic practice in the clinic, as we will see in a moment.

At Cedar Grove, such practices proceed within a context—managed mental healthcare—that is far from value neutral and, as we have seen, incentivizes the cultivation of "good patients," those who are rational, predictable, and oriented toward health. Accordingly, questions of agency and choice come to the fore, both practically and therapeutically. From a practical standpoint, what counts is what a client *does.* If she eats her snack, this action is taken as a proxy for her choice to eat her snack. In other words, agency and behavior become collapsed. From a therapeutic perspective, however, a client eating her snack only counts as healthy agency when she not only eats her snack, and not only wants to eat her snack, but when she *wants to* want to eat her snack. I will return to this mismatch between the views of agency below. Here, the point is that the capacity for this sort of multiple-order self-reflexivity requires at least a temporary division of the subject so that one aspect can reflect on the other(s). As clients learn to cultivate and manage this state of multiplicity as healthy and normal, they develop new ways of thinking about their illnesses and themselves.

PRIMING THE SUBJECT: DEVELOPING ACCOMMODATING AGENCY

Here, I find anthropologist Janice Boddy's work on Zar practitioners in Sudan to be useful.[18] Boddy describes a setting in which married, middle-aged women break with the everyday world of female subordination by becoming possessed by powerful spirits that cause them to act in scandalous ways. Boddy considers how these competing figurations of women's agency (everyday understandings that locate them as inferior and subordinate to men, and the parallel world of the spirits in which they are powerful and even threatening) can—and do—coexist. She argues that it is precisely *because* of this doubling of agency that the women can experience Zar practice as transformative. It allows them to creatively engage with and work through competing models of who they are and who they should be and to come to a largely individualized solution, concretized in each woman's relationship with her possessing spirit. Boddy proposes the concept of "accommodating agency" as a way of conceptualizing this process. Women learn how to live *with* their possessing spirits, she says, and even to collaborate with them. In so doing, these women can paradoxically inhabit contradictory value systems as they carve out for themselves ways of being-in-the-world that are otherwise foreclosed to them.

I find this line of analysis useful for thinking about the practical utility of IFS at Cedar Grove. I suggest that, through the work with IFS, clients at Cedar Grove develop a form of accommodating agency with Ed akin to that described by Boddy. Both recovery at Cedar Grove and Zar possession entail a person identifying a force other than herself who has co-opted her will and bent her behavior to fit its own needs and wants. Both provide a language for talking about the relationship between the person and this entity and a framework for understanding a path to healing. And both hinge on the notion that agency is complex, situational, and contested. Just as Boddy's informants had to learn *how to be possessed,* clients at Cedar Grove must learn *how to live in relationship* with Ed. And Ed is thought to never entirely go away. Clients must learn how to live in an accommodating relationship with him for the rest of their lives.

But this isn't just any relationship. In IFS, and Cedar Grove's version of it, there is clearly a "right" way to organize one's inner system, with wise Self at the helm and the parts—with all their disagreements, polarizations, coalitions, and back-room deals—agreeing (ideally) to work toward common ground for the good of the system. How does this happen? In a rather Rawlsian vision of pluralism and deliberative democracy, parts are encouraged to articulate their grievances and concerns and to engage in active dialogue with other parts and with Self in a process that every part in the system can agree is fair, even if not every part likes the outcome.[19] Parts are then expected to uphold their side of this social contract by stepping back. In return, Self ensures that they have the emotional and physical resources they need to function and that they will be protected against the intrusion of danger. This, according to IFS, is how a healthy self-system functions.

The political resonances of the IFS model are not lost on its founder, and in fact, Schwartz explicitly likens the IFS model of internal systems to a pluralistic view of society. "Pluralism," he says, "involves an attempt to hold unity and diversity in balance, to value the many within the one, to resolve conflict without imposing synthesis or expelling groups, and to celebrate difference. Multiplicity of the mind involves this kind of pluralism."[20] It is taken as a given in IFS that such forms of governance are "naturally" healthy and optimizing.

Within this framework, a client's emergent experiences of mastery and agency in treatment are considered legitimate only when they emerge from a process of deliberative consensus among parts. Clients learn to reorganize their inner worlds as a sort of miniature United Nations, where various parts, each with its own diverse interests and motives, learn to work together for the good of the whole person. As Self becomes the leader, the client (in theory) becomes more compliant with the treatment team, aligning with them against Ed. She becomes more predictable because, supposedly, her impulsive parts are brought under the governance of Self. And because Self is seen to be always already an expression of health, clients who are Self-led are, by definition, thought to be proactively engaged in their own recoveries. What this forecloses are expressions of agency that don't align with treatment team priorities and impulses toward health that may not be legible within managed care structures (remember Carly's black fingernail polish from chapter 7).

In the context of managed mental healthcare, IFS offers clinicians at Cedar Grove a strategy for "rendering subjectivity calculable" by providing a model of the pluralistic subject where patients can be both "sick" and "responsible" at the same time.[21] Clinicians are able to report to managed care companies specific achievements or "failures" in therapy in concrete terms that, in practice, signal much more complex and nuanced understandings of agency. A client is either able to unblend with Ed and act from Self or not. She can either do this occasionally and only with much staff support or do it more regularly and on her own. She can *want* to want to see Ed as a separate part within her but struggle with the technique, or she can *not* want to see Ed as a separate part and roll her eyes at the idea. As a client demonstrates that she is capable of developing an accommodating agency in relation to Ed, she is thought to signal that she is working toward this style of internal governance, and these changes are supported and rewarded through the provision of healthcare benefits.

Importantly, in a for-profit healthcare environment, as clients become more proficient at using the IFS model to understand their eating disorders, they emerge as simultaneously agentic and nonagentic, powerful and vulnerable—multiple, but in a way that they can learn to coordinate and direct. Both clinicians and managed care case managers can then assess progress based less on overt behaviors (though these do remain important) and more on the processes of self-governance a client signals she has internalized.

For example, Trudy, the therapist who led the group therapy session described above, was thrilled with Jill's participation in the group, not only for the potential therapeutic value but also for the practical utility of obtaining additional treatment days from Jill's insurance company. "This is great," she told me. "This is something really concrete I can take to them to say, 'See—she really is trying. She's working hard. Her weights don't show it yet, but she's doing the work and using treatment.' I'll tell them about the part at the end for sure. They like to hear about patients getting pissed at their eating disorder. It makes them believe they're motivated to get better." Regardless of Jill's actual motivation to recover, she had to leave treatment after thirty days, the maximum allotted by her insurance plan. She relapsed shortly thereafter.

One challenge of the IFS model is that it risks co-optation by economic models of the liberal, rational subject, which are predicated on the ideals of deliberative process and individual choice. By reframing the client's experiences of mastery and agency as legitimate only when they are the outcome of negotiation, consensus, and collaborative action among parts, this process in its fruition approximates the liberal, rational subject favored by managed care. In "successful" IFS treatment, a convergence develops between a client's experience of her inner life and her managed care company's institutional parameters of moral selves deserving of care. As this happens, the client and clinicians learn the contours of acceptable and unacceptable forms of internal orientations and are guided toward those that coincide with the rational patient-actor model consistent with predictable profit margins. In the end, "recovery" from eating disorders through IFS may be as much about social-izing clients to become appropriate subjects of the managed care economic model as it is about healing the eating disorder itself.

Despite this critique, I want to emphasize that my analysis of IFS as a technology of political and economic subjectivity does not mean that it does not help people find relief from eating disorders and many other conditions. It absolutely does. I use elements of it in my practice with my own clients.[22] In my experience as an anthropologist and as a therapist, I can say with con-fidence that IFS can and does seem to help many people. And while this chapter may add fuel to arguments that psychiatry is little more than a tool for re-educating disruptive subjects into dominant structures of power, this is not my intent, nor do I think that is nearly the whole story.

Certainly, models of the self, even those that appear to run counter to traditional psychiatric conventions, nevertheless emerge within moral ecolo-gies that favor the subjectivities that sustain them. As sociologist Nicholas Rose argues, even those psychotherapies that contain subversive potential remain inextricably tangled up with the economic and social structures within which they emerge.[23] This, however, is quite a separate issue from whether or not they "work," in the estimation of the people who use them. In fact, one might argue that some degree of resonance between models of self and the broader social systems in which they operate is a necessary condition for such therapies to be effective.

THE PART OF ME THAT HATES "PARTS":
CLIENTS' REACTIONS TO IFS

On the whole, clinicians and families seemed to have very positive orienta-tions toward IFS and the idea of "separating out" clients from their eating disorders. "It was so much easier to relate to her after we learned to think of it that way," said Betsy, referring to her daughter Miranda (whom we met in chapter 6). "An eating disorder is like a kidnapping. Seriously. Like someone has come and kidnapped your child. And you can't negotiate with the kidnappers. There's no point. You have to be absolute and take action. That's the way it is. It helped enormously to know our daughter was in there somewhere just being held, basically, against her will. That made it easier to deal with the way she was acting and all the anger and ugliness she was directing towards us." Stacey, a Cedar Grove dietician, described a similar experience:

> It can get *really* tiring to sit across from client after client, day after day, obsessing about an extra twenty-five calories here or fifty calories there. Just obsessing and obsessing and obsessing, and fighting about every little thing. Sometimes I just want to scream, "It's just fifty calories! *It doesn't freakin' matter!*" But then I remember that this is their eating disorder talking, not *them*. They're not in control. Obviously, or they wouldn't need to be here. So that helps me bracket it off. And it helps me reconnect with the person in there who is feeling terrified and needs help. That's something I can work with.

Clients, however, had a different sort of experience. Generally, while they did find the language of "parts" and talking about the eating disorder as separate from themselves to be a helpful shorthand, they also often became frustrated at the way this was at times deployed against them to delegitimize their claims to agency or self-knowledge (or both), as some of the opening quotes to this chapter illustrate. Kendall had quite a bit to say on this subject one day:

> I guess, a lot of times, I feel like they think we don't have a mind of our own or that we're only our eating disorders, and we're not. We're each individual human beings who deserve to be treated as individuals and not just clustered, or just as, "Well this is what's happened in the past," or "In all of our clinical trials, this is what is average," or "This is what normally happens." Every person is an individual, and when you don't treat people as an individual, it keeps them stuck in their eating disorder, and isolated, and like, "Well, they don't get me." I'm not just my eating disorder, and just because I disagree with something it doesn't mean it's my eating disorder talking. Sometimes it is, but usually it's actually not. But there's no way to win that argument because the more you argue, the more they say it's evidence that Ed is controlling things. It's pretty infuriating.

For Kendall (whose view was echoed by many other clients), having any of her thoughts, feelings, or intentions that didn't fit standardized norms or expectations (based on theories that have their own complex histories, as we've seen) dismissed as "part of her eating disorder" further exacerbated the experience of being unseen. In other words, she and others felt there was no way to effectively speak back to the hegemonic press of long-standing theories, clinical trials, and norms of practice without it being dismissed as "coming from the eating disorder." I will explore this more in chapter 10. For now, suffice it to say that unlike clinicians, staff, and families, clients did not uniformly find talk about Ed to be empowering, and it often felt to them as if Ed talk became yet another vector of delegitimation and a subversion of their attempts to be seen, heard, and known.

As these dynamics intensify in the course of treatment, clients often begin to experience a sense of radical dislocation, as if the structures that held them together are giving way. This is, of course, part of the point of treatment, to remove the eating disorder as the scaffolding of the self to make way for new, purportedly healthier, structures to emerge. But the experience can be frightening and overwhelming.

FREE FALL

KENDALL: I have basically missed out on my whole adolescence. I have not had thirteen, fourteen, fifteen, sixteen, seventeen, eighteen. You always think of kids going out, having fun with their friends, learning to drive, that kind of stuff. I never had that. I just felt like I really missed out, and I just kind of have a little resentment that I never got that.

REBECCA: What's the resentment towards?

KENDALL: I'm not sure if it's towards one thing. It's just towards a lot. I think it's at myself, at my eating disorder, at my town. At a lot of different people that I can't seem to forgive for things they've done to really hurt me. And sometimes my family. Just everything. I just have a lot of resentment and anger. I realize I have no idea who I am. None.

Before treatment, when in the throes of an eating disorder, clients often feel in full control of themselves and their lives and vehemently reject suggestions that they are not. They often deny the seriousness of their conditions and report feeling invulnerable. "I didn't think anything could really hurt me," Pema said. "It was like, 'My body has already gotten this low. What more can I do? How low can I go? How low can I get my potassium and not have a heart attack?' I wanted to keep pushing my limits." In the course of treatment, these dynamics of control are, in theory, reversed. The goal in treatment is to get clients to understand that they are, in fact, completely *out* of control, that what they thought was control was actually an illusion. Separating clients from the eating disorder is key to this process. "I finally see that my eating disorder was controlling *me*," Anita said. "*I* wasn't in control. At all. It was Ed. I was completely *out* of control, but I didn't know it." Part of realizing they are out of control involves accepting a degree of vulnerability that many initially find quite intolerable. "I didn't want to believe that anything could really hurt me," Malory told me. "Which sounds crazy because all I was doing was hurting myself. I see that now, but I didn't then. It was like, 'How much of this can I take and remain functional?' Of course, what I thought was functional was definitely not." "I didn't want to accept that I was seriously damaging my body in a potentially permanent way," Jennifer said. "Not really. I mean, I wanted to hurt myself, to punish myself for all the things I felt guilty about. But there was this disconnect between that and thinking I could really die from what I was doing, or that my bones might never be the same, or that I might not be able to have kids."

At this point, in treatment, without the eating disorder to structure their behaviors, their affective lives, their relationships, and their senses of agency and identity, most clients fall apart emotionally. They can become erratic, frantic, and desperate, as this exchange demonstrates:

MARJORIE: I feel very hopeless, and I don't know if I'm ever going to get better, and there's those moments where that eating disorder is so strong that it's just, I don't want to gain any weight. I don't want to do this. But then I don't want to go back to the way I was living. I've had one of those moments tonight where I told the staff that I wanted to leave and I didn't want to be here, and to take the tube out of my nose right now. And then they said, "We can't let you go. If we do, we're going to have to call an ambulance." It's hard because I'm like, "Well, I willingly checked myself in here, so I should be able to leave." But then meeting with Dr. Casey today and starting groups again today, I feel the support and that it's a really caring environment, and then it makes me want to stay here.

REBECCA: What is that like for you to stay and not just go, what is that like?

MARJORIE: I guess I kind of felt like no choice because would I want the ambulance to come and probably put me in a psych ward? And I've been in the psych ward before. They don't know how to treat eating disorders, and I'm definitely not going to get better there. And this is definitely, obviously, a more caring, supportive environment. I guess I feel stuck, but

I don't want to sound like oh, I'm just giving into treatment because it's my only choice. Because it's not always like that. Because I mean, we need that push, I guess. For when that other side takes over, and there's another side where you feel safe here. You want the treatment and stuff. And it's just a battle.

In IFS terms, we would say that Marjorie is experiencing a polarization of two parts—the part of her that wants to recover (which wants to stay in treatment), and her eating disorder (which wants her to leave). Marjorie's task, according to the clinic program, is to recognize these as two parts of herself, both of which want her to be free from suffering and struggling, but which have very different ways of accomplishing this. The part that wants recovery seeks resolution through staying in treatment and getting well. The eating disorder part wants her to flee the immediate context that is causing her discomfort (treatment). The clinic wants Marjorie to connect with Self as something outside and beyond these parts and to let it lead her. She is at a point, however, where she is not sure how to do that and feels hopeless about moving forward.

As clients learn to accept their physical vulnerabilities (which many had patently denied or even purposefully challenged) and to recognize that they have become out of control with their eating disorder (which many had experienced as a source of comfort and safety), many of them enter a state of existential crisis. "Everything is falling apart," Bethany said. "It's like [the game] Jenga, when you start pulling out the blocks and the whole thing collapses. Not that I am ready to just give up the eating disorder and be healthy all of a sudden. It doesn't work like that. But it's like the things I thought were keeping me safe are the same things they say are hurting me. I don't know what to do. I understand what they're saying, but at the same time I'm terrified to not have my eating disorder anymore."

It is worth noting that such existential distress in the face of change is not unique to people with eating disorders. Very few people enjoy feeling out of control and vulnerable, certainly not as an ongoing, existential way of being. But this kind of existential dismantling does take on particular significance for people who feel like they have no grounding outside of the very behaviors that are being systematically blocked while in treatment. "It's like the eating disorder becomes the glue that holds them together," Dr. Casey explained. "You take that away, and they fragment. The center doesn't hold." Edie described this feeling one day, about three weeks into her treatment:

EDIE: Right now, I still very much want to cry and go home and say "That's it," you know. "This isn't helping." I don't know the answers, and I think it's just gone on so long. It's got so much wrapped into it that I can't understand everything that's in it, and everything that causes it. And I have no idea how to counteract it yet.

REBECCA: It sounds like you're feeling a little hopeless about it at the moment.

EDIE: Yeah. I'm trying to think of a good metaphor, and I can't really. Except being in the middle of a hurricane or a tornado or something. Not a hurricane because I guess there's an eye in the middle of a hurricane. But this kind of sense of so much swirling around and so much that is not easy to grasp onto, it's like "What's going on?" Kind of like drowning, or falling.

As we can see from Edie's description, this stage of treatment, while it does seek to institute clarity regarding the eating disorder versus the self, also removes structure and familiarity. This is an extraordinarily uncomfortable and disorienting process, and clients are often eager to rush through it and on to recovery, a tendency the clinic calls a "flight into health"—when someone who has been ill "decides" to be well and wants to leapfrog over the intervening processes and move directly to recovery, insisting that they are better. A flight into health is not necessarily disingenuous on the part of the client; it can signal a real desire to be well (or at least to no longer be sick), but it can also cause people to minimize or underestimate how much work must be done to actually get them to that point. "Inevitably, they relapse," Dr. Casey explained, "because they haven't really done the work they need to do. It's great that they want to be well, and we can build on that. But they still have to do the work and to practice new behaviors and attitudes. As much as we say it's up to the client to decide to get well, it's not really a 'one-and-done' decision. It takes time and unfolds over weeks or months or even years."

Such flight-into-health impulses are compounded by the fact that by this point (usually about three to four weeks into treatment), most clients have largely stabilized medically and may have gained several pounds, evidence insurance companies often use to designate them "ready to discharge," regardless of the fact that, emotionally, they are at their most vulnerable.

How, then, to persuade clients not only to enter into this state of radical existential uncertainty but to *remain* there and work their way through it slowly, rather than either going back to the eating disorder or taking an unrealistic flight into health? And how to persuade insurance companies to continue to pay for care beyond the barest indicators of medical stability?

In the next chapter, we turn to the ways clients are gradually retethered to experiences and practices outside the eating disorder and how they begin, slowly and tentatively, to construct new senses of self, identity, and meaning.

Calculated Risks

AUGUST 1987

I lie sprawled on my stomach on the floor of my room, the diet magazine splayed out before me. The powder blue carpet scratches roughly against my skin, the raw areas on my elbows a testament to the many hours I've spent in this very position and this very spot, the protected corridor between the exercise bike and the window seat of my bay window.

My body is longer at age seventeen than it was when I was eleven, but so many other things are the same. I can't believe I'm in this place again—anorexic. The descent this time was so fast.

As I turn the page, perusing the recipes, the cat sidles up to me and rubs her soft body against my arm, her paws crinkling the magazine pages. "GO AWAY!" I growl, pushing her roughly with my forearm. I have zero tolerance for affection since things got bad again, even affection from a cat. It makes me want to jump out of my skin. The cat turns and rubs the other side of her body against me. Ugh! I struggle up off the floor, joints hurting and feeling slightly lightheaded, and toss the cat out of the room, slamming the door behind her.

Back down on the carpet, I smooth out the pages of the magazine. I begin adding up calories. Safe. Numbers. OK. I'm OK. I'm still OK.

NINE

"Fat" Is Not a Feeling

DEVELOPING NEW WAYS OF PRESENCING

My eating disorder has raised me, in a way. This is kind of like a rebirthing.

—LAUREN,

a 25-year-old woman diagnosed with anorexia

I don't know why Shelly picked that day to show me. As far as I could tell, it was a regular day, like any other. But as she walked past me into the therapy room, she turned, looked at me pointedly, and said softly, "I want you to see something. Close the door." "OK," I said, curious, but also a little wary. Shelly regularly self-harmed, and as she slowly lifted up the bottom hem of her t-shirt, I wondered if perhaps she was going to show me a new injury that needed medical attention. But what she showed me wasn't new. Just above her waistband, I saw the large, jagged letters, tight-skinned and shiny with old scar tissue, pale and almost shimmering in the overhead light. They were as clear as day, etched into her abdomen: F-A-T. My eyes found Shelly's, and she looked back at me, trying to judge my reaction. "Tell me about it," I said softly. We sat down, and Shelly kept her gaze on her hands, twisting them into a knot in her lap. "I did that about two years ago, because that's how I always feel—fat," Shelly said. "But in group yesterday, Dr. Casey kept saying that 'fat' is not a feeling. She said we should explore here in treatment what's really going on, what we're really feeling underneath. But honestly," she said, looking up at me, "I don't *know*. I have *no clue*. I don't have any idea what else I may be feeling. I guess there's stuff in there, but I don't know what it is or how to access it. All I know is that, for as long as I can remember, I've felt *fat*, and I just want to obliterate myself."

Once clients have become practiced at identifying their eating disorders as distinct from themselves and have begun to sense the possibility of agency and identity separate from their illness, the next tasks of treatment focus on helping them build alternative structures and avenues of being-in-the-world.

The tasks in this stage are aimed at helping clients prepare for life outside of the clinic.

In chapter 3, we looked at how eating disorders function to facilitate and modulate experiences of "being there" across a number of levels: the physical (the body grows and shrinks), the affective (one numbs out, one's senses and emotions are heightened, or sometimes both), the cognitive (thinking becomes fuzzy and difficult, one feels spacey), the interpersonal (one retreats from social interaction), and the social (life becomes centered on the eating disorder as engagement with other activities diminishes). Eating disorders become a means of "tinkering"[1] with being-in-the-world in different ways across different circumstances and situations. They become a strategy for being present—or absent—to oneself, to others, and to the world. Treatment at Cedar Grove seeks to systematically dismantle this eating disorder "technology" and replace it with new ways of organizing the self, new ways of experiencing the body, new ways of managing relationships to others, and new ways of operating in the world—in my terms, new ways of presencing.

But this process of presencing in a new way is not self-evident. It entails learning new propositions about what constitutes the body and the mind, and how material and immaterial aspects of existence are related and may affect one another. This is no small task. It is a wholesale reformulation of one's existential and metaphysical understandings of the nature of being human.

BEING/HAVING/SEEKING A BODY

Having a body is both a given and a goal in the clinic. It is a given in the sense that biomedical indicators—the body's pulse and respiration, its temperature, its blood pressure, its weight, its lab values, its need for caloric sustenance—take center stage. But the body is also a goal in that one of the core features of an eating disorder is extreme ambivalence about embodiment and difficulty being in one's body—that is, feeling oneself as grounded in the fleshiness of existence. Being in the body can trigger intense panic for a person with an eating disorder for a variety of reasons, some of which are idiosyncratic to each person. Molly's reflections give a sense of why this might be the case: "When I'm in my body, I just feel so gross, so completely and utterly disgusting, like I am swimming in shame. It clings to me and suffocates me. I can't stand it. That's what 'feeling fat' really is for me. It's more feeling myself in my body that is so intolerable." When I asked her why she thought being in her body felt so horrible, she replied, "I'm not sure. All I know is that it is terrifying. I can't even describe it. It's a kind of panic that's hard to describe unless you've felt it. But I know that I *have* to get out of there." "Get out of where?" I asked. "My body. I have to get out of it somehow. Cutting helps with that. Or restricting. It disconnects me, and then I feel safer." I heard similar things from other clients in the clinic, who described being in their bodies as "awful," "unbearable," "painful," "absolutely not OK," and "the worst thing I could ever imagine."

Helping clients become accustomed to being in their bodies was an important part of the therapeutic program at the clinic. Movement therapy (dance), yoga, and mindful eating were three techniques specifically designed to help clients connect with their physical bodies in ways that were meant to be integrative. Understandably, these were some of the least liked activities by the clients, who often dreaded them. But learning how to understand and experience the body in new ways reaches far beyond these particular activities, and was fundamental to treatment at Cedar Grove.

FEELINGS VERSUS MATTER: A BODY IMAGE GROUP THERAPY SESSION

About a week after Shelly showed me her stomach, I was with the clients in a body image group run by Gemini, a therapist who had worked at Cedar Grove for several years.

The group therapy room had big picture windows along one side, and the soft spring early afternoon light streamed in as we formed a circle to begin the group. Gemini began the session by giving each client a huge piece of paper and setting out a pile of markers in the center of the circle. "I want each of you to draw your silhouette," she told the group. "A life-sized drawing, based on your own sense of your body. It's OK if it's not perfect. What's important is that you draw it to reflect how you experience yourself. As you do so, I want you to label the parts of your bodies you don't like and write on the drawing the kinds of messages you tell yourself about those areas, like 'fat,' or 'disgusting,' or 'beautiful'"—"Yeah right," giggled Jemma—"whatever it may be. Write on the part the kinds of words and messages you direct to it. Then I'll tell you what to do next."

The clients grabbed markers and spread out around the room, laying their papers down on the floor to begin their work. As they got busy, the room grew quiet, aside from the occasional squeaking of markers and the ringing of phones from the main office.

In the silence, thick with intensity and focus, I glanced around the room at the hunched figures bent down over the papers. Carly was wrapped in a blanket, her bony elbows jutting up toward the celling as she worked. Kendall was lying on her stomach with a pillow under her hipbones to cushion them from the hard floor. Allison was on her knees, inching around the paper as her image took shape, biting her lip and looking displeased. As my eyes moved to the clients' emerging drawings, words jumped out at me, almost leaping off the paper. "HIDEOUS." "GROSS." "UGLY." And not surprisingly, "FAT."

Once everyone was done, Gemini gave further instructions. "Now, find a partner. Flip the paper over and lie down while your partner traces the actual contours of your body on the other side." Audible groans erupted from the group. "I know, I know, this is hard!" Gemini said. "It's really vulnerable, and it means letting someone get close to you. And I know you all worry about what the outline will look like. But trust me. There's a point to this."

The clients did as Gemini asked, taking turns lying on the reverse of their drawings and allowing their partners to trace the outlines of their bodies.

"Now," said Gemini once they were done, "with the paper still flat down on the floor, write different *feelings* you have and where you feel them in your body. *Actual* feelings. Not assessments or judgments like we did last time. Feelings. Emotions. Where do you feel them in your bodies?"

The clients got to work. Carmen and Polly wrote "anger" in their stomachs. Alicia had "fear" in her throat. Shelly had "loneliness" written in her hands.

"Now," instructed Gemini, producing a role of masking tape, "go tape this up against the big picture windows over there. Put your first drawing toward the glass and the tracing of your outline facing into the room."

As they did so, and the light streamed through the paper, both images appeared. The clients could see not only how vastly different their body image drawings were from the actual contours of their bodies but also how the places that they particularly identified as "problem areas" (gross, disgusting, fat) were similar to the places where they identified holding feelings.

"Whoa," said Polly under her breath.

"Do you see? It's your feelings that inflate and distort your sense of your body," Gemini pointed out. "Do you see that? See, Shelly? You have 'anger' and 'guilt' in your stomach, and that's exactly where you had written 'Fat.

Horrible person.' Do you see?" Shelley nodded, amazed. "And Lisa, look here. You feel 'sadness' in your legs and that's the area where you wrote 'disgusting' on your body image." Lisa nodded, surprised. "Remember," continued Gemini, "'fat' is not a feeling. It stands *in* for feelings. Every time you tell yourself something about your body, ask what *feeling* is really going on. Our bodies are like a language, and body image is the way people with eating disorders talk to themselves about their feelings. As you get better at identifying and talking about your feelings directly, your body image gets less distorted. Recovery is about inhabiting your body in new ways."

NEW UNDERSTANDINGS OF AFFECT AND EMBODIMENT

The main goal of the body image exercise was to get clients to begin to understand that what they experience as "fat" is actually produced by *feelings* and that by containing and holding these feelings within their bodies, they are making their body image feel inflated. "Fat," then, is not a feeling (or not *only* a feeling); rather, accumulated or unexpressed *affect* makes you feel *as if* you are fat.

This idea that feelings can "inflate" matter links affect to flesh in a particular way. Affect, in this view, animates matter, activating it, bringing it alive, and affording it a sort of agency. It circulates, binds, can get stuck, or be foreclosed. It can overwhelm. How one regulates affect literally shapes the flesh, and vice versa. If holding affect in the body leads to feelings of inflation and bigness that are out of proportion to the physical, material body, it follows that contracted matter can contain fewer feelings. This, in fact, is how people with eating disorders often experience themselves, and it is also how they learn to make sense of their behaviors in treatment—at Cedar Grove, clients learn that their eating disorders allowed them to starve or purge out their feelings, leaving no room for them.

Julia, for example, talked about how her eating disorder allowed her to manage her anxiety, not simply by numbing it but by redirecting it:

JULIA: My eating disorder for me is about acting on the anxious urge to not eat.

REBECCA: So when you're feeling anxious and you don't eat or you purge over and over, what does that do your anxiety?

JULIA: It helps, but I get especially the urge to restrict when I'm really anxious because I'm just—it's almost physical. I'm not thinking about food because I'm really stressed out about something else. I mean, [if] you know you're going to give a talk in front of a thousand people, the last thing you want to do is eat a full meal. Certain things just come in to settle me down. [The eating disorder] gives me something that I know I can do right. Binge and purge. And I don't have to think about it. I can zone out and not think about whatever else is stressing me out.

REBECCA: And how long does that feeling last, that kind of zoning out?

JULIA: It depends, it's not too long. Maybe half an hour. Before you get discouraged again.

REBECCA: But it sounds like it buys you a window of time.

JULIA: Or it feels like it does that. Yeah.

Eating disorders become a way of inhabiting the world by modulating affect, which can create safety and help manage interpersonal interactions.

But affect, clients learn, is not finite, and it is not self-contained. It is interpersonally generated and circulated. You can get rid of feelings temporarily by starving or purging, but there are always more that must be either felt or dealt with. The irony, then, is that the smaller you get, the more feelings you aren't allowing yourself to feel directly, which makes you feel fatter and fatter and makes you reach more and more to starving or purging to manage them. This fuels the drive to lose ever more weight, and the spiral continues.

DOUBLE BINDS

In recovery, clients are encouraged to let feelings out and let care and attention in—to let things in general flow. They're told not to hold on to hurt or anger or sadness, not to "stuff" their feelings. Yet at the same time, they are told they cannot and should not give outside voice to absolutely everything they feel. This would be just as dysregulated as holding everything in and would cause others to have to hold the affect that was being off-loaded. The emphasis, then, is on continual self-monitoring and self-modulation. The boundaries of the affect-body are encouraged to leak but in a more or less consistent fashion that must be carefully calibrated at all times.

This self-regulation has high stakes in the clinic. Financial resources, certainly, but also emotional resources, in terms of staff time and attention, are limited, and clients are continually policed and reminded that they are always at risk of being "too much"—too needy, too expensive, too much work. Even as they are induced to gain weight and to let their affect out and care in, relationships of care in the clinic communicate to them that they are already "too big" and "too hungry" for time, attention, and resources.

This situation perpetuates another double bind in terms of the subject of affect and the "ideal self" that is cultivated in the clinic. On one level, eating practices and affective styles are viewed in the clinic as synergistic, and this is identified as a core of the problem: they should be disentangled as part of the process of recovery. It is the point of therapy to separate out affect and food. Clients are encouraged to think of food as medicine, for example, as something the body needs but that is otherwise devoid of meaning.[2] At the same time, under the conditions of managed care, food and eating are taken as indices of therapeutic progress. Calories consumed and weight gained are held as principal indicators of whether or not someone is getting better. So on the one hand, clients are being told to disentangle their experience of affective self from food, but on the other hand, their behaviors regarding food are being read as proxies for the relative health or illness of that affective self.

These double binds within the treatment context communicate conflicting messages to clients about how to be good patients. Clients' impulses to rein themselves in relationally, to make themselves "smaller" and less demanding of resources, become entangled with urges to restrict or binge or purge, which then mark them as resistant to getting better. Yet giving up control over their eating—sometimes having to consume three or four thousand calories a day to gain weight—and being prevented from purging or exercising opens up affective floodgates for clients over which they have little internal control, leading them to feel overwhelmed and panicky, which likewise positions them as ill.

Of course, this kind of affective dysregulation is precisely what is targeted in the therapeutic recovery process of the clinic. Ideally, patients would eat in a more or less consistent way in the clinic—disentangling affect from food—and would learn new strategies for managing the overwhelming or dysregulated affect that emerges with this loss of control. That's the whole point of recovery. But the managed care system is such that it privileges body weight and program compliance as indicators of recovery. Once someone is eating and has regained weight, she is deemed "recovered" and is discharged from care, even though it is precisely at this point that she is often most affectively *dysregulated* and in need of additional treatment to develop new strategies for managing affective processes.

These double binds are complicated by clients' own ambivalences about care. We will remember that, as they learn to separate out their sense of self from their eating disorders, clients enter a serious and significant existential crisis where "everything is falling apart," as Bethany described it. In recovery language, we might say this is a version of "hitting bottom," which is seen to be a necessary part of the process of tearing down old structures and beginning to rebuild a life from, essentially, scratch. But this process takes on additional significance in the treatment of eating disorders. While, from a recovery model standpoint, clients are perhaps at their most vulnerable at this stage, from a medical model standpoint, they are often significantly "healthier" than when they entered the clinic and may be nearing "readiness for discharge" (as we saw in the case of Caleigh in chapter 6). This tension plays out in particular ways in the context of this illness.

Eating disorders are fundamentally about not feeling worthy of existing or of receiving any sort of care. Imagine, then, being at your absolutely most vulnerable, depleted, and helpless point emotionally (having already felt undeserving of care but now feeling it even more acutely) but knowing that your body is now medically stabilized. These two issues together often lead people with eating disorders to a grueling ambivalence about remaining in treatment.

In the eating disorders literature, this ambivalence is often characterized as "resistance," and in some cases, it is. In many ways, it is easier and more compelling to flee to the relative safety and familiarity of an eating disorder than to feel and sit with the affects, feelings, and sensations that arise in its wake, which can be overwhelming and feel intolerable.

But for most people struggling with an eating disorder, this ambivalence is about much more than simple resistance; it is about wanting desperately to be *good,* which for them means needing as little as possible and not taking more than is absolutely necessary. In such a context, wanting continued care or wanting to recover can feel greedy, gluttonous, and selfish, especially given how much treatment costs and the kinds of sacrifices loved ones often have to make for treatment to be possible. Mallory describes this dilemma:

MALLORY: This week, I have been struggling with thoughts of, "I don't need to be here. I'm not thin enough. I'm not sick enough. I've gained enough weight. I should go home now." Or I struggle with feeling like, "If

I want treatment, then I shouldn't be here." It feels like sometimes people don't want to get better. It's hard to be around people who don't want to get better. I feel guilty saying, "Hey, I know I'm ready to let go of this eating disorder, and I want to recover." It's just really hard for me. I've been having a lot of body image issues this week. I just really struggle in my mind with the idea that I don't need to gain any more weight.

REBECCA: So how do you get through that?

MALLORY: Well, I just try to talk to people. They tell me, "You're still incredibly underweight. You're not at a healthy weight, you are nowhere close." It's just really hard because when I look in the mirror—well, I don't look. I'm trying to avoid mirrors.

REBECCA: I'm just thinking about everything you just said, that issue of either "I'm not sick enough to be here" or "There is something wrong with me that I want to get better."

MALLORY: Yeah, it's like I don't fit in or I'm not really sick because I want to get better. I don't know how to deal with that.

Bettina, a twenty-six-year-old woman diagnosed with bulimia, also described feeling like she didn't fit in because she was actually eating food and wanted to get well:

BETTINA: Sometimes I feel like an outcast, or like I don't even fit in here. I've been really restrictive before. But before I came [into treatment] this time, I would eat food. I just purged everything I ate. But still, I ate. So sometimes I feel ashamed, because everybody talks about how little they would eat in a day and how many days they would go without eating. And I'm just like, "Wow, I really don't need to be here. I'm not sick enough." Because I was eating, but none of it was staying down.

REBECCA: And what does that mean about not being sick enough? Not being sick enough for what?

BETTINA: For the attention, for the care, for people to relate to me. I want people to be able to relate to me.

Both Mallory and Bettina are speaking to yet another profound catch-22 at the heart of eating disorders treatment: To be "good patients," clients must want to get well. But if they want to get well, then they feel that they are not sick *enough* to deserve care (and may be seen this way by clinicians and managed care case managers). If, on the other hand, they *don't* want to get well, they may be seen as sick enough to deserve care, but they may not want it. Moreover, they may very well be construed as "bad patients" and therefore denied treatment. Wanting care, or even merely *accepting* care, can be read as evidence that one is not sick enough to *need* the care in the first place, compounding the sense of guilt and shame at the heart of an eating disorder.

When I asked Amanda, a thirty-three-year-old woman diagnosed with anorexia, what the hardest part of treatment was for her, she responded, "The treatment or care and attention that you get. Sometimes it's hard to really embrace that or even accept even the nurturing part of the treatment directed towards you. It's like, 'Well, that's great and all, but I'm not sick enough to get that. And now I'm going to feel guilty that I'm getting that.' I have this voice inside that just says, 'I don't deserve it, I don't deserve it.'" This is a refrain I heard again and again and again from clients in treatment: I don't deserve to be here; I'm not sick enough; I should leave. It didn't matter if the person was at 100 percent of her ideal body weight or 70 percent. The sentiment was the same.

Now, we might say a dangerously underweight person saying she's not sick enough for treatment is an expression of cognitive distortion. And perhaps it is. But if we simply write off this ambivalence about care as part of the illness—a result of "hungry brain," denial, or resistance—we miss the ways this conviction of not being worthy of care echoes the messages clients receive, day in and day out, from a variety of sources, including the people and institutions that are supposedly providing that care. Clients internalize these messages, and because they resonate so strongly with what the eating disorder already tells them, the messages feel unquestionably true.

Patients become caught in these ambivalences. They are induced to want to get well, to become responsible for their own recoveries. But coming to this place of wanting to get well either prompts the eminent withdrawal of care or is dismissed as a "flight into health" and thus as further denial of the seriousness of the illness. There is no comfortable middle ground, no grey area where clients can sit with and work through their own ambivalences about deserving care. If they are "too good," it is not trusted; or, in some cases, it is read as the opposite, as manipulation (as we will see in chapter 11). Sometimes clients are even induced to *perform* a degree of resistance or pushback for their investment in recovery to be taken seriously, yet they do so at the risk of being coopted into discourses about chronicity.

PUSHING BACK

One place this ambivalence shows up is in noncompliance in treatment. I will say more about this in chapter 10, but here I want to give this exchange with

Lilia as an example of one way this can manifest. At the time of this conversation, Lilia had been in treatment for about four weeks and had recently had an NG tube placed.

REBECCA: So that's pretty unpleasant, I gather—the tube.

LILIA: Yeah, but what I'm worried about is, once I start eating, then I'm going to barf again. Because when I get full . . . Most people stop eating when they get full. When I get full, it triggers the urge to puke. So I'm really worried about that.

REBECCA: Are there opportunities to do that [purge] here? I know they try to keep an eye on things, but well, usually where there's a will, there's a way.

LILIA: I keep stuffing my snack in my pocket and tossing it in the lawn. And people have this vision that you'd have to go into the bathroom and hang your head over a toilet to puke. I can do it sitting up, in a baggie. But I've tried to be honest with them, I mean, because I'm not here to throw my money away. And I had a coffee cup in the closet there, and I've tried to puke in it twice since I've been here, but nothing came up. So, I guess that's a good sign.

REBECCA: I wonder why that is?

LILIA: I didn't eat very much. And, I mean, it's not the kind of food here that is easily upchuckable. [This latter point is true and by design.]

REBECCA: So, what was that like for you? To try to puke but not be able to?

LILIA: Frustrating. But I guess it's good. I do want to get better. I think I do, anyway.

As we can see, Lilia is quite ambivalent about her eating disorder and about treatment. She wants to purge, but she also wants to be honest; she thinks about how to get away with behaviors but is also nervous about getting the tube out because she is afraid she might feel triggered to return to her bulimia. In this case, treatment is both a safety measure and an obstacle. She continues:

LILIA: I just don't know that I really need to be here. I mean, I guess I do.

REBECCA: What do you mean?

LILIA: I don't know. It just seems like I should be able to be normal. Just eat like a normal person, you know? How hard can that be? It's so *basic*. But it's completely foreign to me. I've been doing this [having an eating disorder] for so long, I just don't know how else to be. I wonder sometimes if there's really any point to trying to get better.

So where do clients find the motivation to get better when they aren't sure they want to, or if they even can? Edie shared some of her thoughts on this struggle about four weeks into her treatment:

> EDIE: The restriction kicks in still. This morning, I was supposed to have an add-on on my breakfast. They didn't give it to me, and I didn't say a thing. And if there's stuff on my plate like garnish and stuff that we don't *have* to eat, I don't touch it. I've slept on my own [without sleep medication] three times I think since I've been here. And to be really honest, I'm also a self-harmer. And I've [had] trouble with scratching my arm, particularly when the community is so tense, like last night in community meeting, I couldn't deal with it. I couldn't handle it. So, I was scratching my arm. And the staff, whoever the staff member was, didn't notice. Or didn't say anything. And then I was homesick. I called home last weekend, a really long call. I sat there for two hours begging my husband to let me come home.

> REBECCA: So what does keep you here?

> EDIE: I think not wanting to disappoint my husband is the biggest thing right now. I don't have anything else to grab onto right now because I'm not yet in a place where I can say I really want to recover. So I have to look outside of it. I think about him, and you know, we do want a baby, we wanted that baby so bad and I lost it [had a miscarriage]. And I really want a family, and I do not want to lose that.

Edie says something really important here: "I have to look outside of it." This is a seemingly minor statement, and it's embedded in a lot of anxiety and ambivalence. But it actually indicates a critical step in the process of recovery, because it signals that Edie is beginning to be able to see that there *is* a reality "outside" of her eating disorder.

I can say from personal experience and from my research that when you are in the midst of an eating disorder, there is no "outside." The illness is all-encompassing, all-consuming. As we've seen, it takes over your brain, your body, your psyche, your affects, your sensations, and your thoughts; it controls how you move, how you feel, how you relate, how you process information, and how you understand the world and your place within it. It is, as I have been arguing throughout this book, a means and medium of presencing—and it feels like there is no life, no world, no existence without of it. So for Edie to be able to even imagine an "outside" of her eating disorder is an enormously significant step.

Edie also identifies something she wants more than she wants her eating disorder. In her case, this is a family. For others, it is a career, going to medical school, traveling, writing a book. For me, it was becoming an anthropologist and helping people better understand and treat these illnesses. When clients are able to connect with something outside of their eating disorders that gives them a sense of meaning and purpose, a means of *presencing*—this is where the kernel of recovery lies. Anita and Mallory recounted similar "pivot points" in their process. As Anita noted:

It's like I'm kind of at this stage where I know what my problem is, but I still have those negative thoughts. I just have to counteract them with positive ones. And so I just have to keep doing that. I don't want to be like this forever. I want to go to med school. I have wanted to go to med school for as long as I can remember, since I was a little kid. And there's no way I can do med school and be sick with an eating disorder. I know I can't. And I don't want to give up on that dream. I don't want my eating disorder to take that from me too. It's taken so much already. It can't have that also.

Mallory echoed this concern:

It feels different because I'm an adult now, and I signed myself in. I could choose to sign myself out. And it's like, I kind of feel proud of myself, in a way, because I have chosen to stay. But there was one night where I was like, "I am signing myself out in the morning. I hate it, I hate it, I hate it." Something my mom said to me on the phone is, "If you sign yourself out, you're letting your eating disorder win." And I was like, "Well, they [staff] can't control me. I'm in control." And she told me, "Well, why don't you use your control to your advantage, and use your control in a good way, by choosing to stay in treatment?" Which is what I did and what I'm going to try to continue to do.

I want to be very clear here, though, that recovery is not as simple as making a choice to get better. *Eating disorders are not a choice, and neither is recovery.* It is true that someone has to want to get better for recovery to be successful. But that is not *all* that is needed. It still takes months, if not years, of concentrated effort that must be supported by material, interpersonal, and emotional structures. Choosing to get well from an eating disorder is akin to choosing to run a marathon. You certainly won't run one by accident—your intention and dedication to it are absolutely critical. But that's just the *beginning,* not the *end,* of the process. And it has to be sustained for a long, long time—despite pain, possible injury, intense frustration, and even failure—for the desired outcome to happen. To reduce recovery to a client's "choice" not only radically minimizes the degree of difficulty and effort required but also completely evacuates the moral responsibility of the structures of care (both institutional and social) within which she is embedded.

Sometimes, what propels clients in recovery is so basic it's heartbreaking. It speaks to how excruciating living with an eating disorder actually is. This was clear in the response Karen gave when I asked what recovery meant to her:

> Just like, being able to go to a restaurant, and sit down, and enjoy something that you really like to eat. And carry on a conversation. And when you're full, and you get up and you leave the restaurant, and you don't go purge or think, "Oh God, I can't eat for two weeks." And to be able to just exist and not have your eating disorder with you all the time. Like, when you go to bed at night, not be dreading the next day. I guess that's what recovery is to me. It's having an inner peace. Something like that.

Gillian, a thirty-one-year-old woman diagnosed with bulimia, had a similar answer: "Recovery would just be being able to look forward to the day. Look forward to everyday activities. Look forward to normal activities and not have to plan the day around restricting and binging and purging. Be able to just do everyday things that people without eating disorders take for granted, that when you have an eating disorder, you can't do, because you're controlled by those thoughts."

Anita had this to say: "I just want to get a blizzard from Dairy Queen and not worry about it. Know that that's not going to make me gain weight, that one blizzard. Or if my friends go out for pizza to not order a salad or something. Because, really, I want the pizza and not the salad. So to be able to kind of be in the moment. To have a life, to not think about food all the time."

Bettina's vision of her life to come was quite positive: "I think life is going to be good. There is med school, there is art. I'm going to have my apartment, probably with a roommate, and I'm going to have a kitten, because I'm getting a kitten when I get back. It's going to be a little chocolate Persian. Depending on the personality, I think I might name it Cappuccino."

Jemma, too, was optimistic, but cautious: "I can be at this weight. I know I can do it. I just have to take the tools with me. Of course, I'm going to need a maintenance plan and stuff, or I can't do it, because I won't know how. But, I know that I can do it if I just try, and I have to believe that whether anybody else believes it or not."

While many clients expressed these kinds of hopes about their futures, they were not cavalier about recovery. Many of them still harbored deep fears and ambivalences about whether or not recovery was possible, and they still had to fight the eating disorder thoughts and urges moment to moment. As Julia noted, "That's what I'm hoping, that I'll be able to actually have hope and function in life and live the life that I want. But I don't know, because my eating disorder is so strong. I'm wanting to fight that fear of gaining weight, but it's so strong. I don't have the answer right now, but I know I have to keep going. Yet at the same time, I don't know how to handle that fight." Doubts are common, even when the desire for recovery is strong. This speaks to the continued struggle many clients feel about whether or not they are truly more powerful than their eating disorders.

Many of us have not had the experience of harboring something inside us that we fear may take over our lives at any moment, lying in weight to surge when we are not paying attention or when we are at our most vulnerable. It is a truly terrifying prospect for clients, and one that becomes even more so in the process of recovery, as they start to imagine and experience life without the eating disorder and become aware of just how deadly and destructive it is. And yet the eating disorder is familiar. It does offer a degree of safety, at least emotionally. The brain, body, emotions, and thoughts crave it sometimes, inviting in back in. Fighting it is a constant, relentless, exhausting battle.

LEARNING HOW TO FAIL BETTER

Simply cultivating a new sense of efficacy and new forms of directed intensity by investing in recovery is not enough. Most clients have years, if not decades, of eating disorder history behind them. Starving, bingeing, purging, using laxatives and diuretics, and/or overexercising have become their very modes of embodiment in the world. They have become fully entrained[3] to life with an eating disorder. It has come to regulate their senses, their thoughts, their affects, and their ways of being and relating. Even when someone is fully dedicated to recovery, it takes an extraordinary amount of deliberate practice to unlearn old physiological and emotional patterns and to learn new ones.

This rehabituating takes time, and time is the one thing most people don't have. As I've noted, at this point in the process, most clients have stabilized medically and may be at or near their goal weights. According to the medical model, they are "well," or at least well enough to discharge from treatment.

It is here that (re)lapse becomes a concern. In clinical parlance, a "lapse" occurs when a client temporarily returns to eating disorder behaviors but then gets back on track with recovery. A "relapse" is a full-blown descent back into the illness. In Frankfurt's terms (from chapter 8), we would say that a person experiencing a lapse remains an unwilling addict—she is able to hold onto recovery enough to re-engage in it before the eating disorder takes over completely. With a "relapse," however, the patient becomes a willing addict, turning back to the desire for the eating disorder (or, at least, the relative absence of the desire not to have it), and the eating disorder resumes control.

The simple truth is that people simply do not get better without lapsing or relapsing in some fashion at some point along the way. This may be as relatively minor as skipping part of a snack one day when the staff forgets an add-on (like Edie mentioned doing earlier in the chapter), or it may be as relatively major as binging and purging all afternoon when on a pass. Regardless, bumps and challenges are part and parcel of the process and are understood at Cedar Gove as not only natural but critical for getting better. This is because Cedar Grove clinicians believe that lapses and relapses provide instances of insight into the origins, triggers, and mechanisms of the eating disorder itself. They are seen as microcosms of the illness, mini-instances of how and why the eating disorder behaviors emerged and are sustained. They are invaluable in the larger process of long-term recovery.

What makes a lapse at this stage different from an active eating disorder is that clients in this part of recovery are expected to "present with increased honesty and accountability for their behaviors, urges, and thoughts" and to "openly process struggles both in individual sessions and group therapy," according to the Cedar Grove patient manual. That is, rather than being overwhelmed by a lapse and catapulted full on back into the disorder, they are scaffolded in how to use the lapse to better understand their condition and how to intervene to continue to move toward recovery.

Lapses tend to occur as the containment of the program eases. The clinic assesses a client's readiness for discharge by seeing what she does when she has time away from programming on passes (scheduled time away from treatment). As I've noted, the clinic positions itself as a sort of substitute family and developmental context. As treatment begins, clients are tightly swaddled in care, surveillance, and structure, and these limits are progressively loosened as clients progress through the program—they are afforded more flexibility, more independence, and less oversight. Toward the end of treatment, clients begin to take more and more passes away from the clinic to engage the various skills they have been learning (e.g., affect regulation, boundary-setting, distress tolerance) and practice managing food and eating on their own.

The clinic views passes somewhat like experiments. They are a way to see where a client is in her recovery and whether or not she is "ready" for additional freedoms. While on pass, does she eat her snack as she is supposed to? If not, does she report this to staff when she gets back, or do they only know this because her mom called or because her weight went down? Does she binge and purge while away from the clinic? Engage in self-harm? Spend the afternoon trying on her old size o clothes, becoming increasingly distraught? Anything and everything that happens on a pass gives the clinical team information about what a client is still struggling with and what kinds of supports she needs going forward.

If a client does engage in behaviors away from treatment, she is asked to fill out a "lapse packet," which consists of a series of questions meant to help her reflect on what happened and to learn from it constructively. "It's critical that we don't shame clients if they have a lapse," Brooke, a therapist, told me. "This disease is so shame-based already. And lapses are to be expected as part of the recovery process. We're not telling them that it's OK, but we need to engage it from a place of, 'Let's see what this can tell us about your eating disorder and where you are.'"

Managed care companies tend to see passes as experiments, too, but they view lapses in a very different light, as evidence of treatment "failure." A lapse or a relapse signals to them that treatment is not working and that the investment of healthcare dollars is not producing the expected returns.

There are, of course, different ways to respond to such "failure." Let's say I have an infection of some sort—pneumonia, for instance. I take a low dose of an antibiotic for two weeks, but the pneumonia remains. The treatment has failed (note that we do not say that *I* have failed antibiotic treatment, which is the language used when eating disorders treatment is unsuccessful). So how would the medical system react to this? The response, generally, would be to increase the dosage or try a different antibiotic. Certainly, it wouldn't be to just stop medication all together and then blame me if I remain ill. *But this is precisely what happens with eating disorders under the current conditions of managed care.* Occasionally, clients who lapse or relapse are moved to a higher level of care, but more often than not the opposite happens: their ability to access any care at all is put in jeopardy. "If three weeks in residential wasn't enough, what's to say that two more weeks will make the difference?" one case manager asked me as she was denying benefits for a client who, we discovered, had been skipping her afternoon snack when on pass. "Maybe she's just not ready to get better." In other words, the failure, this case manager was suggesting, was with the *client,* not with the proffered care.

Let me be clear: *Clients do not fail eating disorders treatment. Eating disorders treatment fails clients.*

In this case, I argued to the case manager that the client was still quite underweight, that she remained affectively dysregulated with significant anxiety, and that there were particular family dynamics that contributed to her eating disorder that were being addressed in family therapy. Discharge at this point, I pressed, would almost certainly lead to full relapse. None of this was persuasive to the case manager.

In situations like this, the utility of appealing to biological explanations for clients' behavior starts to become understandable. What finally made the difference in this case was the fact that the client had recently started a new anxiety medication that would hopefully make it easier for her to battle her eating disorder thoughts and urges. Medication changes were often useful for obtaining further treatment authorizations, and so I deployed this one deliberately. After much conversation with the case manager, the medication change enabled me to get the client approved for two more weeks of residential care.

This was a fairly straightforward case. As Suzanna's example shows, however, the situation is often much more complex.

SUZANNA

At the time of these events, Suzanna was twenty years old. She had been transferred to Cedar Grove directly from the hospital where she had been treated for kidney failure as a result of her bulimia. Prior to the hospitalization, Suzanna had been bingeing and purging for up to ten hours a day. She spent hundreds of dollars a week on binge food and, for the past year, had even been engaging in sex work to get money for her binges. She also engaged in self-harm and had scars on both forearms from years of self-inflicted razor blade cuts. She had a long history of depression and frequently felt suicidal, though she had never actually attempted to take her own life.

By the time she made it to Cedar Grove, Suzanna was distraught. She had been in the hospital for two weeks straight, and her urges to binge and purge were extremely high. She felt and acted like an addict desperate for a fix. She paced, shook, and couldn't concentrate because of intrusive thoughts about food. She was a wreck. Eventually, she figured out a way to purge in secret at the clinic, and she began to do so regularly. She was caught when Ziploc bags full of vomit were discovered hidden under her bed. Over the next several weeks, she continued to find new ways to purge, but she began to come to staff directly afterward to tell them what she had done and to process what had prompted the behavior. She participated in groups, saw her therapist, and took her medications. Gradually, although she still struggled with strong urges, Suzanna's episodes of purging began to decrease. She continued to be invested in treatment and began to develop new strategies for modulating her urges. At one point, three months into her treatment, she went seventeen days without bingeing or purging, the longest she had gone in over six years. She began, for the first time, to feel optimistic about the possibility of recovery, even though it still seemed distant.

It was at this point that Suzanna's insurance company determined that her condition was no longer "acute" and that she should be discharged from treatment. When Suzanna heard the news, she panicked. "I can't leave treatment!" she told me, sobbing. "I'm not ready! If I go out there, I know things will go back to the way they were. I can't go back to that life!" The evening of this decision, Suzanna purged for the first time in over two weeks. The following day, she spent the entire three hours of her pass binging and purging. She cut. She became suicidal. The Cedar Grove staff initiated three insurance appeals on Suzanna's behalf, all of which were denied. When pressed by Dr. Casey for an explanation, the insurance case manager eventually revealed that the company had determined that Suzanna was "borderline" (i.e., she had borderline personality disorder, or BPD) and because, in his words, "You can't treat borderlines," they were no longer authorizing coverage.

CONCEPTUAL DYSFUNCTION

Let me pause here to consider in more detail what, precisely, was being communicated between the insurance case manager and Dr. Casey in this interaction. The care manager maintained that Suzanna was no longer eligible for care because, prior to the insurance denial, her acute symptoms of binging and purging had abated. In his view, the cessation of symptoms marked the end of the present episode of her eating disorder. Whatever difficulties remained, he suggested, were due to an underlying, chronic personality disorder, which he deemed to be outside the scope of the managed care company's treatment purview, primarily because "you can't treat borderlines"—that is, the company's view is that there is little evidence-based research on which to design standardized treatment interventions for this condition. Ignoring for the moment that this is factually untrue (there is actually quite substantial literature on the efficacy of dialectical behavior therapy for treating BPD), what the care manager seemed to be communicating is that he recognized that Suzanna was not "well" but did not consider her sick *enough*—or rather, not sick enough in the *right way*—to warrant further care. Because BPD is traditionally considered to be a chronic, lifelong condition (as opposed to an "episodic" condition, like an eating disorder is construed to be), Suzanna could presumably do nothing about it. Once a borderline, always a borderline. Given managed care's privileging of the role of rational choice in achieving health, treating someone with BPD—who is viewed as having an explicit absence of rational choice—*for* BPD made little sense to this particular case manager.

The Cedar Grove clinicians strenuously disagreed. The cessation (while in treatment) of Suzanna's eating disorder symptoms did yet not represent, in their view, an authentic shift in Suzanna's state of being. She was simply contained. If they could keep Suzanna engaged in recovery, they argued, she could continue to get better. But if, as the managed care company insisted, treatment support was withdrawn prematurely and Suzanna was not treated for these more chronic, underlying issues, she was doomed to relapse.

The conflict here between the managed care company and Cedar Grove has to do with different assessments of Suzanna's agentic efficacy (both past and potential) in her recovery and the models of authenticity on which such assessments are based. Both the managed care company and Cedar Grove agreed that Suzanna had worked hard to gain control of her self-destructive behaviors and cease binging and purging in treatment. Both agreed that she exercised constructive, self-preserving agency in this regard. They had differing views, however, on whether this process is seen as contiguous with working through the psychological and emotional issues underlying those behaviors and whether that even matters.

By characterizing Suzanna as borderline (and therefore "untreatable"), the managed care company's case manager was asserting that the two are not contiguous but rather that they entail different sorts of processes with different likelihoods of success. Suzanna's eating disorder symptoms had improved, bringing her actions more in line with the value of health as self-preservation. From a *procedural* standpoint, which is the position endorsed by the managed care company, Suzanna had developed new capacities for autonomous action vis-à-vis her eating disorder, and treatment was therefore a success.

From an *epistemic* viewpoint, however, which is that held by Cedar Grove, the fact that Suzanna's significant psychological difficulties persisted even though her eating disorder symptoms decreased indicated precisely the opposite—that treatment was not even *complete,* let alone a success. In fact, an increase in other symptoms is often to be expected when the coping mechanism of the eating disorder subsides. The Cedar Grove clinicians argued that Suzanna's eating disorder *was* contiguous with these other difficulties and objected to the procedural view that behavior consistent with an ideal of health necessarily indicated an endorsement of that ideal. They contended that while healthy behaviors are important, they should not be taken to indicate a fundamental shift in a client's ability to embrace self-preservation but must instead be viewed with caution and within a more long-term understanding of the recovery process as difficult and often full of setbacks.

BORDERLINE TALK AND THE ETHICAL AMBIGUITIES OF CARE

The managed care company's denial of coverage for Suzanna posed a real dilemma for the Cedar Grove treatment team in terms of what to do next. They were confronted with a client who was rapidly deteriorating, yet they could not continue to effectively treat her. Although many of Suzanna's behaviors were consistent with BPD (e.g., bingeing and purging, cutting, mood swings), the question of whether she had the condition had never been a focus of clinical concern. She came to Cedar Grove with a raging, tenacious eating disorder, severe depression, and difficulty living day to day, and treatment had primarily focused on these issues. Yet clinicians could not entirely dispute the insurance company's assessment. Suzanna *did* engage in self-harm. She *did* have problems with impulse control and *did* act erratically. All of these are possible indicators of BPD. In fact, the very symptoms the treatment team asserted as evidence that Suzanna needed continued treatment served only to further support the insurance company's diagnosis of BPD and their denial of coverage. "We're stuck," said Kelly, Suzanna's therapist, in a treatment team meeting. "This is a no-win situation." How, they wondered, should they proceed ethically in this situation?

What happened next seems puzzling at first glance. Although the Cedar Grove staff still vehemently opposed the insurance company's position, over the next several days (as the insurance appeals were playing out) I noticed that in everyday conversation they began talking about Suzanna in new ways. In fact, it seemed that clinical discussions about her symptoms involved a sort of doubling. When Suzanna increased her bingeing and purging after the insurance denial, clinicians viewed it (as before) as evidence of an ongoing, raging eating disorder. But they were increasingly discussing these behaviors with an edge of suspicion, as if it were part of a manipulative strategy on Suzanna's part to circumvent the insurance decision by appearing "sick enough" to warrant continued care.

Now, one might wonder (as I did) why Suzanna would have to *try* to look "sick enough" for care if, as the treatment team agreed, she was nowhere near ready for discharge. When I asked about this, Kelly, Suzanna's therapist, explained that the problem was that Suzanna "needed to feel attached and dependent on us" and, as a result, was unable to accept the insurance decision without becoming unhinged. This, in Kelly's estimation, meant that Suzanna's symptoms were, indeed, more a product of her *personality issues* (e.g., BPD) than her *bulimia* per se. As Suzanna's symptoms increased, so did this sort of "borderline talk" among the clinicians. When Suzanna returned late from a pass because she had been out purging, or when she told staff she was feeling suicidal, I began to hear comments in the clinical area like, "Now you're really seeing that borderline part of her," and, "That's her borderline side coming out."

Why would these clinicians appropriate in such an apparently uncritical way the very language deployed by the view they opposed? I want to be clear that I am not arguing that the insurance company exerted some sort of hegemonic influence over clinicians' opinions of Suzanna's illness. And I do not think the clinicians' assessments of Suzanna's symptoms actually radically changed. What *did* change, though, is the degree of clarity the team had about what constituted, for *them*, ethical treatment for Suzanna, and this is where "borderline talk" emerged as important. Clearly, Suzanna was on a self-destructive rampage. Clearly, she needed further treatment. And clearly, her insurance company would not pay for it. Suzanna and her family did not have the resources to pay out of pocket, so she had no other options. From what I saw, the borderline talk in Suzanna's case—and in several others

I followed—became a way for clinicians to work through the ethical imperatives of care in a no-win situation.

Specifically, borderline talk engages the conflicts between procedural and epistemic authenticity in a singular, if disturbing, way—by rendering epistemic authenticity itself impossible. If Suzanna's behavior is construed as manipulative in large part precisely *because* she has been identified (based on her BPD and eating disorder diagnoses) as a manipulator, then it becomes difficult for the clinical team to *ever* perceive her as acting authentically, regardless of her actual motivations. In a context where authenticity (procedural, epistemic, or both) is understood as foundational to autonomy and psychological health, this rendering of Suzanna as *incapable* of epistemic authenticity—because she is thought to have no authentic self from which to act—configures her as largely outside the purview of reasonable clinical intervention. It therefore upholds an evaluation of her treatment based on her outward actions alone. Under such circumstances, it becomes not only acceptable but also *ethical* to discharge her from treatment until and unless she is prepared to invest in her own care, with the burden for demonstrating this readiness now resting squarely on her.

We can see how, in cases like Suzanna's, invoking borderline talk enables a provisional resolution of the authenticity problem by rendering any reliable subjectivity at all unattainable for a given client. This, of course, requires clinicians to negate the very thing they claim legitimates their existence as trained professionals—the self as an entity deserving of care. At the same time, this practice affirms and supports the ends of managed care organizations. In this regard, we might be tempted to conclude that clinical processes are co-opted in the classic work of ideology, which conceals its effects and persuades participants to advocate for their own subjection. And indeed, one interpretation could be that, through borderline talk, the philosophical and ethical incoherence of the American healthcare system becomes displaced onto individual clients, who then carry the symptom of the system—it is *the client,* not the practitioners or the healthcare industry, who is rendered fragmented, conflicted, and incapable of decisive action.

But what goes on at the clinic is more than just a simple machination of ideology. The clinicians I worked with are in many ways quite aware of these dynamics and work actively to resist them in all sorts of ways all the time in how they chart or in how they report information to (or withhold it from) insurance companies. Yet the positioning of the clinic within the American healthcare landscape complicates the pathways of ethical action open to them.

In this regard, these clinicians are not simply interpolated by managed care ideology. Nor are they always successfully resisting it. Rather, by brokering plural ideologies of the subject, they become active participants in redefining the boundaries and meanings of "eating disorders," at least in this clinic and with these clients. In the process, they affirm an understanding of themselves as ethical professionals who remain instrumental in the project of healing.

What does all of this have to do with processes of reconnecting? I offer Suzanna's story here as a way of illustrating how disruptions and disconnections in the broader system of care get read back onto patients as evidence of their own *personal* dysfunction in ways that then legitimate the *withholding of care* as an ethical treatment response. Clients must therefore devise ways of working around these dynamics while trying to reconnect to a life outside the eating disorder. To do this, they must become expert tinkerers.

TINKERING AND THE MODULATED SELF

In her study of gambling and gambling addiction in Las Vegas, anthropologist Natasha Dow Schüll argues that addiction and therapeutic interventions for addiction coexist within the same circuits, as both gambling machines and therapy practices "gear their interventions around a model of the self as an ever-changing configuration of behavioral potentials responsive to external modulation."[4] That is, there is an "unexpected resonance of . . . technologies and techniques" in how gambling machines and therapy interventions understand the subject to which they are directed.[5] Specifically, both bank on the proposition that anything can addict and anyone can become addicted, though they position themselves on opposite sides of this phenomenon (those who create gambling machines purportedly want people to become addicted to them, whereas those involved in the therapy industry want to treat addiction). At the same time, as Schüll points out, the mere existence of gambling machines and gambling addiction materially supports the industry of gambling addiction therapy, creating something of an uneasy alliance. And this alliance cultivates a particular kind of subject, one who "should vigilantly *manage* themselves."[6]

What Schüll is getting at here is the synergy between addiction and treatment in the kind of subject they create and, indeed, require: a subject who is forever modulating, tinkering with, and fine-tuning her experience through the use of technologies—material technologies, like gambling machines, or practical technologies, like CBT and other therapies. Such an orientation is consistent with Nicolas Rose's vision of the "active and responsible citizen" who "must engage in a never-ending monitoring of health," "a constant process of modulation, adjustment, and improvement."[7]

In this way, Schüll notes, recovery techniques are borrowed from a more general set of self-making tools, shaping an "ethics" of the self[8] where there is "an economy of adjustment rather than abstinence; compensation rather than commitment; maintenance rather than transformation."[9] That is, rather than working to maximize quality of life as in an entrepreneurial selfhood model, recovery produces "not a consumer sovereign who masterfully pursues a pristine, coherent, and unconflicted set of desires, but a subject whose desires constantly shift in response to environmental feedback, and who constantly recalibrates action in relation to those shifting desires—modulating action not to *maximize* but to *maintain.*"[10] In this way, Schüll argues, the predicament of compulsive machine gamblers "offers clues to aspects of normative neoliberal subjectivity that analyses framed solely on models of entrepreneurial selfhood miss."[11]

Taking these insights into Cedar Grove, I wish to make two points. First, we can see that both the medical model and the recovery model embrace the notion of an entrepreneurial self who seeks to maximize health. While they differ on which strategies should be employed to get there (e.g., the medical model advocates techniques of control, whereas the recovery model promotes techniques of "letting go") and on what the trajectory of the process should look like (the medical model sees the path as linear, while the recovery model views it as cyclical), both constitute a recovering patient-subject who is agentic, self-directed, and supremely responsible for the self. Yet in both models, there is a parallel recognition that the patient-subject is always already an adulterated subject, one who is impaired, "sick," and incapable of self-care. This places patients in a situation where they are expected to be self-directing and responsible, but where their efforts in this direction (coming, as they do, from an impaired subject) are discounted, undermined, or pathologized. I will take this up in more detail in chapter 11. Here, suffice it to say that the ambivalences and double binds that emerge at Cedar Grove resonate with Schüll's observations about the injunctions to entrepreneurial selfhood and the problems with this formulation.

Specifically, the kind of "tinkering," "modulating" self that Schüll identifies takes on particular significance in the context of eating disorders. We will remember that people with eating disorders are often described as being obsessed with control and that a key dynamic in the treatment setting is to induce clients to give up this control to the clinical team. How, then, does this sit with the kinds of expectations of entrepreneurial selfhood contained in both the medical and recovery models?

Schüll's analysis suggests that close attention to modulation and maintenance becomes an avenue of development that is often missed by theorists of entrepreneurial selfhood, and this is an excellent insight. Indeed, despite the entrepreneurial ethos of the medical and recovery models, this tinkering/ modulating practice is what is foregrounded in the eating disorders clinic. Weights and labs are tinkered with through changes to a client's meal plan or medications. Mood is tinkered with through the use of pharmaceuticals. Behavior is tinkered with through the deployment of rewards and punishments. Clients, who used their eating disorders as their primary tinkering tool before coming to the clinic, learn to adopt new tools over time: they are mentored in how to track their urges and behaviors, keep food logs, chart their moods, and keep track of their medications. In this way, the self as responsible for itself remains a primary ethos, and the self that is exquisitely attuned to minutia and ready to act to maintain balance is the most valued.

Yet clients are told that the desire to control is part of their illness. It is Ed. Wanting to control themselves so extensively is evidence of pathology. We can see, then, the hair's breadth line that separates ill clients from clients enacting an "ideal subjectivity." When I asked Brooke, a Cedar Grove therapist, how clients should navigate this apparent predicament, she said, "Well, it's a different sort of control. You can feel the difference. From the outside, I mean, and maybe from the inside. Ideally from the inside, too. Eventually. There's a different sort of energy around control that's pathological and control that's part of recovery." When I asked her to elaborate, she explained, "Control that's pathological is motivated by anxiety or fear. Fear of the unknown, fear of the unexpected. It's a kind of clamping down. Control that comes from a healthy place is motivated by a desire for life beyond the eating disorder. It's more of an opening up." This is a real, if extremely nuanced, distinction, and the degree to which clients can reliably master the "right" kind of control during their brief time in the clinic is dubious at best.

In Suzanna's case, control holds an ambiguous place. On the one hand, she is construed as being entirely out of control in terms of her behaviors, which include bingeing, purging, crying, and pleading). This is viewed by the insurance company and clinicians alike as problematic—she is demonstrating her "failure" in treatment by engaging in them. She *should* be able to control herself, but she is not doing so. On the other hand, her attempts to *exert* control over her own treatment course and its outcome are viewed as manipulative, as an indication that she is overstepping her bounds, and *also* as evidence of her failure in treatment. Suzanna is faulted for simultaneously not exerting *enough* control and exerting *too much* control. The only appropriate expression of control in this case would be for Suzanna to demonstrate a certain kind of docility by abiding by treatment limits and accepting insurance company decisions without complaint or push back. Clinicians find themselves in a bit of a bind here, too, as they both accept the premise that clients should abide by limits and also recognize that insurance companies make decisions that don't have the clients' best interests at heart. It is here that strategies such as borderline talk emerge, as they enable clinicians to transpose the ethical question into a clinical one and justify the withdrawal of care as a form of best practice.

Clinicians, then, have a range of strategies available to them for navigating these contradictions. But how do clients experience and make sense of these tensions? Clients, as I've noted, are often acutely ambivalent about whether or not they are deserving of care, which in turn impacts their desires or hopes for recovery. Most articulate a deep, profound longing for a life free of torment and struggle. And make no mistake—living with an eating disorder is absolute torture. But so is living with overwhelming anxiety, desperation, panic, trauma, and soul-crushing depression. And that's what often awaits clients when the eating disorder subsides, at least at first. Simply expecting clients to "choose to get well" without addressing the underlying causes and conduits of the eating disorder is completely unrealistic and exculpates moral responsibility for the kind of responsive care that is necessary for this to occur. Often, clients are left to figure these dilemmas out on their own, and this leads them to deploy strategies that can reinforce characterizations of eating disorder clients as manipulative, resistant, and difficult.

WHAT *DOES* HELP: REVIVING CONNECTIONS

I've known what recovery is. I know that the first time I went inpatient that [it] was probably the most effective thing. That was just due to the other people there, and their attitude, and making connections with them. I think that's what's most important, is being able to make a connection with whoever's trying to help you. Not feeling judged by them and not feeling that they're treating you as an eating disorder instead of a person. For me, that's really, really important. And that's like Trudy here, and Brooke, and there's others, but particularly those two. You can tell them anything.

—THERESA,
a thirty-two-year-old woman diagnosed with bulimia

Many things help in the process of recovery: structure, programming, skilled clinicians, adequate facilities—all of these are important. But by far the most important thing clients pointed to as making a difference in their recoveries were the connections they built with caregivers.

As Kennedy explained, the fact that the Cedar Grove program could be individualized to a given patient's needs and that services were delivered with compassion were two of the most important dimensions:

> This is the first treatment center [where] I felt like it wasn't just a job to people [i.e., staff], that they actually care. And that support has helped me to stay here, because with the refeeding and everything, it's so hard. I would just want to flee and go back to my eating disorder. But this place gives me some hope. And even the nutritionists here, it's hard with the increases, and I know I battle with Nadia, but Nadia wants to sit down and take the time and talk to you. If I needed it, she would spend an hour with me. At other places, nutritionists never talk to you. They just said, "You're getting an increase, that's it."

Even though, as I've noted, clients did not always feel that they were seen, heard, and respected as human beings, they emphasized the importance of this kind of intersubjective recognition, and many pointed to it as a critical component of their recovery. Anita noted, "Usually, I feel like my voice is actually acknowledged and heard here and it's OK to use my voice. In my past, I was too scared to voice anything for fear of the reaction. But I feel safe here expressing myself, and I feel that it's OK to give my opinion and that there's nothing wrong with me, as a person. And people will actually listen and take time to consider my feelings or my thoughts. I feel like a human being."

Darcy shared a similar sentiment: "You feel that you can—when you have you have a problem or a struggle, you can go and tell somebody. Because you're just not going to get punished. You're going to get that support. You're going to get, 'OK, what's really going on here?' It's not just taking away privileges and things like that. It's, 'OK, you're struggling. It's OK to struggle. You're going have those slips and falls.' But then it's, 'Let's look and learn from them. What we can do differently?'"

In a conversation with Edie just before she was discharged, I asked her what she had found the most helpful in her treatment at Cedar Grove. She replied,

> I think actually talking to the program director and Dr. Casey in person and seeing how knowledgeable they are and how kind they are. They really seem to

care, and what they say makes sense. I think that that was a big thing for me. I don't feel like I'm just a number going through. That and then some of the staff members have been really awesome. Claire, I love Claire. And Denise and Amelia. They're really good, and I like them. And I have found the groups here much more helpful than either time at [another treatment facility]. They're trying to teach us these different strategies and different techniques. And they're so knowledgeable about the different techniques. Even the nutritional groups—they approach in a much deeper way. I just get a lot more out of them.

In short, the sense of personal connection clients felt at Cedar Grove was the single most important thing they pointed to in keeping them invested in recovery through their most challenging times.

Clinicians attributed the relationships they built with clients to Cedar Grove's relatively small size, its residential (versus hospital-based) setting, and the expertise and personal investment of the staff. Dr. Casey, in particular, was hugely influential for many clients, who saw her as a highly knowledgeable and deeply compassionate professional whom they (almost) uniformly trusted to have their best interests at heart, even when they didn't always like what she was telling them. Although Dr. Casey was the head of the clinic (and therefore very busy), she was involved in the day-to-day running of the program, got to know each client personally, and served as a role model for clients that would be difficult to replicate in a more sterile or less personal environment.

CLIENTS' IDEAL TREATMENT

Toward the ends of their stays, I asked clients to imagine an ideal eating disorders treatment scenario. Kelsey's answer sums up the general sentiments they expressed:

I think more understanding and sympathy and care from the staff, like what I've experienced here. I would not want it to be like [another treatment center,] where the staff was really cold, and even when you left, the staff members weren't even allowed to hug you, or if you were having a bad day, to show any feelings towards you.

I think that helps a lot to know that people care and that they're just not watching you and it's not just a job. And if they speak harshly with you it's not your fault—eating disorders can be manipulative, so they still have to be on guard and not let everybody get away with things that some people do.

I think everybody should have individualized treatment because every-body has different circumstances. Treatment centers do have to be cautious of being too accommodating with some people. But I think a lot of times treat-ment centers just use a certain mold of how they treat patients. And that's not exactly effective with everybody.

I also think that there should be more compassion and not so much focus on the weight, because that's not the real issue. I believe that taking it slower and really working on the real issues is what's going to help. But unfortu-nately, insurance companies aren't going to go for that. And I'm not saying—obviously you cannot lose weight or maintain the same weight. You have to be gaining. But some places require three or four pounds a week. That's just typically very uncomfortable. It takes time to heal, and they say the last piece to get better is your body image, but then so much the focus of a treatment is gaining weight when that's not really the problem.

I'm sick of seeing girls come back to different places and not get the right treatment. I think there needs to be better awareness about things and how to treat this.

As Kelsey's reflections make clear, building these sorts of therapeutic rela-tionships necessitates personal and individualized care that makes the client feel "more like a person than a patient." It is within such caring but profes-sional relationships that clients begin to learn how to presence without their eating disorders.

REFLECTIONS

The alternative affective practices presented to clients (e.g., mindfulness, dis-tress tolerance, using words to express feelings) take time to develop and perfect. Even when they "work," they are not as immediate as bingeing and purging or restricting for managing affective states, so getting client buy-in is often difficult. But more than this, these alternative affective practices do not exist in a vacuum—while they might "work" in theory, in practice they unfold within relationships and institutional structures that call forth the very kinds of affects that eating disorders emerge to attenuate in the first place. While clients might be persuaded to reach for alternative strategies for managing these feelings, the feelings themselves (e.g., the sense being unwor-thy of care, desperation, acute anxiety) are continually reproduced within the treatment context itself. And even when clients do engage alternative strate-gies, assumptions about clients' propensities for manipulation lead clinicians to view their behaviors with skepticism and suspicion. Clients become caught in a situation wherein the conditions for an eating disorder are perpetuated and even heightened while alternatives for successfully navigating these conditions are diluted or thwarted.

This generates and is generated by what I call *affective recursions,* which amplify themes of deprivation and scarcity across multiple levels, from the physiological to the interpersonal to the institutional. I take this up in the following section.

Looking for the Exit

DECEMBER 1987

A deep, painful, bone-chilling coldness inches up my thighs as my knees grind into the bathroom's concrete floor, deep in the bowels of the Burton-Judson Courts basement, my dorm at the University of Chicago. I try in vain to force out the food I have shamefully just consumed. How much extra was it? God, I don't even know. That's how pathetic I am. I don't even know how much extra I ate. I just know that I have to get it *out*. Why won't it come out? Other people can purge. I can't even do this right.

I know my friends are concerned. They watch me at meals, worry etched on their faces as they assure me that what I've chosen to eat looks reasonable and is not "too much." I have no sense of that at all. I used to know exactly how much I was getting. But restricting like that is not feasible anymore. Not that I don't want to, but my body is in full rebellion. Bodies do that, eventually. They eat whether you want them to or not. I think it is the last desperate, flailing gasp of a starving organism before it dies. And I might still die, one way or another. I haven't decided yet.

Yesterday, I bought the pills.

Recursions

In section 3, we looked at the processes of unmooring, recalibration, and reconnection and the kinds of tensions and frictions produced in the context of managed care. In this section, I consider how relationships of care in the clinic are structured by economic priorities and what kinds of implications this has for the constitution of eating disorders—and eating disorder patients—as objects of concern.

Cedar Grove, as we have seen, is a particular kind of affective institution that attends to and shapes the affective lives of people within it. Its job is to change, regulate, modulate, inspire, corral, channel, and transform clients' troubling affects, emotions, and sensory experiences into health-seeking and health-promoting ones. It is designed to do so *in and through* the affective and emotional labor of Cedar Grove clinicians and staff and the relationships of care they build. In everyday life in the clinic, affects circulate, accumulate, become blocked, or get diverted in relations between and among people (between clients and clients, clients and clinicians, and clinicians and clinicians), literally constituting the boundaries of health and illness as people engage in the communal life of the clinic. I argued in chapter 3 that eating disorders—and recovery from them—are *affective practices* in Margaret Wetherell's sense of the term, constituting and reshaping clients' affective subjectivities through everyday embodied engagements.[1]

But this affective recalibrating does not happen in a vacuum. It happens under the conditions of American managed mental healthcare, in which themes of scarcity, deprivation, and deservedness prevail, settling into and animating practices, interactions, and interventions. By threading themes of scarcity, deprivation, and withholding through these various levels, both eating disorders and processes of recovery in Cedar Grove draw on similar foundational logics, even as they purportedly enact divergent modes of being. Understanding the shared logics of eating disorders and managed care, as well as the various different ends to which they unfurl, allows us to better understand the ambiguities and contradictions at stake in everyday practice in the clinic and the kinds of improvisations clinicians and clients must make in attempting to navigate them.

TEN

Running on Empty

RELATIONSHIPS OF CARE IN A
CULTURE OF DEPRIVATION

"I relapsed, Rebecca."

Anita slouched on the couch, as if it took too much effort to hold herself upright. I had first met Anita the previous summer, when she was in treatment at Cedar Grove for the first time. Now she was back. Looking at me forlornly, she slowly moved aside the long gray-blue sweater that had been wrapped around her body. I swallowed hard, trying not to show my reaction. Even through her leggings I could see the full outline of Anita's pelvic bones. Her stomach was so shrunken in that she seemed to almost disappear into the couch. Her ribs jutted forward as if straining to break free of her skin. After over twenty years of working in the field of eating disorders, I had seen many people with anorexia, and I was quite accustomed to the physical manifestations of extreme starvation. But something about seeing Anita that day shocked me out of my habituated orientation, as if I'd been doused with a bucket of ice water. I saw anew what this illness does to people, what it takes from them, the shell that is left behind.

My gaze met hers. "Rebecca, I'm sorry," she said, and her eyes filled with tears. "I tried to stay healthy, I really did." Her voice pleaded for me to believe her. "I don't know what happened. I didn't mean for it to get this bad." I sat down on the couch next to her and held her hand while she wept.

Talking about this incident later that afternoon with Claire, one of the clinic nurses, I voiced my feelings about seeing Anita back in treatment and expressed my concern for her well-being. To my surprise, Claire let out a snort and rolled her eyes. "Oh please," she said. "Don't you see what she was doing? She was totally *manipulating* you, trying to get you to feel sorry for her because she's so sick. You can't validate that. It's exactly what she wants."

I found this comment perplexing, and the more I thought about it, the thornier the issue appeared. There was no question that Anita was—literally—deathly ill. But Claire maintained that the fact that Anita wanted (or maybe needed) acknowledgement of her suffering and the fact that she solicited it through an appeal to the consequences of her illness were aspects of the very same illness that was causing her suffering. In such a scenario, Claire was telling me, explicitly *not* acknowledging Anita's suffering therefore constituted some sort of care. Under what conditions does "care" come to mean the explicit withholding of a response to suffering?

In this chapter, I use the cases of Anita and others to explore how relationships of care in the clinic materialize—and elide—different ways of being for both patients and clinicians. This is an interpersonal and intersubjective process that has deep historical roots and proceeds within the current structures of quantification, rationing, and deprivation produced in the managed care system. My goal is to think through how relationships of care and a culture of withholding coexist and to explore the kinds of frictions, foreclosures, and erasures this creates.

I begin with some words about becoming a Cedar Grove clinician and what kinds of skills are necessary to work successfully in this context. I then turn to what I call "halo features"—the elements outside the bounds of the official diagnostic criteria that help clinicians determine what they think is "wrong" with a client. This leads into a discussion of transference and countertransference, or the ways affective responses to—and from—clients shape clinical assessments. I end with a discussion of two commonly recognized "problems" in eating disorders treatment—manipulation and noncompliance—and use these to demonstrate how particular kinds of agency—the socioculturally mediated capacity to act[1]—for clients are produced while others are foreclosed.

THE "GOOD ENOUGH" CLINICIAN

Eating disorders hinge on paradoxes.

They are about being seen and known but also disappearing from view. They are about feelings of strength and control but also of helplessness and hopelessness. They are about independence and self-determination as well as inextricable interdependence and feelings of deep indebtedness. They are about assertiveness and aggression as well as supplication and submission.

Understanding these paradoxes is critical to treating these conditions. Yet they can be confusing and even maddening for clinicians, and working with eating disorders requires special kinds of training and capacitation. Only a small portion of this skill base comes from book-type learning, which is accessible to anyone who cares to put in the time and effort to do it. Anyone, after all, can learn about electrolyte imbalances and BMI. The vast bulk of this skill set has to do with things that are much less tangible but significantly more important, including, principally, the ability to sit with ambiguity, to navigate multilayered interpersonal dynamics, and to manage one's own internal affective life.

How do clinicians learn these skills, and how do they put them in practice? Some of these skills may come naturally or from their own lived experiences; others are learned through extensive training and experience. People are drawn to different kinds of work for a variety of reasons. While some direct care staff at Cedar Grove are there primarily because they are fulfilling practicum requirements for a social work or counseling degree, most work in the eating disorders field because they have a specific interest in and passion for working with this population. That may come from having had a personal experience with an eating disorder (themselves or a loved one), or they may have chosen this field simply because, as one staff member told me, it "is among the most complex and challenging issues to work with because it crosses so many different domains—biological, psychological, interpersonal, family. It's a whole person-in-context kind of thing. That makes it interesting."

Wherever they begin in terms of their skill base, staff must be deeply committed to working with eating disorders if they are to become "good" clinicians. Maintaining a consistent "therapeutic" attitude with eating disorder clients requires special skill, and the challenges are many. Good eating disorder clinicians cultivate a unique blend of patience, capacity for attunement, healthy suspicion, solid personal boundaries, relevant medical knowledge, self-awareness, warmth, openness, humor, and a tough skin. They have to be able to deal with emaciation, feeding tubes, and vomit; people who panic at being touched; people desperate to be seen but just as desperate to disappear; people who want attention 24–7 and others who won't give you the time of day; perfectionism; blatant disregard for rules and limits; attempts at splitting (pitting staff or clients against each other); and gossip and critique. They are yelled at, pleaded with, sought out for comfort, and singled out for ridicule. They are the targets of rage and the butt of jokes. They are sources of support and sometimes the objects of clutching attachment. They are rivals and friends. They are the person with whom clients enact their most profound and debilitating attachment difficulties. And they have to remain grounded and adept enough to provide a safe "holding environment"[2] for all of this to unfold. Over time, skilled eating disorder clinicians develop a particular sensitivity, not only to explicit eating disorder behaviors but also to other features thought to be associated with them.

HALO FEATURES

As we saw in chapter 4, diagnostic criteria, insurance coverage, and best practices research are three critical components of how clinicians learn to see and think about what is "wrong" with the patient. But these are not fully determinative. Equally important are the kinds of affective responses clinicians themselves have to different patients and what these are believed to tell clinicians about patients' ongoing struggles.

Danielle, a Cedar Grove therapist, described this space on the underside of diagnosis:

> You get a feel for people after you do this job for a while. There are many different flavors of eating disorders—not just anorexia versus bulimia or binge eating disorder. No two people with anorexia are exactly alike. They may have similar issues in some ways, but [the issues] are deeply embedded in how they are in the world. It's not just about food. The food reflects how they manage themselves interpersonally. It's really about relationships. How they relate can tell you a lot about what they're dealing with and what the eating disorder is about for them.

In other words, diagnosis goes only so far, and clinicians believe their affective and interpersonal engagements with clients tell them at least as much about what the client's struggles are as do disordered eating behaviors or measuring changes in weight or lab results.

But this alternative "gut wisdom" approach can also lead to significant frictions. The American managed healthcare system privileges behavioral factors and biometric data in diagnosing and treating eating disorders, and these factors have a direct effect on whether or not treatment is allowed to continue. Under such regimes, a clinician's "feel" for a client is deemed much less important than what the client's lab results say or whether her weight is moving. Yet these feelings are what enable clinicians to connect with clients and help them engage in recovery, although it also opens clinicians up to interpersonal struggles and pushback from clients. Clinicians, then, consider their interpersonal relationships with clients to be both critically important and structurally devalued, and their affective investments in clients to be both vitally necessary and personally and professionally risky.

To navigate demands that they be both emotionally *available to* clients and emotionally *protected from* them, clinicians often draw on their own personal reactions to clients—what we might variously call "countertransference," "clinical intuition," "expertise," or "gut feelings"—in sorting through ethical dilemmas.

Critical to this process are what I call "halo features," those features—like manipulation, difficulty with interpersonal boundaries, or a focus on control—that flicker at the edges of official eating disorder diagnostic criteria but are not part of clinical definitions. Halo features allow clinicians a degree of flexibility in where they draw the boundaries of "pathology" for a given client in a given situation, as these features enable them to lump certain things together as part of the illness while excluding others as they see fit. Whether and how they do this depends on the particular interpersonal relationships at play as well as the set of circumstances involved.

Importantly, halo features are identified in and through a therapist's own intersubjective sense of the client and the situation. In the case of eating disorders, the way that halo features are identified and engaged allows clinicians to regulate their own emotional closeness and distance with clients while figuring such responses as caring acts dictated by the nature of the illness itself.

CLINICIANS' COUNTERTRANSFERENCE RESPONSES TO CLIENTS WITH EATING DISORDERS

In some ways, the claims on eating disorder clinicians are similar to those made on people working in mental health more generally. But there are special considerations in working with eating disorder patients. Although the presenting problem of an eating disorder may be one of not eating, bingeing, and/or purging, an eating disorder is thought to comprise much more than these specific behavioral components. It encompasses a person's way of affectively engaging with the world, both in terms of her own inner being and her relationships with others. What this means practically is that dynamics such as connection, attachment, relatedness, and attunement are precisely the arenas where people with eating disorders struggle to make their way in the world and therefore need the most concentrated therapeutic attention. This makes any sort of interpersonal engagement in the treatment context both challenging and potentially transformative.

In psychotherapeutic terms, the ways of relating that a client brings with her to the therapeutic relationship generate *transference,* meaning that she transfers her ways of being-in-the-world into the therapeutic dynamic (and transfers feelings and expectations from specific significant others onto the therapist), recreating experiences of interpersonal communication and affective bonds she has experienced elsewhere. Therapeutically speaking, transference in and of itself is a good—or at least productive—thing; it is seen as essential in doing the therapeutic work because it creates within the therapy something of a parallel to the client's lived experiences in the outside world, which can then be explored and understood within the holding frame of the therapy relationship.

In a milieu model, such as that used at Cedar Grove—one that views the whole clinic as the site of therapeutic action (versus just therapy sessions or groups)—transference not only occurs between a client and her individual therapist but also happens on a variety of levels all at the same time: with the individual therapist, to be sure, but also with direct care staff, nurses, physicians, dietitians, and other clients, who all have their own transference issues arising. This makes for a complex dynamic of both here-and-now relationships and transference concerns that become heightened in such a concentrated therapeutic environment.

Navigating this under the best of circumstances would be challenging enough, but eating disorder therapists must also contend with their own *countertransference* reactions—the responses that the therapist has to a client based on the therapist's own transference dynamics.

Eating disorder clients are notorious for evoking strong countertransference responses in caregivers. There are several different reasons for this. First, the common misapprehension that eating disorders are about food (as opposed to interpersonal connectedness and problems with knowing how to exist in the world) ill prepares many caregivers for the issues at stake and what to expect in their relationships with eating disorder clients. Second, misunderstandings about what the food behaviors are about can generate interpretations that make the behaviors appear hostile, willful, or elective. Third, eating disorder patients are generally quite high functioning in many ways. They tend to be intellectually astute and extremely bright. Many are quick-witted, politically engaged, and socially aware. This can make it easy to forget how much they struggle in certain areas of their lives, how vulnerable and wounded they are, how intensely they can lash out when hurt, and how profoundly they can withdraw. It can make such reactions look like a choice or an intentional drama rather than what they are—deeply felt pain, shame, and fear. This can lead to further misattunement in the therapeutic environment. And finally, the physicality of eating disorders makes a difference, especially in anorexia. Something visceral is triggered when we encounter someone who is dangerously underweight. This is why images of starving children are used to raise money—it wrenches us in a deep and perhaps instinctual way to see someone in that state. To be a caregiver and to want to give care to someone who is visibly starving only to have that care rejected or interpreted as intending harm can be extremely difficult.

Eating disorder clinicians, then, must be able to keep their focus on what is happening *for the patient* and to remain fully mindful of transference dynamics without discounting their own responsibility in the here-and-now interpersonal interaction. While they may struggle with some aspects of interpersonal engagement, people with eating disorders are often acutely attuned to the emotional vibes of people around them and are adept at maneuvering within difficult social circumstances to try to get their needs met. This can feel highly manipulative and even aggressive to others, but it is not usually intended as such; instead, it is a manifestation of survival skills developed within challenging emotional environments where the direct expression of needs was not allowed or was actively punished. While expressed emotion may be high (mostly among bulimic clients) or practically absent (mostly among anorexic clients), multiple emotional registers are actually active in clients all at the same time. Successful eating disorder clinicians must become adept at reading all of these at once and sensing the layers of interaction unfolding, while at the same time managing their own emotional reactions and responses to them. This is no small task, and clinicians sometimes falter.

GINNY

One Friday, Ginny, a nineteen-year-old client diagnosed with anorexia, with a history of compulsive exercising and self-harm, had a pass to leave the clinic for the afternoon. She wasn't supposed to have one. Permission should have been pulled because she hadn't met her weight goal for the week, but somehow that never happened. So she left. While on pass, she went running. She cut herself with wire. She didn't eat.

Sharon, Ginny's therapist, confronted her about this behavior on Monday, and Sharon recounted the conversation at Wednesday's staff meeting:

SHARON: You knew you weren't supposed to have passes this weekend. You knew you hadn't met your weight goal. We talked about this in therapy on Thursday. So why did you go?

GINNY: Well, the pass was still in my chart, so I went.

SHARON: But you knew better. You knew we had set that limit.

GINNY: I don't know! It was there. I took it.

SHARON: I think we need to look at why you have difficulty with the limits of the program.

GINNY: Fuck off!

"Oh, that's crossing the line," interjected Dr. Casey. There was agreement from around the table.

"Ginny told me, 'I need a therapist I can cross boundaries with,'" Sharon continued. "She asked to be switched to Trudy."

"Well *that's* not going to happen," Joan, a therapist, scoffed. Trudy was, at that time, a relatively new therapist, known to have a kind and gentle disposition. The staff was concerned that Ginny wanted to work with Trudy because Ginny thought she could push her around and intimidate her.

"Let's offer her Brenda as an option," Dr. Casey suggested.

"Why?" asked Abby, another therapist. "Why gratify that for her? Shouldn't we make her work within the limits that Sharon is setting for her?"

Julia, another therapist, piped in. "Give her enough rope to hang herself. When she starts to see Brenda as 'bad'—which she inevitably will—we can at least tell the family that we tried to be flexible."

"She's really panicked about gaining weight," Sharon added. "She's been hiding food. I have a really somatic countertransference to her. In session I feel prickly, I get butterflies in my stomach. It feels very borderline."

"No doubt about it," confirmed Dr. Casey, and others nodded their heads.

"Wait a minute," said Dr. Vargas, a psychiatrist who consulted on a few cases but was not a full-time employee at Cedar Grove. "Aren't we forgetting something? There was major confusion with the case notes and staff communication, and that's why her pass was still active. Should we really be blaming her for taking the pass? I would have taken it, too, if I were her."

"But she *knew* better," countered Dr. Casey. "This is classic manipulation with her. She knows the limits but just doesn't want to follow them. She'll find any way to get around them."

"Then let's stop making that easier for her," challenged Dr. Vargas sardonically.

This was not the last time miscommunication and confusion among staff came up in Ginny's case. Just two weeks later another incident occurred.

Ginny had, as was discussed at the meeting, been switched to Brenda, who reported to the team, "Ginny is scaring me. She's being really nice. She's doing assignments. She's leaving nice little notes on my desk. It's weird. I'm waiting for the other shoe to drop."

"You know," said Dr. Casey, "as I get to know the family more, I see that Mom is often the one causing problems. Why are we labeling Ginny? Maybe it's just regular adolescent behavior. But I think Mom has the same disorder. She [Mom] clearly has mood problems, very black-and-white thinking."

"I'm pretty worried about what will happen with this family," offered Tamara, another therapist. Others around the table agreed.

Rhonda, a dietician, spoke up next, "She was supposed to have a meal increase on Sunday night, but she refused it."

"Wait. So why is she still getting passes?" asked Amelia, a direct care staff member.

Apparently, there had been another miscommunication among staff about passes, so Ginny had been able to go on a pass even though she wasn't completing her full meal plan.

"Insurance is going to yank her out," Rhonda said. "She doesn't have that many days left. We need to really focus on weight gain."

"How should we handle this?" Dr. Casey asked the group. "Do we just let insurance run out and explain to the insurance company about the borderline family?"

"She wants to be able to use the bathroom with the door closed," Rhonda added, "and to have meal passes with her family. I don't think she's ready for either of those."

"Agreed," said Dr. Casey. "But I say we go ahead and give it to her, and if she doesn't comply we'll have more to use in terms of justifying discharging her."

"She has gained seven and a half pounds since admission," Rhonda noted.

"That's something," said Dr. Casey. "But my tolerance for borderline dynamics is really low."

There are a number of things going on here. First, Ginny is blamed for capitalizing on staff mistakes. This contradicts both medical model and recovery model expectations because Ginny both flouts medical authority and acts against her own recovery goals. But we also see how Ginny is, in effect, *set up to fail* as that enables clinicians to work ethically within managed care limits. In this situation, the clinicians are feeling powerless in the face of both the eating disorder (or more specifically, the "borderline family" that is thought to be perpetuating the eating disorder) and the insurance company, and they essentially decide to step back and let the client crash and burn.

How is this configured as "good care"?

I want to emphasize again here that Cedar Grove is a highly respected facility and its clinicians are well-trained, passionately committed, and deeply caring professionals. They are good people who genuinely want to do the best by their clients. The question, therefore, might be better phrased as: How do good, caring clinicians come to this sort of a decision? What sort of conditions must align for this to be rendered as "good care"?

In the meetings described above, clinicians had to balance information across at least three different axes: trust (should they trust the client or not?); control (should they be more restrictive or less?); and temporal focus (should they focus on the here and now or the future?). In doing so, they had to keep in mind several key propositions: (1) knowledge is always partial, incomplete, and speculative; (2) judgments must be based on a balance between hard data and interpersonal knowledge; (3) knowing what is best for the patient involves a triangulation of information and disciplines and making best judgments; and (4) reliance on research and "best practices" is a way out of situations with ambiguous answers. In other words, when clinicians were faced with contradictions between the medical model and recovery model propositions, the standard seemed to be: numbers could be trusted but patients could not; autonomy and expressed emotion were only viewed as "healthy" when they aligned with protocol; and failed treatment was justified, but noncompliance was not. In other words, it was the staff's job to do the best they could, but it was the patient's job to not be sick. This puts patients in an untenable situation, given that they are in treatment precisely because they are struggling with an illness.

I don't mean to suggest that Ginny was necessarily "right" for taking passes she knew she was not supposed to have. Rather, I am interested in how such exercising of agency was interpreted by staff as part of Ginny's eating disorder. We can see here how the boundaries of Ginny's eating disorder (and those of other patients) are defined by adherence to the *protocols*. If you follow the protocols, you are not in your eating disorder. If you break them, you are in your eating disorder. *But protocols themselves are not clear.* They are ever shifting and not consistently enforced—in part due to attempts to accommodate to various insurance expectations, and in part (at least in Ginny's case) due to human error. Yet the client is held responsible for not anticipating these limits and complying with them. There was never, as far as I could see, any reflection on the part of the staff on how this dynamic mirrors common family dynamics in eating disorder families—in this case, Ginny became the identified patient of a dysfunctional system twice over.

As clinicians had to consistently navigate between the recovery model and the medical model while at the same time managing the particular paradoxes and challenges of working with eating disorder clients, they sometimes made human mistakes. This is understandable. What interests me is not the fact that clinicians are fallible humans doing the best they could but rather the patterns into which such humanness organizes itself, how this creates the reality of a given client's "eating disorder" as a phenomenon within the context of treatment, and the implications this has for patients.

Specifically, when patients' perceptual, rational, emotional, and/or behavioral capacities are thought to be impaired as a result of their illnesses, patients become systematically delegitimized as reliable agents of knowledge and action through a looping effect. In such cases, patients essentially become *objects* similar to other materialities rather than *subjects* whose perceptions matter in the enactment of an illness. Clinicians then learn to read clients' interpersonal engagements not as expressing legitimate subject positions but as further data about their illness to be fitted into a diagnostic paradigm. Despite what clients may try to assert about their own intentions or experience, clinicians' own feelings toward clients become especially critical to these unfolding enactments, shaping how clinicians read ambiguous situations for clues about clients' diagnosable conditions. In effect, clients become exiled from their own experiences in ways that can mimic the features of the illness itself.

This ontological delegitimation is pronounced in the case of eating disorders, where patients frequently are perceived not only as being incapable of accurate reality testing but also as being (as Claire perceived Anita to be in the opening vignette of this chapter) deliberately manipulative or playing on others' emotional investments to obtain desired ends.

Characterizing clients' behavior as manipulation in the managed care context—where access to treatment is precarious and unpredictable—does particular kinds of affective and pragmatic work. Specifically, it renders clients as, paradoxically, both hyperagentic and agentically challenged in ways that delegitimize them as full subjects and therefore as subjects deserving of care. This makes the selective withdrawal of attention and effort into a locally meaningful therapeutic act. Ethical care for eating disorders, then, emerges and takes shape in the clinic through a struggling out of differing kinds of truth claims from differently legitimated actors.

It is clear, for example, that Claire (the nurse mentioned at the opening of the chapter) and I had different understandings about where to draw the lines around "Anita" and "anorexia." For me (and, I believe, for Anita), anorexia was something Anita and I were both reflecting on in our interaction; it was present in the sense that it was extant in Anita's lived experience, but it existed in the interaction as the relatively distanced object of our discussion. For Claire, on the other hand, anorexia was actively structuring the very terms of Anita's relating to me, which therefore justified her characterization of Anita's claims to empathy as part of the illness itself. Similarly, Ginny's eating disorder was thought to dictate not only the "noncompliance" she demonstrated by taking passes when she wasn't supposed to but also her solicitousness when trying to build a relationship with her new therapist.

In other words, in clinical settings, some people's realities are considered "truer" than others, and in psychiatric conditions this can loop back onto itself, becoming part of local power dynamics. This requires us to pay special attention to how practices of truth-making intersect with such notions as rationality and agency in different contexts. At Cedar Grove, this paradoxical rendering of care (that withholding care is a form of care) mirrors the paradoxical construction of Anita's and Ginny's agency as both ubiquitous and impossible.

In thinking about how the withholding of responsiveness to Anita could be construed as care, we need to understand the practices by which people become authorized (or not) as legitimate subjects in eating disorders treatments and how different worlds come into dynamic—and uneven—engagement in the constitution of the "what is" of an eating disorder.

CONSEQUENCES OF VIEWING EATING DISORDER CLIENTS AS MANIPULATIVE

Claire's admonition that I should not have responded to Anita's expressed suffering and the staff's indictment of Ginny both hinge on the notion that eating disorder clients are notoriously manipulative. In clinical terms, "manipulation" can mean many things, but it can broadly be defined as using subtlety, dishonesty, deceit, and/or other strategies of persuasion to attempt to get someone to act or feel a certain way without that person being aware of what is happening. Manipulation is usually considered to be a hallmark of a personality disorder (such as BPD); it is viewed as a feature of one's "character" rather than an occasional strategy. It is regarded as an expression of who one *is*, not just something one *does*, and is thought to structure interpersonal relationships in certain ways. Specifically, it leads to viewing the "manipulator" as an illegitimate agent, an unreliable subject, or both.

I wish, however, to be very clear. The clinicians at Cedar Grove were, from all indicators I could see and sense, compassionate and caring professionals who genuinely wanted to help clients get well. As in most mental health settings, they sometimes struggled with issues of workplace stress and occasional burnout, but this in no way characterized the general atmosphere of the place. When clinicians described patients as "manipulative," then, it did not generally stem from cynicism, hostility, or disregard, though these sentiments may have been present to some degree. Rather, such attributions emerged from a very particular and mindfully thought out way of relating to those clients who were thought to be, as one clinic psychiatrist described it, "agentically challenged" in fundamental ways, a perspective grounded in decades of assumptions about eating disorders that have persisted despite shifts in theoretical and clinical priorities (see chapter 2). That is, clinicians at Cedar Grove understood eating disorder clients to have developed problematic strategies for getting their needs met, such that personal agency was refracted through interpretive and behavioral lenses that distorted and contorted it into destructive patterns. For this reason, "gratifying" a directly expressed need of a client—like Ginny's request to be switched to Trudy—was almost always considered to be bending to a form of manipulation and was therefore to be avoided or actively shut down.

This view of eating disorder clients is by no means unique to Cedar Grove. In the clinical world, clients with eating disorders in general are thought to be characteristically manipulative and are frequently characterized in the literature as secretive, dishonest, sneaky, sly, and gamy.[3] Such assessments often sit at odds with clients' own experiences, yet they have profound practical implications for the trajectory of treatment. Specifically, viewing clients as manipulative legitimates a relational strategy within which the nonacknowledgement of clients' claims to agency and/or authenticity can be construed as optimal care. Following is another ethnographic example that can help illuminate these dynamics.

HEATHER: TWO VIEWS

One day, Heather, a twenty-two-year-old woman diagnosed with bulimia, seemed to be in a particularly good mood. "I just feel really good," she told me when I asked her about it. "I feel really on top of things. I've got my plan in place, and I'm ready to move on." Heather was talking about her discharge plan, in which a client sets out her goals for recovery and her specific life plans after discharge. Usually, it is completed the week prior to discharge, once the end of treatment is in sight. Heather, however, had been at the clinic for only two weeks and was facing a projected stay of two months. Although she knew it was premature to be working on her plan, Heather told me she wanted to show the treatment team that she was taking her recovery seriously and was thinking realistically about the challenges ahead.

When I saw Heather a few days later, she was distraught. She sat on her bed and hugged her knees, tucking them under her chin. Sobbing quietly, she told me that the treatment team had not only rejected her discharge plan but had told her she would likely stay an extra month past the original estimate. She was devastated. "I just don't understand," she told me. "I just wanted to show them I'm trying to be responsible and take my recovery seriously, and I feel like I'm being punished."

After the interview, I spoke with Jim, Heather's therapist, and asked about the treatment team's decision. "Yes, Heather did submit a very complete and detailed discharge plan," he told me. "Very complete. In fact, we thought it was a bit obsessive." When I asked for clarification, Jim said, "It seemed like she was trying too hard to please us, which is one of her issues: to be seen as a 'good girl' and to get what she wants through the back door. A kind of manipulative thing. And that's at the heart of her eating disorder. So we didn't want to gratify that."

Here, again, we have two very different interpretations of the same set of events and, more specifically, different understandings of how to think about Heather. Underlying this disjuncture is the proposition that the treatment team is ultimately able to better discern the truth of Heather's actions than Heather herself is—a proposition grounded in a philosophy of the person that holds that outward behaviors speak a truth about a client's inner experiences that she may not be aware of or may even categorically reject.

While it is certainly true that people may not always be directly conscious of their motivations for behaving in a certain way, it seems that something more complicated is going on here in terms of practical theories of self. Heather understood her writing of her discharge plan as a concrete demonstration to the treatment team that she was fully and willingly engaged in the recovery process. For her, intention and action were aligned and consistent, and her outward behaviors articulated her inner dispositions in a fairly direct way. The clinicians, on the other hand, understood Heather to be eclipsed by her eating disorder. They understood the discharge plan as evidence of how far removed from authentic action she really was. For them, Heather's true (albeit unconscious) intention was to manipulate the treatment team into thinking of her as a model patient. Although this intention aligned with the action of writing the discharge plan, in their view Heather's behaviors distorted and misrepresented her real intentions, thereby rendering the action itself inauthentic and evidence of pathology.

ASSUMPTIONS ABOUT MANIPULATION VERSUS AUTHENTICITY

Anita's moving aside her sweater, Ginny's taking of passes that she knew she was not entitled to, and Heather's creation of a discharge plan were constitutive acts. That is, they created certain realities. The therapists, clients, and anthropologist all had different interpretations of what those realities were, but we all agreed that something changed in those moments. Ultimately, if paradoxically, the apparent ability of Anita, Ginny, and Heather to actively advocate for certain aims was seen by the clinicians as evidence of the fact that these women were, in actuality, fully immersed in their disease. Although these clients were, in some ways, enacting the kind of proactive agency they were being induced to develop, this "hyperagency" ("trying to control the world," as clinicians often described it) was read in the clinic as evidence of a lack of *legitimate* agency, as it was thought to indicate that they were under the sway of their illness. Patients, therefore, were constituted as always already manipulative, such that the exercise of any sort of nonmanipulative agency, even when clients are compliant with treatment expectations, is deemed a logical impossibility.

Ironically, then, clients often have little recourse under such conditions aside from inhabiting the "manipulative" stance accorded to them at the outset. Indeed, Heather had to strategically alter her enthusiasm about preparing for discharge in order to better approximate what the clinicians expected of her and to hopefully secure an earlier release date. Anita had to learn to not solicit empathy and concern quite so directly but instead try to eke it out with no one being the wiser. Ginny had to learn to be grateful and solicitous with her new therapist, although this, too, was viewed with suspicion. In such situations, the only "healthy" agency a patient can exhibit is one that mirrors expectations of subterfuge (thereby risking accusations of manipulation) while recognition of her needs is denied.

If Ginny's, Heather's, and Anita's behavior is construed as manipulative in large part precisely because they're seen—by definition, being eating disorder clients—as manipulators, then it becomes difficult for the clinical team to ever perceive them as acting authentically, regardless of their actual intentions. In a context where authenticity is understood as foundational to psychological health, this puts clients like Heather, Ginny, and Anita, as well as the clinicians themselves, in a tricky spot in terms of how to evaluate when or if clients are "getting better" and how to respond clinically as a result.

What is important about this in terms of relationships of care is that the client herself is simultaneously erased as an agent in this dynamic and figured as powerfully agentic and therefore pathological. In enactments of illness, not all agents in a system are created equal, especially when issues of agency are themselves considered diagnostic of the condition of concern and where regimes of care hinge on understandings of agency that become foreclosed. This can have tangible consequences in terms of how resources are allocated or withdrawn.

Sometimes, however, the problem is not the withholding or denial of care but the fact that clients refuse the care that is offered.

"Can you tell me about your decision to stop taking your medications?" I asked the young woman sitting across from me in the therapy room. At the time of this conversation, Kelsey, a twenty-four-year-old woman diagnosed with bulimia, was a client in the Cedar Grove outpatient program. Her decision to abruptly stop taking her mood stabilizer (for bipolar disorder), potassium supplements (to prevent cardiac arrhythmias due to hypokalemia from purging), and antianxiety medication (for generalized anxiety disorder, panic disorder, and traits of obsessive-compulsive disorder) concerned me on a number of levels. Medically, I was concerned that she could have a cardiac or neurological event. Psychologically, I was concerned about a recurrence of her suicidal depression, panic attacks, and debilitating anxiety that had been present before she went on medication. And I also wondered why she decided to stop all her medications *now*. She had been working hard in therapy and had recently made some important strides. Why would she choose *now* as the time to cut off something she had previously viewed as a necessary component of her recovery?

Kelsey is certainly not alone in her ambivalence toward psychiatric and other medications, nor is this ambivalence unique to people with eating disorders.[4] Yet medications can take on particular significance for some eating disorder clients, as I discuss in a moment. What I have learned from these clients resonates with contemporary American cultural understandings of the body as flawed but perfectible through pharmaceutical interventions,[5] with moral responsibility for managing the body located firmly within the individual.[6] Yet these clients' experiences also point to an underside of this trend. The logic of "pharmaceutical reason"[7] presumes that people naturally strive for optimal health and use medications to improve their quality of life by alleviating pain (physical or emotional), optimizing performance, or otherwise enhancing mental and/or physical capacities. But what about those for whom health is as terrifying a prospect as cancer? I will return to this fear of health in a moment, but first I wish to highlight the importance of understanding medication use as a *relational practice* between the individual and the medicine[8] (as well as the prescriber) and consider what this can tell us about relations of care in Cedar Grove more broadly.

The concept of medication use as a relationship becomes more intelligible when we remember that pharmaceuticals exist expressly to *do things* to our bodies. They are *meant* to alter us. Medications, then, inherently contain a sort of agency in their capacity to transform, enhance, alleviate, or stabilize. People who use medications regularly, especially medicines that transform not only one's body but also one's sense of who one *is,* often develop intimate and highly complex relationships to these drugs and their transformative capacities.[9] Viewed in this way, we can see that, beyond the effects of the substances themselves, people's behavior in relation *to* their medications— especially psychiatric medications—can become powerfully significant avenues for shaping their understandings of themselves and their experiences of the world around them.[10] Taking medications as prescribed cultivates and solicits a subjectivity of active self-care within logics of health that presumes a desire to "get better."

Against this backdrop, I have come to understand the use of medications in the clinic as *a form of intimate touch.* In the absence of almost any physical contact at Cedar Grove (for therapeutic as well as potential liability reasons—the two are related), medications become a key mediator of intimacy and care. They pass from the hands of one person to the hands and eventually the insides of another, carrying health-promoting compounds meant to nourish, repair, regulate, or strengthen. So when a patient refuses to take her medication, much more is going on than noncompliance with protocol. It is a *relational* act that is multivalent and potent in its communicative power. Like other forms of absenting, however, refusing medication leaves a gap in signification that is often filled in by others in ways that radically miss the mark.

Food Is Medicine / Medicine Is Food

One of the standard mantras of contemporary eating disorders treatment in the United States—and certainly at Cedar Grove—is "Food is medicine." Eating food, patients are told, is like taking a pill, something presumed to be symbolically neutral. Framing food as medicine is meant to help patients view food through a utilitarian lens, stripped of its hefty symbolic and cultural meanings.

This reframing of food as medicine does, indeed, seem to help many patients, at least to some extent. It seems to help them separate out the nutritive purpose of food from the desires and pleasures associated with eating. And if food is medicine—and if it is good and important to take your medicine as prescribed—then the enjoyment of food becomes slightly less guilt-laden, since pleasure becomes viewed as simply a side effect of the food/medication rather than the driving reason for this "indulgence." This approach fits well with many analyses of eating disorders that view these illnesses as centered on issues of sexuality and bodily pleasures and see restricting food or bingeing and purging as ways of controlling those desires or denying them all together.

Over the years, however—both at Cedar Grove and in my private practice—I have observed a parallel phenomenon that is openly acknowledged among clinicians yet, from what I can tell, is entirely absent from the clinical or social science literature, aside from its inclusion as a form of "treatment resistance." Many eating disorder patients have extremely ambivalent and complex relationships with their medications, which often begin long before they encounter the "food is medicine" discourse in treatment. They may take their medications as prescribed for some time but then begin restricting them, taking a smaller dosage than prescribed, or skipping them all together. Some take their medications but then purge them. Some hoard their medications, finding comfort in having stockpiles of drugs and using them in what they plan to be a final, terminal medication binge. Notably, it is not only psychiatric medications that become enlisted in the restriction and binge-purge dynamics of these clients. Other supplements, like multivitamins, potassium, calcium, or even insulin, are also sometimes used in this way. While clinicians may promote the view that food is medicine, these practices seem to suggest that, for some people with eating disorders, *medicine is food,* or at least that there is a commonality that bears exploring.

How might we understand this phenomenon? And what might it tell us about relationships of care in the clinic?

Andie

Andie was nineteen years old when I met her at Cedar Grove. Short, with shoulder-length dark brown hair and brown eyes, Andie would not immediately be identifiable by the average person as "sick." She seemed, at first glance, to be a very together, self-assured young woman. But she was not.

Andie had been through eight weeks of residential care the year before at a clinic in another part of the country and had since relapsed badly. Her parents had spent all of their savings on that treatment program, so Andie obtained a personal loan from a bank to pay for the $1000 a day stay at Cedar Grove. Technically, Andie fit the diagnosis for eating disorder not otherwise specified (now called other specified feeding or eating disorder). Since health insurance plans often exclude treatment for this condition, however, Andie was admitted under the diagnosis of bulimia nervosa, which was, at that moment, indeed perfectly apt. Before coming to the clinic, Andie binged and purged several times a day, some weeks leaving her apartment only to buy more food. She had dropped out of college (she excelled in academics, so this was especially devastating for her), stopped seeing friends, and isolated herself from her family. She had been struggling with her eating disorder and grinding, debilitating depression and frantic anxiety for five years. Andie also engaged in regular self-harm, slicing her arms and thighs with razors and burning words into her skin.

Andie had tried various medications during her previous treatments and during the intervening year before she arrived at Cedar Grove. The standard antidepressants did not work for her. The physical activation associated with these medications made her mind and body race, making it very difficult for her to focus and triggering panic attacks. Anxiolytics helped with her anxiety but tended to make her depression worse. She had been on various mood stabilizers but developed horrible side effects that were both intolerable and dangerous. Finally, after many weeks of trying different combinations of medications in different dosages, she found one that worked: Neurontin (an antiepileptic that has been shown to have mood-stabilizing effects), Lexapro (an antidepressant), and Paxil (an anxiolytic).

Andie made some strides in the clinic, but she quickly gained a reputation among the staff as a "difficult client." She certainly did not make their jobs easier. She argued with the dietician about her meal plan. She pushed back against rules about computer use, bedtimes, and access to bathrooms. She sometimes refused to go to groups or therapy. For a period of time, she refused to eat at all, and an NG tube was placed to deliver liquid nutrition directly to her stomach. And she periodically refused all medications. This last issue posed a real problem for the staff. Legally, they could not force her to take medicine against her will. Yet when she didn't take them, her moods became increasingly unstable, and her panic attacks returned, both of which impeded her ability to engage in treatment.

The staff interpreted all of these behaviors, especially the medication refusal, as indicative of Andie's underlying personality disorder (she had been diagnosed with borderline personality disorder during a previous stay at another clinic) and as evidence of her "immature" mode of relating that used defying authority figures as a means of asserting independence. Certainly, they understood that Andie's issues were complex and not easily reducible to a single dynamic. Nevertheless, the issue of Andie's refusal to take her medicine came to assume center stage in her treatment at the clinic, indexing for the staff her willingness to commit (or not) to recovery. Power struggles flared up frequently between Andie and the staff, and neither she nor they willing to budge an inch. It was overall a very unpleasant and unproductive situation.

When I first met Andie, I was at the clinic solely in the role of ethnographer. As such, I occupied an interstitial space; I was neither a staff member nor a client, but I participated in activities sometimes considered proprietary to each. In this sense, I was positioned largely outside the power structure of staff and client, which is likely what enabled me to develop a rapport with the otherwise guarded and sullen Andie during groups and meals and through general socializing in the clinic.

As I watched the evolving tensions between Andie and the staff, I sensed there was something more going on for Andie other than simply "treatment interfering behavior" (as it is called in the clinical literature) or adolescent stubbornness. On those occasions when she refused to go to group and instead sat in the common area, I began to join her and chat. Among other things, we talked about her experiences of treatment so far, what she was finding helpful or unhelpful, and why. This naturally included discussions about medications.

On one level, Andie readily admitted to me, she refused to take her medications simply because the staff wanted her to take them, and she was feeling angry and defiant. But there was much more to it than that. Andie hated the panic attacks, and the depression was deeply frightening to her. Yet she still refused her medications. On one occasion, after I helped talk her through a panic attack, I asked her why she was still reluctant to take her medications. As she caught her breath and tried to calm herself down, she told me that she had actually wanted to start her medications again the previous day but had found that she could not. She literally had not been able to get herself to take the pills. She had asked the nurse for her morning medications, sat down with them and a glass of water, and told herself over and over to take them, yet she felt completely paralyzed by anxiety and fear. She sat there for thirty minutes before giving up and returning the pills to the nurse. "Why couldn't you take them?" I asked her. "I don't *know*," she said, in a voice full of frustration and bewilderment. "I have no idea. I *wanted* to take them. I had them in my hand. I kept willing myself to just put them in my mouth and swallow them, but I just couldn't do it. I couldn't. I have no idea why."

Days went by, and Andie continued to struggle with taking her medications. She maintained that she wanted to take them but could not. I asked her what would happen—what would feel different to her emotionally—if she were able to take her medications that evening. After a long pause, she said quietly, "I would feel like I failed." "Failed at what?" I asked. "Would it feel like you were giving in and letting them [the staff] win?" "In part," she answered, "but that's not what I meant. It would feel like I was letting my *body* win." When I asked her to clarify, Andie explained that taking her medication was an acknowledgment that her body *needed* something and she was providing it willingly. This was something she could not tolerate. The anxiety and overwhelming guilt and shame of participating in the enhancement—or even the prevention of further decline—of her physical functioning completely paralyzed her. And the longer she was off her medications, the more intense these feelings became.

Once Andie was able to articulate that the core struggle for her was less about defying the staff and more about her own crushing shame over willingly attending to her body's needs, she and the staff were able to come up with a solution. Andie found that she could tolerate accepting the medications if they were ground up and fed through her feeding tube. This way, she could rationalize to herself that the agency at play was not her own but the staff's; they were "making" her take them. Even so, allowing herself to accept these "feedings" (as they are called in the clinic) was very difficult for her, and she felt an enormous amount of guilt about it at first. After about a week, and with a great deal of struggle, however, Andie finally became able to take her medications by herself again.

After she had left the clinic, and after I had completed my clinical education and training, Andie began to see me for individual therapy in my outpatient practice. We met twice a week for almost three years until she graduated from college and moved to another state. While in outpatient therapy, Andie often struggled with medication restriction or taking her medications and then purging them. Usually, this meant that she would purposefully skip a dose here and there or stop taking one of the medications for a few days, but none of this significantly altered her welfare. On these occasions, we were able to talk about her medications in the terms she herself first identified—as a form of bodily nourishment about which she was extremely ambivalent.

On more than one occasion, however, her medication restriction was much more extreme. Periodically, Andie would come into a session and tell me that she had stopped taking all of her medications—just stopped taking them, even her multivitamins and calcium. When I would ask her why she had stopped, her initial answer would be something like, "I don't know, I just didn't want to take them anymore," or "I'm tired of taking pills every day," or "I don't think they're working, so why should I bother taking them?" While there was undoubtedly truth to these statements, they seemed rather flimsy justification for risking the kinds of emotional and physical suffering Andie faced when the depression and anxiety hit. But each time, no degree of my reminding her about how horrible things got for her when she was off her medications or how vital it was for her to take care of her basic functioning made any difference. She knew all of that. In fact, she had enough insight to know that this was precisely *why* she was doing it—for her, it was a form of self-harm, self-sabotage, and punishment for feeling better. Each time, she had to descend to rock bottom—to the point of acute suicidal misery— before she would finally begin taking her medications again.

It is clear that medication restriction held a particular significance for Andie beyond a desire to be obstreperous. And her medication restriction was not a roundabout means of suicide—despite the potential danger of restricting her potassium supplements, she was very careful to take just enough to prevent a full-blown medical crisis.

In therapy, as we focused on her *relationship to* her medications, Andie began to see how she restricted her supplements to keep her potassium at deprivation level in the same way she restricted her food to keep her body at starvation levels. Following this line of discovery, Andie came to see that the core issue for her was that she wanted to punish herself for continuing to be alive. She experienced herself as a worthless, loathsome, utterly repulsive human being. She hated herself with such vehemence that the idea that she might do something—like eat or take medications—that allowed her to exist felt morally wrong and intensely shameful to her. Yet she could not quite bring herself to commit suicide. She had overdosed on medications on two separate instances, but in neither case had she taken enough (thankfully) to kill her or produce lasting damage. So she had settled for what, in her mind, was the next best thing—subsisting in a state of constant deprivation.

HEALTH AS MORAL FAILING

It is clear that much more was going on for Andie than simple acting out or noncompliance, as medication refusal is often characterized in clinical settings, and in fact we see that the main motivations for her medication restriction have much more to do with her own internal processes of fear, shame, and guilt than a desire to manipulate others. For Andie, medication refusal was primarily about cultivating and maintaining a moral subjective stance that structured her entire philosophy of being. Andie's ambivalent relationships with medication indexed intense existential struggles about how to survive in a world where one's very existence feels irredeemably wrong.

Creatively tinkering with psychiatric medication use as a means of regulating inner experience is by no means uncommon. Anthropologists Janis Jenkins and Elizabeth Carpenter-Song discussed this at length in their work on "pharmaceutical selves."[11] And, as anthropologist Eileen Anderson-Fye and social worker Jerry Floersch found in their study of psychiatric medication use among college students, altering one's moods and focus to achieve an idealized state—a simulacrum of the "normal"—can be a primary motivator for students who experiment with dosage and timing, often devising their own personalized regimens.[12]

What is notable about Andie and Kelsey (from the beginning of the chapter), however, is that the "idealized state" they sought was quite different from the elevated mood, reduced anxiety, or enhanced capacity to focus that Anderson-Fye and Floersch found to be goals for the students in their study. In fact, Andie and Kelsey were willing to risk descending into horrific depression or becoming wracked with anxiety and panic to restrict their medications. So why were they doing it? And what can this tell us about how relationships of care unfold in the clinic?

One might suspect that restricting medications could be an effective way to get attention or to generate crises that made others feel obligated to come to the rescue. These motivations were certainly part of the picture for Andie and Kelsey, but they were not the most compelling for them. In fact, they were both highly secretive about their medication restriction and went to great lengths to hide their emotional struggles from others so that their behaviors would not be discovered. Furthermore, their restriction extended to multivitamins, calcium supplements, and potassium supplements, clearly suggesting that the focus of this behavior was something other than direct mood alteration through the substance of the medicines themselves.

Rather, the "idealized state" both Andie and Kelsey sought was the *awareness of depriving the body of what it needs to function optimally.* For these clients—and several others I have worked with over the years—restricting medications became one way of maintaining a state of constant deprivation, of not allowing oneself to thrive. It was about cultivating a subjective stance that is acutely morally charged. What we saw with Andie, in particular, was enormous ambivalence and shame about taking proactive measures to care for her body beyond those required for bare subsistence. In her mind, to actively do something—like take vitamins or psychiatric medications—that would ease her suffering or, worse yet, enable her to thrive felt horribly, morally wrong. Conversely, restricting medications, knowing she was depriving herself of care—even when she couldn't directly feel the physical effects—felt like just compensation for the burden of her continued existence.

This existential angst is a core feature of eating disorders that is often overlooked in approaches that focus on cultural pressures about weight and body image or the social sanctioning of female desires and appetites of all kinds. While these cultural pressures are vitally important in understanding how and why eating becomes a key mechanism through which these concerns are expressed,[13] the driving issues for people with eating disorders are far more fundamental. At heart, eating disorders are not about *wearing* a size 0; they are about *becoming* a size 0, about feeling unworthy to exist and about the experience of sustaining an existence as a nonentity while relentlessly punishing oneself for the unforgivable crime of remaining alive.

Controlling food and eating is one obvious avenue for expressing and enacting this angst, but it is certainly not the only way. For example, people with eating disorders almost always have very specific restrictions and rituals concerning fluid intake (including water), although this is given scant attention in the clinical literature except as a complicating factor. They also regularly engage in all sorts of behaviors of withholding care from the body—such as refusing to use an umbrella in the rain. Since medication use is increasingly viewed and promoted at a cultural level as a means of self-care, a form of empowerment, and a step toward a better and more enjoyable life, medication *restriction* can become a powerful way of enacting and experiencing a moral practice of deprivation for these clients.

With this in mind, understanding eating disorder clients' refusals of care through the lens of moral self-management rather than seeing it as acting out or resisting treatment pivots our orientation to these behaviors and opens new opportunities for constructive collaborative work with these clients. Refusals of care in eating disorders treatment must be understood as part of a broader existential and moral project in which these clients are deeply embedded. This does not make it OK—people still need care, and the structures and beliefs of the eating disorder must be actively challenged. But understanding such refusals of care in this way reframes the dynamic, changing it from an oppositional one to one where collaboration is possible without either side losing face or integrity.

Bringing the issues of (counter)transference, halo features, manipulation, and noncompliance together, we can see how eating disorder clients are configured within regimes of care such that "healthy" agency is rendered nearly impossible and clients become caught in double binds from which it is very difficult to escape. "Care" comes to be characterized by deprivation and withholding in ways that reinforce the core dynamics of the illness while at the same time habituating clients to such practices as reflective of their deservedness. It is critical to note that this is not due to a lack of compassion or concern among caregivers. Rather, such practices are situated within broader structures that condition both the possibilities and contours of "good care" on the ground. Clinicians' understandings of care are inseparable from the larger frameworks within which they operate and from which certain kinds of practice derive their legitimacy. This is what we turn to in the next chapter, where we will see how the things that heal—therapeutic relationships—are precisely those that are most damaged by the structures of care that govern them.

Breaking

DECEMBER 1987

I dump out the pills on my nightstand and count them by twos. Two, four, six, eight . . . twenty. That should be enough. Will it be enough? I weighed eighty-nine pounds that morning. Not that much, but up five pounds from a few days ago. Oh my god, I am so out of control. How did I let this happen? I started eating, that's what happened. Maybe if I just go back to what I was doing before, the toasted (slightly burnt) rice cake crumbled up into the low-fat yogurt midmorning and another before bed. That's less than four hundred calories. I could do that.

Stop! I can't do this anymore! I can't. I can't go back to that. And I cannot live like this, totally out of control. I already ate two Giordano's pizzas today. Two! By myself! My skin feels tight and sore, like it always does now that I've started eating. My ankles are puffy, and I can leave indentations in them with my fingers when I squeeze them. It has been less than a week since I started eating, but I can see where this is going. Fat? Surely. But it's worse than that. My whole life is disintegrating, fragmenting, falling completely fucking apart. There is no way out.

Except this.

I look at the blue, oval Unisom pills on my nightstand surface. It is night-time. Wednesday. Sometime between Thanksgiving and Christmas break. It is my first fall at the University of Chicago, and the brutal cold is quite a change from the north Florida weather I grew up with. I love the seasons, but my anorexic body shivers and shakes almost constantly trying to stay warm, even under multiple layers of clothes.

I hear people laughing outside in the courtyard as they play in the snow below. Laughing. Joyful. I feel like an alien in a world I no longer understand. I try to peek out the window behind my nightstand, overlooking the courtyard, to catch a glimpse of who is out there and what is so fun. But in the darkness I can't see the source of the joyful noise outside. All I can see is my own reflection—a hollowed-out, brittle, mournful, young woman, deflated in body and spirit like a balloon with the air let out.

I sit down on the edge of my bed, still looking at the pills. I pop open the orange Shasta I have waiting. I prefer Tab, but I am afraid the caffeine might somehow counteract the effects of the pills, and if I am going to do this, I want to do it right. I sit there staring at the pills and the Shasta for several minutes, contemplating them as if they were offerings on an altar. Yet my mind is also strangely empty. I just look at them, steeling myself for what it is I am about to do.

ELEVEN

Capitalizing on Care

PRECARITY, VULNERABILITY, AND FAILED SUBJECTS

In 2015, Cedar Grove was bought by MediCorp,[1] a large for-profit behavioral health management corporation. Founded in 2005, and publicly traded since 2011, MediCorp oversaw just six facilities in 2010. As of June 2017, it operated a network of 587 behavioral healthcare facilities, with a total of approximately 17,300 beds, in thirty-nine states, Puerto Rico, and the United Kingdom. They do not specialize in eating disorders, but eating disorders clinics are among their holdings.

Dr. Casey, who agreed to stay on as the medical director at Cedar Grove under a noncompete agreement for several years, said she and her partners decided to sell the clinic to MediCorp for two main reasons: first, they were growing so much that more capital was needed to fund the expansion, and second, the managed care climate was increasingly challenging to work in. "It was a difficult decision," she told me, "Very difficult. But ultimately, that was the best way for us to stay in business and to continue to deliver care, and even expand our offerings. Many parts of the state don't have any access to treatment at all, so this was a way to try to get into some of those other communities. It's not ideal, but it's the nature of the work these days. You just have to make the best of it."

The sale of Cedar Grove to MediCorp indexes larger trends in the field of behavioral health, where smaller private clinics all over the country are being bought up by large publicly traded equity firms. To take just one example, according to a March 2015 post on the website of the investment behemoth BDO, behavioral health is "a market ripe for growth and consolidation."[2] Citing both increased demand for services (such as the opioid crisis and increasing levels of mental illness across a number of categories) and increased reimbursements for care,[3] BDO identifies behavioral health as a "compelling investment opportunity." An NPR report from June 2016 similarly observed that "investors see big opportunities in opioid addiction treatment," as smaller independent clinics "are being gobbled up by private equity companies and publicly-traded chains looking to do what is known in Wall Street jargon as a roll-up play. They take a fragmented industry, buy up the bits and pieces and consolidate them into big, branded companies where they hope to make a profit by streamlining and cutting costs."[4]

This is exactly what happened at Cedar Grove as it was rolled into the MediCorp holdings. And it was not the only eating disorders clinic acquired by the company. While much of the current acquisitive attention is focused on the opioid crisis, eating disorders have also become a surprising site of development—surprising because eating disorders have long been underfunded by insurance companies on the pretext that they are too expensive to treat and therefore not profitable. But, as a March 2016 story in the *New York Times* observed, the eating disorders treatment industry is "booming," with more than seventy-five centers currently operating in the United States, compared with only twenty-two a decade ago.[5] This increase has been fueled by the Affordable Care Act and other legislation that has facilitated some kinds of coverage for eating disorders, and also by investment by private equity firms like MediCorp.

While this transition to corporatized behavioral health has had the advantage of making more treatment available to more people, there are huge red warning flags suggesting that quality of treatment is being sacrificed for profit. "For the most part, the people who are running and working in these programs believe they're doing the right thing," says Dr. Angela Guarda, the director of the eating disorders program at the Johns Hopkins Hospital in Baltimore. "But it's a slippery slope. Money can cloud your view."[6] Such concerns have led to increasing calls for transparency in marketing and data reporting.[7]

The effects of this situation on the ground are monumental. "The whole landscape of eating disorders treatment is changing in this country," Amelia, a therapist who left her job at Cedar Grove to start a private practice in 2016, told me:

> It's not just MediCorp or Cedar Grove; they're part of a trend. All of the [eating disorders] treatment centers around the country are getting bought up by these big conglomerates, these management companies. And they don't know the first thing about eating disorders! Nothing. They're in it to make money. What they do is keep the cost of treatment the same, but they squeeze

everywhere else, "economize." Which generally falls on the clinicians. For example, I was told that things I did as part of my job were now to be considered "volunteer activities." But I was still required to do them. And then they added more tasks to my job description. It's ridiculous—that's why I left. I couldn't handle it anymore, and the way it was affecting care. It was just getting worse and worse.

So now all the experienced clinicians are leaving. So you know who you have delivering services? The PLPCs [provisionally licensed professional counselors] and PLCSWs [provisionally licensed social workers], people who are just out of school and don't know what they're doing. And then they're the ones training the direct care staff. And it just cascades. The whole quality of treatment has really declined. It's shameful.

As healers who dedicate themselves to treating eating disorders, eating disorder clinicians are situated at the nexus of legitimation and expertise on the one hand and stigma and defeat on the other. How they orient themselves to their practice illustrates a great deal about the precarious figuring of eating disorders within the larger landscape of American psychiatry, and the contemporary industry of psychiatry itself.

PRECARIOUS POSITIONS AND THERAPRENEURS

In such an atmosphere, therapists have to learn to think in new ways about their careers and how to position themselves in the new marketplace. "It's not like before, where you go to school, get trained, and you just do your job, you know, doing therapy," Catherine, another private practice therapist with ties to Cedar Grove, told me. "Now, [eating disorders] treatment centers are being bought up, and things are changing. You have to be flexible, to have the additional skills to say, 'Hey, I'm valuable. Look at all these different [therapeutic] modalities I'm trained in. Look at how you can utilize me.' You need to be able to say [to insurance companies and potential clients] that, you know, 'We have this many people certified in such-and-such evidence-based therapies.' You have to constantly be seeking those trainings and those certifications, because you need to stay in the game."

Brooke, a Cedar Grove therapist, for example, was trained as a licensed professional counselor. This credential used to be sufficient for getting a job at a place like Cedar Grove, and it's what got her in the door. But since she started working at the clinic, Brooke has also obtained certifications in art therapy, Internal Family Systems Therapy (IFS), sensorimotor psychotherapy, eye movement desensitization and reprocessing (EMDR), and dialectical behavior therapy (DBT). None of these modalities was created specifically for use with eating disorders, but each has been part of various research studies that found them to be effective for related issues, such as trauma, anxiety, and borderline personality disorder. These certifications made Brooke especially valuable, and she eventually became clinical director at Cedar Grove.

Training in a new therapy modality is both time-consuming and expensive. I know this firsthand, as I have obtained certification training in Internal Family Systems Therapy (ten months, at a cost of over $3,000), sensorimotor psychotherapy (ten months, over $2000), and dialectical behavior therapy (two years, free thanks to a forward-looking program sponsored by the Missouri Department of Mental Health). And this was just to attain level one of these modalities, each of which contains multiple levels that all require additional courses and supervision (for a fee) for full completion. The cost of such training is beyond the reach of many therapists, who must often save for years or take out loans to pay for courses, although some clinics, like Cedar Grove, take advantage of group rates to pay for select employees to get trained in a modality.

Trainings are not the only certification a therapist can pursue, however. For example, the International Association of Eating Disorder Professionals (IAEDP) has a certification program that grants the title of Certified Eating Disorder Specialist. It requires candidates to have an advanced degree and licensure in a clinical field, log 2,500 patient hours supervised by an IAEDP approved supervisor (for a fee), take five IAEDP courses (available online for a fee), pass a certification exam, provide a written case study, and submit three letters of recommendation. While this kind of certification does produce highly trained eating disorder specialists, it is not without its share of problems. The IAEDP program requires therapists to enroll in continuing education, participate in their (costly, though highly respected) symposia, and pay a yearly fee to maintain their credential, leading some to reject the classification on principle. "I already paid for all the coursework and supervision to meet the criteria," Amelia complained. "Why do I have to pay a yearly fee? It's ridiculous." Such arrangements are not unique to eating disorder organizations; they are part of a broader phenomenon in mental health. The result is a constant retooling and recapacitation within an alternate economy of certifications that positions clinicians as forever pursuing an elusive and receding goal.

In this way, therapists at Cedar Grove—and Cedar Grove as a therapeutic institution—are part of a phenomenon particular to the post-managed-care mental health scene that I call *therapreneurism*. Therapreneurs perpetually retool themselves and their practices, balancing the often-contradictory demands of serving their clients' emotional needs and making enough money to make ends meet. Therapreneuial practices include obtaining specialized training in various therapy techniques; taking evening or online classes on building a practice; participating in networking events; maintaining an online presence through websites, blogs, and commentaries; advertising; and branding oneself as a therapist who specializes in a particular kind of client or problem. In other words, the logic of therapreneurship holds that good therapists (or clinics) are those that are economically successful, as long as they are also savvy about the system. Just being skilled at providing psychotherapeutic care is not enough—one must also know how to "work the system," network for referrals, ensure placement on insurance panels, and secure appropriate reimbursement for care.[8]

Yet the relationship between economics and intimate bonds is "vexed,"[9] as financial exchange can render emotional and affective connection in cold and calculable terms that are far removed from their original intent. One therapist wryly described the work of psychotherapy to me as "merging with strangers for pay." In short, therapreneurs constantly refine and retool their capacities for care as well as their capacities to make a living, two goals whose objectives are often diametrically opposed but whose contradictions are elided by the focus on therapist development.

This displacement of contradictory affective modes onto the "capacitation" of the therapist (or clinic) forms the heart of therapreneurism. Successfully navigating a managed care system predicated on for-profit principles can directly undermine the emotional labor thought to be central to psychotherapeutic practice. "The worst is when you know how much someone is struggling, and they actually want to come in and get help, but their insurance won't pay," Janet, a Cedar Grove intake coordinator, told me. "It kills me to have to turn away someone who really wants help, but I don't have a choice. We'd go out of business if we helped everyone who wanted or needed it." In this way, therapreneurism incentivizes what economic anthropologist Karen Ho characterizes as a "naturalization" of the economy, which obscures the affective contradictions between the precarity of the managed care system and the promise of client recovery.[10]

But therapreneurism does more than this. In everyday practice at the clinic, therapreneurism materializes what anthropologist Kathleen Stewart calls the "precarious ordinary," where individuals (or clinics) become overwhelmed with uncertainty engendered by the privatization of risk.[11] Under such conditions, feminist scholars Julie Ann Wilson and Emily Chivers Yochim note, "practices of everyday life become synonymous with risk management" as people develop a hypervigilance and focus on "nailing things down" in an attempt, as philosopher Lauren Berlant characterizes it, to maintain their sea legs.[12] In other words, therapreneurial activities give people a sense of control, a sense that they are doing something proactive in the face of increasingly corporatized healthcare management.

This experience of radical instability, unpredictability, and vulnerability is an example of what philosopher Judith Butler calls "precarious life."[13] Precarity is a concept originally developed in the 1980s to describe the state of increasing insecurity (material, social, affective) under the conditions of late capitalism and neoliberalism. In describing the "precariat" (those living under the conditions of precarity), theorists have tended to emphasize economic and labor instabilities particular to late capitalism, or the "multiple forms of nightmarish dispossession and injury that our age entails."[14] As "the politically induced condition in which certain populations suffer from failing social and economic networks ... becoming differentially exposed to injury, violence, and death,"[15] precarity is "life without the promise of stability,"[16] where lives, leading nowhere, get lived nonetheless.[17] Under such conditions, people struggle to find certainty, even imposing it violently if necessary. In other words, conditions of precarity precipitate action and attempts to fix or stabilize what is otherwise falling apart.

Anthropologies of precarity have tended to look in two directions: first, at what happens when people are radically dispossessed through such things as unstable labor markets, which leaves them unable to meet basic needs and without a sense of security and furturicity; and second, at the emergence and functioning of structures and practices directed at ameliorating the effects of such processes. Anthropologist Andrea Muehlebach argues that these two dynamics are related and that the same forces that instigate precarious life also produce a particular "structure of feeling that privileges empathy, care and compassion."[18] In other words, the breakdown of old structures of stability and security go hand in hand with the emergence of new practices by which people attempt to care for themselves and one another in the midst of these changes.

Healthcare in the contemporary United States is a particular example of both the "breakdown" aspect of precarity and the "buildup" of what happens in its wake. Over the past half-century, heath costs have skyrocketed even as the availability and accessibility of services has decreased. This increased precarity of health coverage has been particularly pronounced in the area of mental health treatment, which, beginning in the 1980s, has been dramatically defunded and stripped of its infrastructure and is now reaching a crisis point. For example, in 1955, the United States had 560,000 psychiatric beds. Following the establishment of President Reagan's deinstitutionalization program in the 1980s, which accelerated discharges from hospitals and lead to the cancelation of many services, the situation has significantly deteriorated. According to a June 2016 report by the Treatment Advocacy Center, the United States now has 37,679 psychiatric hospital beds, down 13 percent since 2010. Spending has also been dramatically reduced. States cut $4.35 billion in public mental health spending between 2009 and 2012, though some states have made modest increases since 2012. "It's not like the patients have gone away. It's the treatment resources that have gone away," said Renée Binder, past president of the American Psychiatric Association.[19] The Treatment Advocacy Center recommends 40 to 60 psychiatric beds for every 100,000 people; the national average is 11.7. The group estimates that the country needs an additional 123,300 state psychiatric beds, though it is urging the federal government to do its own assessment. "Fewer beds and no more community services is a lethal combination," says Ron Honberg, a senior policy adviser at the National Alliance on Mental Illness.[20] Mental health is in many ways the arrow point or leading edge of precarity within the broader American health system.

Within the arena of mental health, some conditions have fared better than others. For example, between 2008 and 2017, government spending on schizophrenia research rose from $249 million to $268 million. Similarly, there has been a dramatic increase in autism research spending, which has gone from $118 million in 2008 to $243 million in 2017. Funding for Alzheimer's research has exploded, jumping from $412 million in 2008 to $1,361 million in 2017. Other conditions have not done as well. Research funding for eating disorders has declined from $29 million in 2009 to an estimated $23 million in 2018.[21]

In a time of precarity, why might some conditions get more support and others get less? In her book *Precarious Life,* Butler notes that some lives are deemed more "grievable" than others.[22] That is, some lives are more valued, their loss considered more profound, than others, which are viewed as *un*grievable. What makes a life grievable (or not) under conditions of precarity?

One of the main factors in grievability is the degree to which an individual is thought to embody his or her full potential as a contributing citizen. To *not* fully realize one's productive potential is to inhabit a state of debility. Yet as a social process, debility is not static. Under the conditions of neoliberalism, with its emphasis on individual initiative and perseverance in the face of adversity, debility can be seen as the condition of possibility for advancement, both for the individual and for society. That is, "debility," queer theorist Jasbir Puar notes wryly, "is profitable for capitalism," because the always perfectible body/self is ever induced to engage in technologies and practices aimed at helping it reach its full potential.[23] In other words, Puar argues, because debility is theoretically correctable, the existence (or appearance) of debility provides the impetus for a striving toward "health," broadly conceived, making debility a net positive force in terms of capitalist markets associated with self-improvement.

I argue, however, that this is not equally true for all forms of debility. Eating disorders are, in this view, decidedly *bad* for capitalism because, supposedly, their sufferers don't actually *want* to get better, so resources consumed by them purportedly disappear into a black hole. In other words, the calculus Puar describes only holds for those who *seek health,* or at least a form of health recognized as legitimate. In this view, some groups—like people diagnosed with eating disorders—are identified as beyond redemption, as generating a drag on the system, as ungrievable, in Butler's terms.

From this perspective, we might say that eating disorder patients represent "failed" neoliberal recruits within the contemporary managed healthcare landscape—they adopt many of the tools of neoliberalism (a desire for autonomy, industriousness, a willingness to sacrifice short-term comfort for long-term gain) and excel at them to the point that they fold back on themselves, coming to produce their opposites (dependency, debility, a time horizon that has become truncated and focused on the next bite of food). They "fail," then, by succeeding too well. This makes the question of "getting better" a dicey one. What does "getting better" mean in such a situation?

This has been a driving question of this book, where we have taken the theme of precarity into the culture of the eating disorders clinic, asking how structures and conditions of ontological insecurity come to constitute a particular affective space within which understandings of eating disorders—themselves structures of (physical and emotional) precarity—do very particular kinds of work. Specifically, I have been interested in how conditions of precarity produce mechanisms for attempting to fix and stabilize daily life in the clinic and how these mechanisms figure eating disorders as certain kinds of realities and eating disorder clients as certain kinds of subjects of care.

As I've thought through these issues, my analysis has followed critical human geographer Nancy Ettlinger's in that I view the analytic value of precarity as lying not in its condition as an end-point phenomenon but rather in the context-specific ways precarity emerges and the dynamics through which it is engaged.[24] That is, as Ettlinger says, precarity is not a macroscale feature unique to post-Fordist production or post-9/11 terrorism but rather an enduring feature of the human condition that "inhabits the micropractices of everyday life."[25] It is "a condition of vulnerability relative to contingency and the inability to predict" that "crosscuts spheres of life; it infuses life."[26] In this way, precarity "inhabits everything from the global political economy to the vicissitudes of employment, health, social relationship, self-perception, . . . the spaces in which individuals think and feel and interact."[27] In other words, precarity conditions affective worlds from the *inside* and the *underside,* not just from above. In response to such conditions of vulnerability, Ettlinger argues, emerges the urge to construct "illusions of certainty."[28] These micropractices of precarity and denial work hand in hand, as in their desperation for certainty people "misrepresent complex realities and act on those misrepresentations, in turn re-creating precarity."[29] Precarity, therefore, is always accompanied by a "grop[ing] for certainty," in what Ettlinger calls a "reflexive denial" of its own reality.[30]

For example, Ettlinger identifies three main logics that emerge to help people withstand the stress of precarity: classification, homogenization, and legitimation. Classification, she says, insulates specific groups from other specific groups, while homogenization reduces the differences within groups. Legitimization is "the means by which identities and power relations bound up with classification and homogenization are justified and possibly institutionalized."[31]

We have seen each of these processes at work at Cedar Grove in the context of managed care. Patients are classified—given a specific diagnosis (anorexia, bulimia, binge eating disorder, or other specified feeding or eating disorder)—which both differentiates them from others not in that category and also "suffocates difference" within categories.[32] This classification and homogenization is further amplified by the emphasis on evidence-based practice (itself predicated on processes of classification and homogenization), whose findings lead to claims such as "the best intervention for bulimia is outpatient cognitive behavioral therapy," as if all people with bulimia were exactly the same and would respond in exactly the same way to a given intervention. The circulation of "truth" between diagnostic regimes and evidence-based practice leads to the third logic, legitimization. If evidence-based practice research shows that the "best" treatment for bulimia is outpatient cognitive behavioral therapy, this is what insurance companies use in developing their protocols for treatment. This has very real material effects on people's lives. If the best treatment for bulimia is outpatient cognitive behavioral therapy, then why—barring medical instability—should someone with bulimia ever be admitted to residential care, regardless of her particular circumstance? Even if she is bingeing and purging twenty times a day, the research shows that bulimia is better treated through outpatient care. If a person is not getting better as an outpatient, then clearly the problem lies with her, and diverting even more resources to that person, who obviously isn't motivated to get better, does not make financial sense.

In this way, we can see how the essentialist logics Ettlinger identifies work in conjunction with each other to produce more certainty for one stakeholder in this situation—the insurance company—while increasing the experiences of precarity for others—most notably the client, but also the treatment center.

Within such an atmosphere, and with such material and affective realities, relationships of care in eating disorders treatment are especially fraught, charged, and unpredictable. They center, perhaps not surprisingly, on issues of control, responsibility, and vulnerability, as clients' "deservingness" for various forms of care are consistently evaluated and adjudicated.

This generates an *affective atmosphere* of surveillance and scrutiny—coupled with abstraction and erasure, and characterized by dynamics of scarcity and withholding—that recreates the lived experiences of eating disorders themselves. Under of the regime of managed care, resources are purportedly scarce, and clients' needs are, accordingly, characterized as burdens. Insurance companies continually scrutinize and penalize both clients and clinicians for asking for "too much" and not making do with the scarcest resources possible. This produces an affective atmosphere in the clinic of tension, withholding, and scarcity, where clients' needs are forever under suspicion.

In such an atmosphere, clients' needs—for a higher level of care, for more oversight by staff, for additional treatment days—are necessarily figured as problematic because these needs deplete valuable resources that should not be "wasted." *Want* is morally suspect for the same reason, shading over into speculations about secondary gains and longings for regression. *Desire* in any form is intolerable and deemed pathological unless it is a desire for *fewer* resources or attention, though even this can be, and often is, read as an indicator of manipulation. In other words, the affective climate in the clinic (re) conditions clients to minimize and even deny their own needs while at the same time telling them that such minimizing and denial is pathological. Denying their needs will kill them, clients are told. But it also structures the pathway to recovery.

THE CRUEL OPTIMISM OF CARE

Lauren Berlant describes "cruel optimism" as a state of affairs when the thing you desire is actually an obstacle to your flourishing, when you are induced to long for something that harms you.[33] An attachment to an object—a person, a goal, a state of being—becomes cruel, Berlant says, "when the object that draws your attachment actively impedes the aim that brought you to it initially."[34] In other words, cruel optimism persuades us to reach for something that, in the end, undoes its own impetus and causes us harm.

Treatment for an eating disorder under the current American managed care system is cruelly optimistic in Berlant's terms, cultivating hope and aspirational investment among clients and therapists alike while obscuring the fact that the structures that govern care replicate the affective dimensions of the illnesses they purport to treat and thus render recovery unlikely. The "optimism" of treatment is that the person with an eating disorder is told that she can get better if she lets go of her eating disorder and subjects herself fully to the expertise and care of the healthcare system. The "cruelty" comes when care is partial or truncated, not at the level needed, and/or attends only to immediate medical crises and not the extensive dynamics that gave rise to them. It comes when clients who are struggling are labeled as resistant and denied further treatment. It comes when clinicians are blocked from offering interventions their specialized clinical experiences tell them will help. It comes when care itself is so expensive that paying for it without insurance coverage is prohibitive for all but the richest members of society (and even for them, it can be painful). It comes when clients who are ill are accused of simply not wanting to get better. And it comes when care is structured by the very ideologies and practices that make people sick in the first place.

At a clinic like Cedar Grove, cruel optimism characterizes the conditions of care, despite everyone's best intentions. It shapes how eating disorders, and the people who have them, are perceived and the ways in which they are made visible—or invisible—as legitimate subjects of care.

SLOW DEATH

In such a context, clinicians can deliver good care only *in spite of* the structures that govern them, not *because* of them. For example, Susan, a Cedar Grove therapist, had this to say:

> I wonder sometimes why I continue to do this work. A lot of people don't want to work with eating disorders because it's so incredibly difficult. It's a very difficult disease to treat, and honestly, the people are a lot sicker than in other conditions like bipolar or even schizophrenia. Because it's not just about the eating. It's their whole way of being, their whole mode of relating to the world and to other people that is problematic. And there are no meds for it. Some things help, but it's not like these other conditions where meds can really relieve the symptoms pretty dramatically. So it's really, really taxing at times. And people fight treatment, even when part of them wants it. It's just part of the disease. So, there's that aspect to it. And then there's insurance. That pretty much dictates everything we do here, from start to finish. Because without insurance, there's no access to care. So, I can be doing brilliant therapy with someone, but if insurance decides it's time for them to go, they have to go. Ready or not. So that makes it hard to really invest in people.

The challenges of working with this population are exponentially exacerbated by the conditions of managed care, as the following conversation with Zoë, another Cedar Grove therapist, illustrates:

> ZOË: I think the burnout rate is so [high] because I feel we are underappreciated for the intensity of the work that we are doing. The work itself is so demanding and all-encompassing, and the support is sometimes lacking from the higher-ups because we are just a bunch of worker ants, just trying so hard to manage all the tiny little fires and making sure people stay alive. But there's not a lot of time to focus on the therapeutic work.
>
> REBECCA: What's gotten in the way of that?
>
> ZOË: For me, 97 percent of it is insurance. I might go to 95 percent, but I would say that the majority of it is insurance. For me, the burnout is that every couple of months, there are more responsibilities added to our plate, like, you're going to take an extra patient, or you're going to take this extra patient for a couple of weeks, and then you're going to do this group, and then you're going to do more meals, and then you're going to do more groups, and then you're going to do insurance reviews.

When we started doing insurance reviews is when I just couldn't keep up with the therapy anymore because everything was so focused on getting patients certed for more treatment days. Each review was something different. Each review, each reviewer. Like with [a major insurance company]—I had three different people I had to speak with, and each one is focused on something different. One wanted to know how family sessions were going, and they would cert more days if family sessions were productive. Other ones would want to know how the patients were doing in groups, meals, or their labs. Each reviewer was focused on something, and they would only cert or give more days if they met this arbitrary expectation that the reviewer had set.

REBECCA: You have to get to know each different reviewer.

ZOË: You did. It was almost a surprise each time. Each time before, they would want to know what the lab values were. We give them the labs and, "OK, we'll schedule after next week." Next week you'd give them the labs and they'll say, "Well but how was family therapy?" I'd say, "The parents didn't show." They'd say, "I can't give any more days until parents show up." Or they'd say, "I can give you two days." It's Friday, mind you, and we don't have family therapy on the weekend. We have to review on Monday, so they want you to have family therapy first thing Monday morning. But who knows if the parents are available or if they will come? A lot of times, the reviewers were focused on family therapy or group attendance. For some of these critically ill patients, they can't even participate in therapy. Their brains aren't working enough to even participate in therapy.

We see here how Zoë and the other therapists are put in the position of having to fight for care for patients based on things that are largely out of the patients' (or the therapist's) control. Zoë continues:

Or insurance would ask, "What sort of coping skills are they utilizing?" Again, they're in residential treatment. They don't really have to utilize any coping skills because there are not a lot of triggers, and if there are triggers, they don't have the availability to act on them. "When are they going on pass?" the insurance company would ask. Well, their blood pressure is 80/32, they still won't be going on pass. So they would not cert them for reasons like that. It was very frustrating in that they wanted them to do more work in therapy, which is fine except for the fact that they're passing out in the hospital every other day, which the insurance companies don't care about. It is so frustrating. I have burned out so quickly because of the reviews.

Here we see something interesting. Zoë is complaining that, at least in the case she's referring to, the insurance company cared more about the client's participation in therapy than about her medical status, which seems to sit at odds with claims I have been making about the priority these companies place on the medical model as opposed to the recovery model. What is important here is that there is not simply a one-to-one correspondence of insurance companies = medical model versus Cedar Grove = recovery model. The calculus is much more complex, and the aspects of care (medical, therapeutic, behavioral) emphasized on any given day varied depending on which reviewer a therapist happened to get on the phone and on what seemed most salient to that reviewer at that particular time. A more cynical reading—yet one that appears to be borne out by experience—is that insurance companies tended to emphasize whatever dimensions of care seemed to be the weakest or least developed in order to legitimize the denial of certification for additional treatment days.

This "whack-a-mole" dynamic, as one therapist described it to me, took an enormous toll on clinicians and had the effect of impoverishing the delivery of therapeutic care. As Zoë described the situation: "It was a full-time job that they put onto us. I felt like my therapy with each patient was insurance driven, no longer from what I felt like was needing to be worked on." Here, Zoë gives voice to the frustrations and overwhelm experienced by therapists at Cedar Grove. They described feeling co-opted by insurance companies and as if their therapeutic engagements with patients were significantly damaged as a result.

Conditions of cruel optimism like those at Cedar Grove produce what Berlant calls a "slow death," or "the physical wearing out of a population and the deterioration of people in that population that is very nearly a defining condition of their experience and historical existence."[35] Puar elaborates on this, stating that slow death is "how precarity is socialized into the intensification of the 'ongoing work of living,'"[36] with those targeted for premature or slow death being figured as bearers of debility. Such situations, Puar notes, raise the following questions: "Which bodies are made to pay for 'progress'? Which debilitated bodies can be reinvigorated . . . and which cannot?"[37]

The current state of eating disorders treatment in the United States is an exemplar of the slow death Berlant identified, but it operates in slightly different ways for different stakeholders. Sick clients are regularly denied access to benefits they have paid for, discharged against medical recommendations, deemed to have "failed" when they struggle, and even referred to hospice rather than provided with treatments professionals know can work. People with eating disorders have been induced to carry the symptom of a healthcare system in crisis, their conditions throwing into razor-sharp relief the fault lines and blind spots of a structure built on a vision of human life and experience that is both empirically false and actively harmful. But as Zoë and Susan make clear, the slow death is not just that of patients but that of therapists as well, as they are worn down, depleted, and devalued even as they are induced to retool, increase capacities, and take on more work.

So why do therapists stay at Cedar Grove? How do they keep doing this work, day after day, given the situation with managed care? As Trudy told me:

> I stay because I care about these girls, and I care about what happens to them. And every once in a while, you see someone turn the corner. And there is nothing better than that—nothing! And one instance of that can carry me for weeks. It doesn't even have to be a big corner. Sometimes it's a baby step, but you see someone starting to move in the right direction, and you think, "OK, I am really helping this person. I am making a difference." And that's what keeps me doing this work.

Brenda had a similar answer:

> I can't imagine *not* doing this work. It's incredibly difficult, but I stay because it's important, because these patients are so misunderstood and the treatment world is changing so much. I can't fix the system, but I can be the leading edge of that system where the patient is concerned and do my best to make it work for them. And these patients, well, they're challenging, but you get beneath the symptom and they are remarkable. Some of the brightest, most caring people you'll ever meet. They're just in crisis when they're here, and I want to help them get to the other side.

In other words, personal connections and relationships are critical to maintaining investment for therapists as well as for clients, yet these are the elements of care that are most at risk of co-optation.

Care at Cedar Grove, then, is both central and elusive, both an organizing principle and an ever-receding horizon. It is, on the one hand, what the clinic is there to *provide:* its purpose is to care for people with eating disorders by attending to their medical, psychological, and interpersonal needs. On the other hand, however, the resources to provide that care are not held by the clinic itself but are gatekept by managed care companies who ultimately decide who will receive care and who will not, under what conditions, and of what that care will consist. In the managed care framework, the fewer resources a patient needs, the "better" that patient is seen to be, a stance that perilously mirrors eating disorders themselves.[38] Worse yet, sometimes what a managed care company proscribes as "care" (e.g., moving a client to a lower level of care against treatment recommendations) is interpreted by the clinicians or clients as unhelpful or even harmful. The concept of "care," then, operates across several domains simultaneously in the clinic, sometimes folding back on itself to produce oblique expressions or even cause harm. This is what Aryn Martin, Natasha Myers, and Ana Viseu call care's "darker side: its lack of innocence and the violence committed in its name."[39] It matters in a material way how eating disorders and eating disorder clients are understood: the logics of care in this setting perpetuate a paradoxical rending of clients, treatment, and recovery that constitutes care as a continually shifting, mutable, and elusive goal.

Spark

To this day, I can't say for sure why I didn't take the pills. I'm very, very glad I didn't. For all the struggle, pain, and difficulty recovery has entailed, I am profoundly grateful that instead of taking the pills I somehow got myself up, walked across the hall to my friends' dorm room, and asked them for help. They took me to the RA. "I think I need to be in the hospital," I sobbed, and he made the call.

—————

TWELVE

Conclusions

WHERE DO WE GO FROM HERE?

In the contemporary United States, eating disorders are systematically undertreated and underresourced in ways that not only affect diagnosis, treatment, and everyday experiences of care but can have costly, debilitating, and even deadly consequences. The core principles of the American managed mental healthcare system resonate with and amplify the paradoxes, contradictions, and erasures that give rise to eating disorders themselves, producing treatment atmospheres that are highly problematic, even when practitioners have the best intentions. Pervasive stigma against and misunderstandings about eating disorders impede change and make collective organizing around this issue difficult.

What, then, can we do?

Abolishing for-profit healthcare would an obvious first step. Unfortunately, that is unlikely to happen. Given this reality, I suggest several concrete interventions that can move us forward. This list is far from exhaustive—rather, it offers some first steps. And what I provide here is merely an outline, highlighting points of interest on a larger and more complex roadmap to improved care. I will not go into detail about the "how" of these interventions—that would make this an even longer book. My goal here is to flag key points of intervention and leverage. These interventions fall under four main categories—terminology, education, research, and treatment— and reflect many goals of recent policy initiatives, including the Anna Westin Act, the Federal Response to Eliminate Eating Disorders Act (FREED Act), and the Missouri Eating Disorders Parity Bill, albeit with some differences.

Terminology

- **Eating disorders constitute an urgent public health crisis in the United States. Providing treatment for them is a social justice issue.** We need to talk about them unequivocally in these terms.

- Eating disorders have biological features, but **they should not be biologized to legitimate them** as "real" illnesses worthy of care. Doing so dislocates them from their social and cultural contexts and evacuates moral responsibility for the changing practices, relationships, and institutions that foster and amplify them.

- **Clients don't fail treatment; treatments fail clients.** This view does not exculpate clients from responsibility; I am a very strong believer in the importance of clients' active participation in their own well-being. Rather, it redirects our focus, taking it away from blaming clients for structural, ideological, cultural, and relational barriers to providing and receiving adequate care.

Education

- **Train professionals.** Currently, health professionals—even psychiatrists—receive very little (if any) training in how to identify, prevent, appropriately treat, and address the complications of eating disorders. Proper preparation is of paramount importance. All too often, individuals are misdiagnosed and/or treated in ways that make their eating disorder worse, not better (e.g., a primary care doctor once told an anorexic client of mine that she "couldn't possibly be anorexic" because she had eaten an egg for breakfast that morning; another doctor told a bulimic client that she "just needed to control herself better" and everything would be fine). To address this issue, we need to incorporate **accurate** eating disorder instruction in **all residency programs for all medical specialties** in the United States.

- **Train educators.** Similarly, we should establish programs to train educators in effective eating disorder screening, detection, prevention, and appropriate methods of assistance (some programs of this kind are already running; they are discussed later in this chapter).

- **Educate the public.** Public service announcements, information campaigns, and community initiatives aimed at educating the public about the types and seriousness of eating disorders and how to obtain help treating them can reduce stigma and increase the utilization of care resources. **But this should not happen unless adequate treatment is available.** It does little good to know you have a condition if you cannot obtain care to treat it. Awareness about eating disorders and genuine accessibility of care must go hand in hand.

- **Educate policymakers.** Many legislators have little knowledge about eating disorders or are misinformed about what these illnesses are and how they can be addressed. Organizations such as the Eating Disorders Coalition are already tackling this issue at the national level, but until eating disorders are recognized as a major mental illness covered by the Affordable Care Act, state-level policymakers have the most influence over the treatment of eating disorders. They should be educated about these conditions, the current barriers people encounter when trying to obtain care, and how legislative interventions can help improve access to necessary treatments.

- **Educate patients and their families about their rights and the avenues of action available to them.** The National Eating Disorders Association has an excellent blog post on this topic,[1] and a number of websites offer guidance for eating disorder clients and families negotiating with insurance companies. But more resources are needed, including more attorneys who are willing to take on the big insurance companies.

- **Bring eating disorders into already existing obesity initiatives.** Federally funded campaigns to fight obesity should also be required to address eating disorders.

Research

- **Obtain reliable community-based data.** We need reliable data. Current knowledge about eating disorders is primarily derived from very specific populations, namely those who have access to certain kinds of clinical care in locations where research studies are carried out. Not only does this select for those individuals who self-identify as having an eating disorder, but, because of the high cost of healthcare, these individuals tend to be middle to upper class and either have an insurance plan that is good enough to cover eating disorders or be able to pay out of pocket. Excluded from such accounts are people of lower socioeconomic status, those who do not have health insurance, those who either don't seek or don't receive an eating disorder diagnosis, and those who don't live near a major research center. This serves to further reinforce the misperception that eating disorders predominate among wealthy white women, when we know that eating disorders affect individuals of all gender identities, all socioeconomic groups, all races and ethnicities, and all geographic regions.

- **Determine the long-term costs and economic burden of eating disorders.** We need to better understand what eating disorders cost the American public. This should take into account the loss of years of productive life; missed days of work; reduced work productivity; the cost of medical and psychiatric treatment, prescription medications, hospitalizations, and treatment for medical and psychiatric comorbidities; the financial and emotional costs to families and caregivers; and so on. These costs should be factored into insurance company algorithms of what is "reasonable" for them to cover for full eating disorder care.

- **Determine the long-term health burdens of eating disorders.** We need to better understand the long-term health consequences of untreated and undertreated eating disorders.

- **Fund more research on finding innovative strategies** for delivering care, including telemedicine and on-line or app-based interventions.

- **Expand our conceptualization of "evidence"** to include more than randomized controlled trials.

Treatment

- **Require insurance plans to cover eating disorders.** Any insurer that provides health coverage for physical illness should be required to provide coverage for eating disorders.

- **Follow the American Psychiatric Association's standards of care.** Require insurers to follow standards of care established by the American Psychiatric Association's practice guidelines for the treatment of eating disorders.

- **Cover all levels of treatment.** Continuity of care is critical in treating eating disorders. Insurance plans that cover eating disorders should be required to cover hospital care, residential care, transitional living, and outpatient care.

- **Cover all major treatment modalities,** including but not limited to family, individual, and group therapy, nutrition counseling, psychiatric care, and medical treatment.

- **Add eating disorders to the services covered by Medicaid and Medicare, and increase the number of treatment centers and**

providers who accept these plans by paying clinicians reasonable reimbursement rates. Eating disorders treatment should be accessible to people of lower income.

- **Expand our understandings of treatment success** beyond weight restoration, medical stabilization, and behavioral symptoms.

- And last, but far from least, **listen to people with eating disorders.** Ask them what will help them get better. Enlist them in the project of treatment rather than seeing them as adversaries. They are experts on their own experiences and are the most valuable resources in crafting treatments that will work.

Taken together, these actions would significantly alter the landscape of eating disorders treatment, research, and prevention in the United States.

CURRENT INITIATIVES

Some of these improvements are already underway. The FREED Act (put before Congress in 2009, 2010, 2011, 2012, 2013, and 2014) was the first comprehensive eating disorders bill proposed in the history of Congress, and it included provisions for improved research, education, awareness, and treatment coverage. Although it was not passed, the FREED Act was a major advance in terms of educating lawmakers about the seriousness of eating disorders and the need for legislative action. In 2016, key provisions of the Anna Westin Act (originally proposed in 2015) were approved in a bipartisan bill that included a clarification of existing mental health parity law to expand health insurance coverage for eating disorders and life-saving residential treatment; improve early identification of eating disorders; increase training for health professionals; and enhance information and resources to help the public identify eating disorders. In the fall of 2018, the Substance Abuse and Mental Health Service Administration awarded the first grant for a new federal program that would provide $3.75 million over five years to fund the Center of Excellence for Eating Disorders at the University of North Carolina at Chapel Hill. The objectives of the center include:

- Providing the most up-to-date information on strategies related to addressing eating disorders.

- Promoting public awareness of eating disorders.

- Educating and training health professionals in understanding the effective treatment of eating disorders; the physical health needs in individuals with eating disorders; the frequently co-occurring medical and mental health conditions in those with eating disorders; integrated treatment of co-occurring eating disorders, other mental disorders, substance use disorders, and physical health disorders; and approaches for programs to address the needs of individuals living with eating disorders.[2]

These are significant and hard-won gains. But we still have a long, long way to go. Because national mental health legislation (including the Mental Health Parity Act) does not consider eating disorders to be "serious mental illnesses," they are left out of most legislative adjustments unless they are specifically identified. This means advocates within individual states have had to fight for equity in eating disorders coverage, with varying degrees of success.

The history and eventual success in 2015 of the Missouri Eating Disorders Parity Bill (SB145) is instructive. The bill was modeled on recent successful legislation for autism coverage in the state, but for the first several years it never made it out of committee. After multiple iterations and modifications, what emerged was a bill that requires insurance companies to cover eating disorders and provide coverage for patients' therapy and medical, psychological, psychiatric, nutritional, and pharmacy care. Furthermore, the act requires coverage to include a broad array of specialist services if prescribed as necessary by a patient's treatment team. It also specifies that medical necessity determinations must be based on a comprehensive evaluation of a patient's needs and not be based on weight alone. The bill was vehemently opposed by lobbyists for insurance companies, who argued that eating disorders are lifelong illnesses with poor prognoses and that requiring insurance companies to provide care for them would constitute an inordinate economic burden (note how this contrasts with the standard insurance position that eating disorders are episodic disruptions that abate once a patient's weight has returned to an "acceptable" level).

So what was it that finally pushed legislators to pass the bill? Much of the credit goes to Annie Seal, mother of a daughter with an eating disorder (now recovered), who worked tirelessly to spearhead the initiative and spent years making weekly four-hour round-trip drives from St. Louis to Jefferson City to educate and lobby lawmakers. Annie is a powerhouse, and her energy and commitment to equity for eating disorder coverage was the core driving force that finally got the bill passed. Her efforts were augmented by the testimony of clinicians (including Dr. Casey), researchers (including myself), parents, and former clients about the urgent need for change in Missouri. Together, we spent dozens of hours educating lawmakers about what eating disorders are, how deadly they can be, the fact that treatment can be effective, and the barriers to care in the state of Missouri. We testified half a dozen times in front of different state congressional committees, some members of which were openly hostile to the cause. I would like to believe that our testimonies made a difference.

But during a recent talk with a Missouri state lawmaker about the bill, I learned he had a different sort of perspective. "I remember when that former Miss Missouri came to the capitol to speak about eating disorders," he said. "That's when you got all the good ol' boys to pay attention! They all wanted to get a peek at her. Did you see how many people came out of their offices to hear her speak? Enlisting her was a stroke of brilliance."

Unfortunately, that is true. A former Miss Missouri spoke in the rotunda at the Missouri state capitol on behalf of our bill. I was adamantly *not* in favor of enlisting a beauty pageant winner as a spokesperson for eating disorders, but I was overruled. And apparently, I was wrong, at least in terms of the efficacy of the tactic. Maybe it was coincidence, but the year she spoke was the year the bill finally passed.

The Missouri bill has been heralded as a landmark measure, so much so that the National Eating Disorders Association has expressed interest in using it as a template for other states to follow in their own efforts. But note this: as good as the bill may be, *there are no means of enforcing it.* In theory, people can report insurance noncompliance to the state office in charge of regulating insurance companies. But in a meeting with the director of this department, I learned that they can do little more than collect complaints. They have no authority to actually *do* anything to sanction the insurance companies who violate the provisions of the bill. Nevertheless, Dr. Casey and other clinicians have told me they have seen some improvement with regard to eating disorder care in Missouri. At least there is a law they can point to when negotiating with insurance companies. But it is far from enough.

A provision of an earlier version of the Missouri bill that made it through the legislative process was the establishment of the Missouri Eating Disorder Council, of which I am a member. The council "is charged with leading eating disorders education, awareness, and treatment initiatives throughout the state, and promoting increased access to evidence-based therapies and other treatments of proven effectiveness."[3] Two key activities of the council are worth highlighting here. First, the council has made it a priority to improve the availability of eating disorder services in the state of Missouri; currently, these services exist primarily in St. Louis and Kansas City. People living in the rest of the state may be hours away from anyone trained in any aspect of eating disorder diagnosis and care. Second, the council has set a goal to train more clinical professionals in how to diagnose and treat eating disorders. To this end, the council developed the 360 Program, which provides free training for clinicians in the top evidence-based treatments for eating disorders, including family based therapy and interpersonal therapy; an eating disorder "boot camp" for dieticians; a class on early identification of eating disorders; and a course on the evaluation, treatment, and medical management of eating disorders. To date, these trainings have been attended by hundreds of clinicians from the entire Midwest region, and video recordings of them are available for viewing on the council's website. More training programs are in the works. Additionally, the council has focused its efforts on a select number of community mental health centers in the state in order to develop them into centers of excellence for treating eating disorders.

The Missouri Eating Disorders Association is working on another side of the issue, and its mission is to "fight eating disorders, educate communities, and save lives."[4] Its flagship program is an education initiative called Feed the Facts, which educates middle and high school students about eating disorders, their dangers, and how to seek help. The program reaches well over three thousand students each year and is growing by leaps and bounds. A version for educators has been developed for teachers and coaches, and versions for parents and younger children are currently in development. As a member of the board for over six years, I have watched this organization grow and flourish, and through the tireless dedication and hard work of its board members and many volunteers, it is beginning to change the conversation around eating disorders in St. Louis and beyond.

All of this is wonderful and important, and it represents significant strides. None of it, however, addresses the fundamental issue of how to pay for life-saving treatment if an insurance company denies a patient coverage or offers contingent, underresourced care. So pervasive is this problem in eating disorders treatment that the National Eating Disorder Association has an entire web page dedicated to the issue, advising clients and families to "document everything" and "thank and compliment everyone who assists you" at the insurance company, because "you're more likely to receive friendly service when you are polite while being persistent." Importantly, the website notes, "your insurance company is not your enemy. . . . Treat each person as though they have a tough job to do."[5] Be this as it may, it remains the case that clients and families often end up spending dozens of hours arguing with insurance companies to get even provisional access to much-needed and life-saving care.

The bottom line is this: until and unless eating disorders are officially recognized as serious mental illnesses, until and unless we have genuine, enforceable parity for mental health treatment, and until and unless insurance companies are required to follow the American Psychiatric Association's guidelines for necessary care, we can't even begin to address the public health problem of eating disorders in this country. And sufferers will continue to carry the burden of a healthcare system that is perpetually famished.

Afterword

"How's the book coming?" my father asks. He and my mother are on the phone, each on a different extension so they can both talk to me at once. "It's almost done," I reply, relief saturating my voice. "Hooray!" they exclaim in unison. My parents are my biggest cheerleaders. They are wonderful people and good parents.

It may appear from some of the vignettes I've included that my parents are somehow responsible for my eating disorder. They are not to blame. Yes, they did and said some things that contributed to it. But so did friends, teachers, strangers, and a group of truly awful boys who sexually harassed and body shamed me daily and without mercy all through my ninth-grade year. All of that played a part. But my issues started long before I was ten, when I began my first diet. And it wasn't until about five years ago that I fully recognized how deeply these issues ran.

Next to Normal is a musical about a family (made up of a mother, a father, and their teenage daughter) that is deeply emotionally haunted by the death of their young son from illness. The musical takes place fifteen or so years after this tragedy, though you don't know this for the first third of the show because the boy (played by a live actor) is still so present for the characters—particularly the mother—in ways that are heart-wrenchingly tangible and real. The daughter struggles for her parents' approval and to get them to simply see and engage with her in the here and now, but they are so drenched in grief, loss, and guilt that they can't quite experience her, even when she is right there in front of them.

On the way home from seeing the musical, in 2013, I felt something well up inside me and break over me like a wave. I began to sob uncontrollably, so much that I had to pull my car over to the side of the road for fear of causing an accident. As deep, bone-rattling sobs and wails emerged from me, wracking my body, I had a profound realization. It was not something I had repressed but rather something I had never given much import to until that moment.

When I was five years old, my parents told my older brother, Marty, and me they were expecting a baby. I was thrilled and wonderfully excited, and I anticipated the birth with eagerness. I helped fold the baby clothes and get the nursery ready. Every day I hoped it would be the day when the baby would finally come.

But inside my mother, unbeknownst to anyone, the umbilical cord was wound around the baby's neck. When she went into labor and the baby dropped into her pelvis in preparation for delivery, the cord strangled him. The baby died in her womb, on the verge of being born.

My parents named him Ethan.

I remember vividly when my father came to the elementary school to tell my brother and me what had happened. We were expecting to hear joyous news of a new baby brother or sister, but instead he told us that the baby had died. At that point, my memory—which is freakishly detailed for much of my childhood—goes blank for about a year. I have a few scattered memories here and there, but I recall very little. I do remember that family friends came to stay with us for a while, and my uncle. But I have zero memories of my parents during that time.

Now, as a mother myself, I realize my parents must have been in excruciating pain, grieving such a horrible, horrible loss while trying to keep it together for their two small children (I was six and my brother was nine by then). I cannot even imagine what that must have been like. I have no recollection of seeing either of them cry (though I'm sure they did, and I assume I saw it at some point). It's just a big, blank void.

What I *did* remember in the wake of seeing *Next to Normal* was a conviction that started during that time and that became a fundamental bedrock of my emotional life. I remembered that I became absolutely convinced that my parents wished *I* had died instead of Ethan, that they would have been happier if he were alive and I were gone.

I am a thousand percent certain that no one ever said this, or anything remotely like it, to me. I was six years old, and I thought with a six-year-old's mind and felt with a six-year-old's heart. Had I secretly wished for there to be no baby and then felt somehow guilty about the baby dying and thought I should be punished? It's possible, although I don't recall anything like that. Instead, I suspect it was something else.

I was a very lively child—something of a handful, apparently. My parents found aspects of this frustrating at times, but they also took a great deal of delight in me. I remember this well. I wonder, though, if, in the aftermath of this horrible loss, my previously endearing spunkiness and fiery nature might have simply become too much for them to bear, too much to humor, too much to tolerate. I wonder if I saw—or sensed—how devastated my parents were and heard—or sensed—that I was "too much" for them in a variety of ways, and that I should make myself quieter, less needy, less *there*. In any event, this deep conviction I had held that my parents wished I had died instead of Ethan came rushing up after seeing *Next to Normal*. I sobbed in my car for close to an hour before I could finally drive home.

I thought about this nonstop for the next week. I was hesitant to raise the issue with my parents because I didn't want to cause them any unnecessary pain, but I finally decided I had to ask them about it.

"Oh sweetheart, no! Of course we never ever thought that!" my mother assured me (both my parents were on the phone again, as usual). "In fact, we were so grateful for you and your brother! You gave us so much joy in what was a very difficult time."

"And I always wanted a daughter," my father chimed in. "I wouldn't have given you up for anything."

"Did we ever talk about this family trauma in our family therapy sessions?" I asked. "I don't remember it coming up."

"Not really. Just as a thing that happened," my mother replied. "But no, we never looked at it as something significant to the eating disorder."

I find this absolutely astounding. How one could *not* consider how such a devastating loss would alter a family system is beyond me. There is no way it *wouldn't* have changed things in some really profound ways. No matter how skilled or smart or capable they may have been, my parents were, at the time, a young couple with two young children who had just lost a full-term baby. The fact that my father is an ob-gyn certainly must have contributed to the complexities of feelings they experienced, even though there was nothing anyone could have done to change the outcome. For multiple family therapists over many years to not have engaged this event in any significant way is telling, I think, of how the psychotherapeutic community has tended to focus eating disorder interventions on the identified patient (in this case, me) as the problem to be fixed while ignoring other elephants in the room.

I should say that, from what I recall, my parents did everything they were "supposed" to do for my brother and me in the wake of Ethan's death. I remember them telling us it was OK to talk about our feelings, and they bought books like *Transactional Analysis for Kids* (my first introduction to psychotherapeutic philosophies) to help us do so. My teachers and principal at school were kept in the loop and were supportive. I don't believe my parents sought their own therapy support (though I don't know for sure), and if not, that might have helped. But for all intents and purposes, they navigated this time as well as could be expected. My younger brother, Joe, was born about a year later.

I bring all of this up here, at the end of this book, as a way of pointing to the kinds of deep, abiding issues that drive the development of eating disorders and to note that identifying and processing them must necessarily be part of healing these conditions. Did I diet? Yes. Did I watch MTV and wish I looked like the women in the videos? Sure. Did my eating disorder focus on thinness and weight and body shape? Absolutely. *But my eating disorder was not "about" these things any more than a compulsion to flip a light switch sixteen times when entering a room is about electricity.* It was, I believe, about not knowing how to *be* when I had become convinced that my existence was fundamentally, deeply *wrong.* It was a way of trying to not exist while still living.

To be clear, Ethan's death didn't directly cause my eating disorder. But it did lay the groundwork for it. Biology—my temperament and a family history of addiction, anxiety, and depression—certainly played a role, but if the thoughts and feelings I had in the wake of Ethan's death hadn't resonated with other messages I was getting at home and in other areas of my life or hadn't been amplified in a thousand ways over many years (including by myself), I doubt they would have taken hold the way they did.

Similarly, recovering from an eating disorder is not going to happen by focusing solely (or even primarily) on weight gain and behavioral modification. These things are vitally important and must certainly be part of the picture. But they are simply the mechanism of expression. Full healing occurs when someone comes to believe that they *deserve to exist,* that *their being is valuable and good,* that *their presence is recognized by others,* and that *they matter.* There are many ways to get to this place—there is more than one path. But there is one shared feature: *it happens in relationship.* It is absolutely, fundamentally relationships that heal—not therapeutic modalities or treatment plans or goal weights, but *relationships.* And because of this, healing is an ongoing, evolving process. As we change and grow, we discover new sharp edges, new sore spots, new dark recesses, and new vulnerabilities. But it is in these places, the human places, that we become fully alive, fully— finally—*here*.

. . .

You must burn.
Burn higher.
Burn for everything you have ever wanted.
For everything you have ever lost,
for every crack in your heart and every fraction of every irreplaceable
    moment.
Burn high for love. For fear. For life.
Burn as fast and as long as you can.
You must burn, burn higher.
Because nothing in this world will kill you faster than a dying fire.

—Mia Hollow

ACKNOWLEDGMENTS

This project would not have been possible without generous investments of labor, support, and encouragement by many, many, *many* people over a long stretch of time. I cannot possibly thank them all here, but I want to offer some particular words of acknowledgment and gratitude to some of them.

First and foremost, I wish to thank the dozens of Cedar Grove clients who shared their stories and experiences with me. They allowed me into their lives during some of their most vulnerable and difficult moments, when their emotional reserves were depleted and their futures were far from clear. Every single one of them expressed a desire to help others through sharing their journeys and experiences, no matter how painful that sharing might have been or how raw and "unpolished" their words might appear in these pages. To these courageous and generous women, I owe a deep, deep debt of gratitude.

This project would not have been possible without the approval and support of the woman I call Dr. Casey, who not only granted me access to Cedar Grove but was also a remarkable support throughout the research and writing process. Her indefatigable spirit and her insights, wisdom, and experience have been invaluable. I also want to thank the many Cedar Grove clinicians (therapists, nurses, dieticians, and on-line staff), who not only welcomed me into the clinic but also mentored me and shared with me the triumphs and struggles of their work. Thank you as well to the many family members who opened up to me about living with a loved one with an eating disorder and the challenges of trying to obtain necessary care.

A number of undergraduate and graduate students at Washington University in St. Louis have also been instrumental in the development of this project, and I am deeply grateful to all of them: thank you to Elizabeth Riley for early discussions about the data and attempts to frame the manuscript; to Remy Schlossberg for transcribing and coding; to Olivia Emmanuel, Hannah Grogin, Georigica Popcorn, Sienna Ruiz, and Lydia Strakka for help with the bibliography; and to Caroline Grant for reading early drafts of chapters, providing invaluable insights and comments, and contributing to an early formulation of some parts of chapter 6. I'd like to give a very special thanks to PhD student Lauren Cubellis for helping me think through the framing of my argument and getting me out of writer's block. I also wish to thank all the participants of the Ethnographic Theory Workshop at Washington University for extremely constructive and helpful feedback on the book project in its early stages, and the students in several years of my Argumentation through Ethnography seminar, who encouraged, challenged, and inspired me. Thank you to my department chair, T. R. Kidder, and to Dean Barbara Staal for providing me with the protected time needed to finish the manuscript.

Several interlocutors in the academic world of anthropology and eating disorders have been (and remain) a continual source of inspiration, intellectual engagement, and support. In particular, I wish to thank Eileen Anderson-Fye, Karin Eli, Sigal Gooldin, Helen Gremillion, Anna Lavis, Merav Shohet, and Megan Warin for their exemplary work in the field and for continually working toward better understandings of eating disorders in the hope of improving the lives of those who suffer. I am especially grateful to Eileen Anderson-Fye and Helen Gremillion for their careful and constructive engagement with the initial draft of this manuscript and their insightful suggestions for improvement. I am extraordinarily fortunate to have benefited from the insights of these two central figures in the anthropological study of eating disorders.

I also wish to thank all of the current and past members of the board of the Missouri Eating Disorder Association for their encouragement and support throughout the research and writing process, most notably Ali Fields, Lisa Iken-Sokolik, Annie Seal, and Katie Thompson, all of whom have inspired me and given me the courage to continue, even when they didn't know they were doing so.

Kate Marshall, my editor at the University of California Press, has enthusiastically supported this project and expertly guided it through the review and production process, assisted by Bradley Depew and Enrique Ochoa-Kaup. A huge thank you goes to Barbara Armentrout for her masterful review of the manuscript and recommendations for editing. Many thanks to Genevieve Thurston, whose careful copyediting was priceless, and to Amron Gravett, for generating the index.

And finally, I want to thank the following people for their support, encouragement, and inspiration at various stages of research and writing: Christine Bertolino, Chris Hayes, Davinder Hayreh, Fiona Hayreh, Peter Kovacs, Arthur Lester, Linda Lester, and Daegan Marker. You all witnessed various parts of the behind-the-scenes process of this book, supported me through this endeavor, and seem to love me still. Thank you.

NOTES

1. All names used in this book are pseudonyms.
2. Martin, Myers, and Viseu 2015.
3. This leads to the issue of informed consent. In the early part of my work at Cedar Grove (before I entered clinical training), I followed standard the ethnographic procedure of obtaining informed consent from all participants to observe clinical activities, and I obtained separate consent for individual interviews. But the bulk of the work that went into this ethnography is unconventional in the sense that it does not clearly fit under any one ethical umbrella. Technically, my work as a clinician (which started in the winter of 2004) fell under the purview of Cedar Grove, and the use of any information I obtained in the course of performing my clinical role was consented to by clients when they signed their admission paperwork (which includes a clause about how their protected health information might be used for research purposes). I consulted with my university's institutional review board, which assured me this would, indeed, be sufficient to ensure consent. However, this did not feel entirely right to me. I felt it important to obtain additional signed consent forms from any clients with whom I worked individually as a therapist and to obtain verbal consents from clients I knew more casually in other ways (through group therapy, for example). I let all clients know (and reminded them at regular intervals) that they had the right to change their minds and decline to participate in the research at any time and that this would not have any consequences whatsoever for their treatment. I got additional consent for interviews. I also obtained consent from all staff at Cedar Grove and renewed this consent every six months. All identifying information has been removed or disguised to protect the privacy and confidentiality of participants.

In addition to conducting thousands of hours of participant observation and both formal and informal interviews with clinicians, clients, and families, I conducted a series of three semistructured interviews with twenty-five clients at three different points in their treatment process (seventy-five interviews in total). In the first interview (conducted within the first seventy-two hours of treatment), I asked clients to tell me how their eating disorder started and progressed, how they came to be in treatment, and what they found most challenging and most helpful so far. I began these interviews with the prompt, "Tell me about how you came to be at Cedar Grove," and followed the client's narrative from there. The second interview focused on how clients were experiencing treatment and how their understandings of their eating disorder were changing (or not) in the clinic. In this interview, I asked questions like: Looking back now, what do you think caused your eating disorder? What is everyday life like for you here? What do you find the most challenging about treatment, and what is the most helpful? If you could design the "perfect" eating disorders treatment, what would it look like? The final interview focused on clients' hopes and fears regarding recovery beyond the clinic. I asked questions like: What do you imagine things will be like when you go back home? What are your biggest hopes and concerns about recovery? What are other people's expectations of your recovery? Where do you hope to see yourself in a year from now? My purpose with these interviews was to get a sense of how recovery is experienced for clients as they move through the treatment process.

4. Stevenson 2014.

1. INTRODUCTION

1. American Psychiatric Association 2013.

2. Other eating disorders included in the *DSM-5* are avoidant-restrictive food intake disorder (ARFID, previously called selective eating disorder), pica, and rumination disorder. ARFID is similar to anorexia in that both involve restricting the amount or kind of foods consumed to the point of medical compromise, but unlike anorexia, ARFID does not involve disturbance in body weight or shape or fears of fatness. Pica involves eating items that are not typically considered food, like dirt, hair, or paint chips. Rumination disorder is characterized by the regular regurgitation of food that may then be re-chewed, re-swallowed, or spit out. Although not an official diagnostic category in the *DSM-5*, orthorexia is an eating disorder that involves an obsession with "healthy eating" to the point that it interferes with daily functioning and with the individual's wellbeing. Although all of these different eating disorders presented at Cedar Grove, anorexia, bulimia, binge eating disorder, and other specified feeding and eating disorder were by far the most common.

3. Becker, Thomas, and Pike 2009.

4. Lester 2014.

5. Hoek 2006.

6. Arcelus et al. 2011.

7. Hoek 2006.

8. Hudson et al. 2007.

9. Dumit 2006, 577.

10. Dumit 2006, 578.

11. Dumit 2006, 580.

12. Dumit 2006, 578.

13. Dumit 2006, 578.

14. Lester 2016.

15. Dumit 2006, 585.

16. I prefer the term "clients" but use these terms interchangeably.

17. Mulligan 2014.

18. Rose 2005.

19. Mulligan 2014.

20. Luhrmann 2000.

21. For an excellent anthropological engagement with concepts of moral agency, see Myers 2015.

22. Noordenbos et al. 2002.

23. Vandereycken 2003.

24. Fox, McManus, and Reichman 2003.

25. Striegel-Moore et al. 2000.

26. "*Glamour* Magazine Exclusively Investigates Managed-Care Organizations Who Refuse Treatment for Anorexics," Business Wire, July 12, 1999, www.thefreelibrary.com/Glamour+Magazine+Exclusively+Investigates+Managed-Care+Organizations...-a055122563.

27. Ibid.

28. Horgan et al. 2015.

29. Hudson et al. 2007; LeGrange et al. 2012.

30. National Institutes of Health 2018.

31. American Psychiatric Association 2013.

32. Kalisvaart and Hergenroeder 2007.

33. Levine and Smolak 1996.

34. Gaesser 2002.

35. Mellin, Irwin, and Scully 1992.

36. Collins 1991.

37. Sullivan 1995.

38. Arcelus et al. 2011.

39. Eating Disorders Coalition 2016.

40. Steinhausen 2009.

41. Steinhausen 2009.

42. National Institutes of Health 2018.

43. See the website of the Eating Disorders Coalition at www.eatingdisorders-coalition.org for information about mental health parity and state and federal legislative initiatives regarding eating disorders.

44. Angell 1993.

45. Warren et al. 2013.

46. Throughout this text, I follow Laura M. Ahearn's understanding of "agency" as the socioculturally mediated capacity to act. See Ahearn 1999.

47. Warin 2009.

48. Levinas 1996.

49. Legrand and Briend 2015.

50. Levinas 1979.

2. RETHINKING EATING DISORDERS

1. Gull 1874.

2. See Mintz and DuBois 2002 for an excellent review of this literature.

3. This is not always seen as a bad thing. In the case of fasting nuns in the Middle Ages or Buddhist monks seeking enlightenment, for example, rejecting human social ties has been viewed as essential to reaching spiritual heights. Similarly, Gandhi's hunger strikes communicated with striking clarity his rejection of the colonialist regime and the moral structures that kept Indians subject to British rule, and they became a model of civil disobedience. Rejecting food, then, can be socially valued when it is associated with abstaining from worldly pleasures and temptations in pursuit of loftier goals and when an individual's motivations for doing so are thought to be clear and trustworthy. Through this rejection, a person can actually become part of a different sort of social group of similar seekers.

4. Bell 1985.

5. Caroline Walker Bynum's *Holy Feast and Holy Fast: The Religious Significance of Food to Medieval Women* (1988) is a classic text exploring these issues.

6. Morton 1694.

7. See Brumberg 2000 for a deeper exploration of these issues.

8. Object relations theory versus ego psychology versus self psychology, for example.

9. The Minnesota Model (based on the principles of Alcoholics Anonymous and centered on practices of abstinence) became the most widespread and influential approach of this kind. See Anderson, McGovern, and Dupont 1999 for a good review of the history of this model. See White 1998 for a more comprehensive look at the history of the treatment of addiction in the United States.

10. See Illouz 2017 for an excellent and provocative history of and engagement with the self-help movement.

11. Lock and LeGrange 2015.

12. James Lock's two-day training "FBT for Eating Disorders," presented on September 26–27, 2016, in St. Louis, Missouri, also supports this.

13. See, e.g., Medway and Rhodes 2016.

14. Klump et al. 2001. See also Bulik et al. 2007 for a good review of the genetics of eating disorders.

15. Keys 1950; Fairburn 2008.

16. Chavez and Insel 2007.

17. Bordo 2004.

18. American Psychiatric Association 2013.

19. See, e.g., Bordo 2004.

20. Orbach 2005.

3. EATING DISORDERS AS TECHNOLOGIES OF PRESENCE

1. See Swartz 1985; Palazzoli 1985; and DiNicola 1990 for representative articulations of this perspective.

2. See, e.g., Nasser 1988; Swartz 1985; Gordon 1988; and Prince and Thebaud 1983.

3. See Keel and Klump 2003 for one of the first comprehensive review articles on the cross-cultural aspects of eating disorders.

4. While at first glance the acculturation hypothesis seems to be well supported by the data, there are a number of significant problems with the causal reasoning used, particularly in the way culture is talked about. See Lester 2004 for a full discussion of these issues.

5. Key theorists include Caroline Giles Banks (1992, 1996), Helen Gremillion (1992), and myself (Lester 1995, 1997, 1999, 2000), as well as others. In her study of people practicing anorexia, for example, Megan Warin (2009) argues that eating disorders enact and structure interpersonal relationships around dynamics of disgust and abjection. Lavis (2016) considers how not eating—rather than thinness—is the driving motivation in anorexia, mediating practitioners' relationships with others as well as with anorexia itself. Karin Eli (2014) examines the interpersonal dimensions of relatedness in inpatient eating disorders treatment by exploring how patients variously consider themselves both similar to and different from others on the unit. Helen Gremillion (2003), who conducted research in a treatment center, contends that treatment "feeds" anorexia by replicating many of the practices of the disorder under the guise of intervention (e.g., hyperfocusing on calories and weight) while also mirroring family dynamics that are thought to give rise to the condition. Sigal Gooldin's (2008) work on anorexia in Israel highlights how the visible presentation of a skeletal body can evoke particular kinds of interpersonal reactions in a society still haunted by the Holocaust. And Merav Shohet (2007, 2008) illustrates how clients narrate identities though the language of recovery. Other anthropologists have examined the cultural and social conditions under which eating disorders might develop and flourish, as well as factors that might contribute to their prevention (see, e.g., Becker 2004, 2007; Lester 2007; Anderson-Fye 2004; and Pike and Borovoy 2004).

6. Annemarie Mol (2002), for example, argues that atherosclerosis is "enacted," or brought into being, in different ways in different settings, from the laboratory to the doctor's office, constituting a "body multiple." Julie Livingston (2012) argues that cancer as a disease emerges and exists not in a festering tumor or in tissue samples on a slide but rather *between* people as they negotiate obligations of care.

7. Like Mol, I consider how eating disorders are enacted in different institutional settings. Unlike Mol, however, I am interested in interpersonal relationships as well

as technological and material practices as sites of production. Like Livingston, I am interested in how eating disorders exist between people but operate in ways that do specific ethical work. Like Gremillion, I engage questions of gender and power in an eating disorders treatment center, but as an anthropologist and clinician, as well as a former eating disorder patient, I tell this story from a range of positions and perspectives with a theoretical orientation that focuses more on the *how* and the *why* of such relationships rather than on the *what*. Like Warin, I understand eating disorders as centering on issues of relatedness and intimacy, but as a therapist and psychological anthropologist I place the self and psychological processes more centrally in my analysis, and this changes the contours of the engagement. Like Eli, I focus on how eating disorders function to navigate intimacies and relatedness in an eating disorders clinic, but I am interested in the range of relationships that emerge (including with clinicians, families, and insurance companies) and how they enable various conjurings of eating disorders as a means for working out ethical and interpersonal claims. Like Gooldin, I engage the visceral dimensions of eating disorders and keep the material body at the center of my inquiry (ironically, this is not common in the eating disorders literature, where the material body often disappears from the discussion), but as my research is located in the United States I consider the massive impact of managed care on the structuring of this process once people have made contact with the healthcare system, and how entanglements of the healthy subject with the moralizing ethos of capitalist market forces shapes experiences of illness and care. And like other authors of cross-cultural studies of eating disorders, I am interested in the role of culture in the development and treatment of disordered eating, but I take a view of culture as emergent and embedded in interpersonal relations rather than as something located outside of or separate from the illness itself.

8. Here, I follow the line of Zahavi 2001.

9. See, e.g., Gutman, Hutton, and Martin 1988.

10. See, e.g., Deveaux 1994 for an excellent orientation to key feminist critiques.

11. Most notably Heidegger and Derrida.

12. See, e.g., Jacques Lacan, Julia Kristeva, and Jessica Benjamin.

13. See, e.g., works by Martin Buber, Matthew Engelke, and Tanya Luhrmann.

14. See, e.g., Sanchez-Vives and Slater 2005, Riva et al. 2007, Loomis 2016.

15. To continue the metaphor for a moment, what often happens in eating disorders is that people who, for a whole host of reasons, "transmit on AM," grow up in families whose "radios" are tuned to FM. An eating disorder becomes a sort of converter that people use to render AM frequencies into FM sound. Often, this generates a lot of static, a great deal of noise, and a whole lot of confusion and frustration on both sides. This is not anyone's fault. The parents may be perfectly good "radios" who are expertly adept at tuning in to FM stations or to a certain range of frequencies. The child may be a perfectly good "transmitter," transmitting beautifully and clearly on AM or on a station outside her parents' range. In either case, they are not able to *tune in to each other,* except through the eating disorder, which is a garbled and distorted kind of tuning in that leaves the person with the eating disorder feel-

ing unseen and misunderstood and loved ones wondering what happened to their daughter/wife/sister who seems to have disappeared into her disease.

16. Riva et al. 2007.

17. See Mitchell 2014; Benjamin 2017; Stolorow and Atwood 2014; Stolorow 2011; and Orange 2010.

18. Massumi 2007, 2016; Thrift 2004, 2008.

19. Ahmed 2014; Blackman 2012; Wetherell 2012.

20. Anderson 2009, 2016.

21. Ahmed 2014.

22. Wetherell 2012.

23. Food, too, is animated by affect. As anthropologist Megan Warin (2003) shows, "eating" for a person with anorexia (or bulimia) does not necessarily mean only the oral ingesting of food—it can include the invasion of smells, sights, sounds, and touch through the senses of body. Food enters the nose, its scent snaking its way in through the nostrils and down the back of the throat. It enters through the eyes, as they feast on its appearance. It enters through the skin, its "miasmatic calories" (Warin 2003) seeping into the body's surface should it happen to make contact or even get too close. Even the ears are a point of entry, as hearing sounds of cooking or of others eating can be threatening and contaminating. The eating disordered "bodyself" is permeable and vulnerable at all times to the accidental incorporation of food (and affect) from the outside. Like affect, then, food has both material and immaterial instantiations.

But food is not just *similar* to affect—it is a bearer of affect in a very real sense. It changes how our bodies and brains feel, depending on the meanings, the setting, and the relationships involved. In eating disorders, ritualized embodied practices develop that manage, create, block, improvise, control, and regulate the way one affects and is affected and, consequently, the textures of existence.

24. MacLeish 2012. See also MacLeish 2015 for the full ethnography.

25. MacLeish 2012, 57, 58.

26. MacLeish 2012, 56.

27. Taussig 1991, 147.

28. Seremetakis 1996.

29. MacLeish 2012, 58.

30. MacLeish 2012, 64.

31. B. Williams 1981.

32. Olivia had a long-term boyfriend, but although the two had a very loving relationship, it had become nonsexual for the five years before Olivia entered treatment.

33. Rand 1957.

34. In fact, far from wanting to regress, Olivia had very strong fears of being infantilized or feeling subordinate in treatment. She identified more with the doctors and clinical staff than with the other patients, and this caused a great deal of social difficulties for her in the clinic.

35. Douglas 1966.

1. Much like the way humanitarian workers in Haiti must construct "trauma packets" to get funding from nonprofit agencies (James 2010).

2. James 2010.

3. Mol 2002.

4. Woolgar and Pawluch 1985.

5. This is not uncommon, particularly in clients with bulimia. Sometimes partial or day treatment can make things worse because clients spend the day connecting with challenging and even traumatic affects and experiences and then leave the safety of the treatment center. They may increase their coping behaviors to deal with the emotions that have been triggered. Clients with anorexia are at least eating during program hours.

6. Reed and Eisman 2006.

7. Reed and Eisman 2006.

8. Although managed care organizations implemented increasingly restrictive measures to hold costs down, their own profits continued to rise, and by the mid-1990s, these organizations had developed a significant image problem (Keckley 2004). The public backlash reached a peak in the 1990s and laid the groundwork for the 2008 Affordable Care Act. In the context of Bill Clinton's initiative for health-care reform in 1993, a bright light was centered on the health insurance industry. Revelations about insurance companies' fee structures and profit margins compounded many Americans' already fraught encounters with HMO bureaucracy, and public opinion of these organizations began to shift.

This shift was fueled by specific practices within the managed care industry that many Americans found distasteful at best and criminal at worst. As part of the move to a for-profit system, many HMOs developed a variety of control mechanisms to regulate the use of benefits and minimize expenditures on care. It was during this era that gatekeepers were introduced (individuals had to see a primary care physician before being referred to a specialist). Also, utilization review processes were put in place whereby a staff of physicians and nurses at the insurance company reviewed the care provided by physicians in their network to determine if it was indeed reasonable and necessary. Before performing an expensive procedure or obtaining an expensive test, doctors would have to get permission from the patient's insurance company. Failure to get this authorization could result in the insurance company refusing to pay. Once a patient was under a doctor's care, the utilization review staff followed her progress to make sure the physician wasn't providing more care than necessary.

Another important cost-saving mechanism was the prohibition on covering treatment for preexisting conditions. This policy allowed health insurance companies to avoid paying for treatment for individuals who, arguably, needed it the most, focusing instead on insuring individuals who could establish that they were healthy at the time of obtaining insurance.

This prohibition made things especially difficult for people with chronic illnesses such as asthma, diabetes, arthritis, or even cancer. The issue at hand became whether and how an illness episode was classified. If a person was deemed to be "recovered" from their illness at any point, any reemergence of the illness would be excluded from coverage based on the preexisting conditions clause.

Such practices led to what is commonly called the managed care backlash—public outcry against HMO practices that was fueled in the 1990s by publicity about the concept of the "medical loss ratio," or MLR.

The MLR is the percentage of every dollar taken in as premiums by managed care organizations that goes to pay for the provision of care. It is notable that this is characterized as a "medical *loss*," as if medical costs constitute a loss of what would otherwise be available to managed care organizations as profit.

Historically, the MLR for nonprofit HMOs has averaged around 95 percent. The MLR for Medicaid is also 95 percent, and for Medicare it's 98 percent. In the case of for-profit HMOs, the MLR typically ranges from 70 to 85 percent. This is a critical number—for a for-profit company to be competitive for stockholders, it must be able to promise a certain return on investment. The lower the MLR, the more money that is available to be paid out as profit. There is therefore a very strong incentive for for-profit HMOs to maintain low MLRs and higher profit margins.

In the 1990s, newspapers began publishing the MLRs of various HMOs. Negative perceptions of HMOs skyrocketed, and the managed care backlash fueled an increasingly insistent demand for something to be done about for-profit healthcare run amok. After the failure of Clinton's healthcare plan in 1994, however, little was done to curb the health insurance industry until 2008, and managed care organizations operated largely with impunity.

9. Tanenbaum 2003.

10. Reed and Eisman 2006, 16.

11. Tanenbaum 2003, 294.

12. Sackett 2000.

13. See Bothwell et al. 2016 for a brief but thorough overview of the rise of RCTs as the gold standard in medical interventions research.

14. Reed and Eisman 2006, 18.

15. Reed and Eisman 2006.

16. Lambert and Okiishi 1997; Norcross and Hill 2004.

17. Increasingly, state and federal agencies are devoting enormous resources to encourage practitioner adoption of evidence-based practices. In the state of Missouri, for example, the Department of Mental Health offered free training and supervision (for up to two years) to any licensed clinician wishing to become competent in the delivery of dialectical behavior therapy, which has an evidenced-based track record of being able to reduce hospital admissions for individuals with borderline personality disorder.

18. Reed and Eisman 2006, 20.

19. Wang et al. 2005.

20. Hoek and Van Hoeken 2003.

21. Gremillion 2003.

22. Hahn 2011.

1. See, e.g., Gremillion 2003; and Brodwin 2013.

2. See Lester 2014.

3. Two were openly gay men, and one was a heterosexual man with a live-in girlfriend. These personal details are important, because they signal that these men were not sexually available. See the discussion on boundaries in chapter 10.

4. Brodwin 2013.

5. See Warren et al. 2012 for a review of this literature and a qualitative analysis of burnout among eating disorder professionals.

6. Dialectical behavior therapy takes a cognitive-behavioral approach and integrates it with perspectives from Eastern philosophy and practices of mindfulness. Originally developed to treat borderline personality disorder, it is useful for helping clients become more balanced, learn to self-regulate affectively and behaviorally, and become more effective in their interpersonal lives. Interpersonal therapy is largely based on psychodynamic and family systems theory, and it focuses on interpersonal relationships as the locus of difficulty. Acceptance and commitment therapy brings together cognitive-behavioral approaches and mindfulness in ways designed to increase psychological flexibility and the acceptance of (rather than overreaction to) negative feelings. Internal Family Systems Therapy brings together family systems theory with a dynamic understanding of the self as multiple rather than singular (see chapter 8).

7. See, e.g., Kemps et al. 2006; McCormick et al. 2008; and Grunwald et al. 2001.

8. Garner 2008.

9. If a client is suspected of water-loading or otherwise altering her weight, she may be subjected to random weigh-ins at other times of the day.

10. Best practice recommendations note that clients who achieve a weight of 90 percent or more of their ideal body weight before being discharged have the best chance of long-term recovery (Rosen 2010).

11. This system afforded a great deal of flexibility. Someone could be plated, for example, at 75 percent with two add-ons, at 80 percent with no add-ons, or at 50 percent with one add-on, and so forth, depending on what a particular client needed at a particular time.

12. Although the food rituals associated with eating disorders have not been much theorized in the clinical literature, they are what drew me to studying eating disorders in the first place. See Lester 1995.

13. It is important to note that while the pro beliefs might perpetuate an eating disorder, this doesn't mean they are necessarily *wrong*. For example, in Molly's case, her illness really *did* keep her parents focused on her rather than on fighting with each other, and as she got better they returned their attention to the problems in their marriage.

1. Debord 1977.
2. Steinhausen 2002.
3. Dawson, Rhodes, and Touyz 2014.
4. Geppert 2015.
5. Manderson and Smith-Morris 2010, 3, 13.
6. Adams, Murphy, and Clarke 2009.
7. Manderson and Smith-Morris 2010.
8. Innis and Innis 1972.
9. Sharma 2014.
10. Adams, Murphy, and Clarke 2009, 247.
11. Adams, Murphy, and Clarke 2009, 246.
12. Adams, Murphy, and Clarke 2009, 247.
13. Time can also be read backward. Lab values can be indicative of purging in the preceding few days. Unexpected weight gain or loss can indicate that a client binged or restricted while on pass.
14. Adams, Murphy, and Clarke 2009, 247; italics in the original,
15. Adams, Murphy, and Clarke 2009, 247; italics in the original.
16. Strathern 2000.
17. Adams, Murphy, and Clarke 2009, 248; italics in the original.
18. Adams, Murphy and Clarke 2009, 248.
19. Adams, Murphy and Clarke 2009, 248.
20. Adams, Murphy and Clarke 2009, 249.
21. Adams, Murphy and Clarke 2009, 249.
22. R. Williams 1977.
23. Orr 2006.
24. Adams, Murphy, and Clarke 2009, 249. See Masco 2014 for an anthropological engagement with how the US government has cultivated and responded to various "states of terror" following World War II by generating what Masco terms "national security affect."
25. Engel 1977.
26. Anthony 1993, 527.
27. Schrank and Slade 2007.
28. Resnick et al. 2005.
29. Peebles et al. 2007.
30. See, e.g., Dawson, Rhodes, and Touyz 2014.
31. Vitousek, Watson, and Wilson 1998.
32. Jones, Marino, and Hansen 2015; Corstens et al. 2014.
33. Barber 2012.
34. Bellack 2006.
35. Adams, Murphy, and Clarke 2009, 251; italics in the original.
36. Adams, Murphy, and Clarke 2009, 255; italics in the original.

37. Adams, Murphy, and Clarke 2009, 258.

38. Livingston 2012.

39. Oshana 2007, 1.

40. Oshana 2007.

41. Gutman, Hutton, and Martin 1988.

42. This is the term used in the eating disorder research and treatment world.

43. Lester 2016; see also chapter 8 of this book.

44. This model of empowerment through submission takes on special nuance in the case of eating disorders (see Lester 1999).

45. Ahmed 2014.

46. Gremillion 2003.

SECTION 3. DYNAMICS

1. Van Gennep 1960.

2. Turner 1967.

3. Seligman 2014.

4. Douglas 1966.

5. Douglas 1966, 35.

6. See Jackson 2005 for a similar engagement of liminality among chronic pain patients.

7. These movements and their attendant tasks emerged from my ethnographic observations over many years as well as from field notes, treatment team meetings, therapist trainings, and dozens of interviews with clients and staff. While these are not local categories in the sense that they are not explicitly identified by the Cedar Grove program, I am confident that clients and staff alike would recognize them as reflecting the arc of the treatment program at the clinic.

8. I do not look at what happens before or after treatment (aside from providing some clients' own reports). For an excellent look at how people live with eating disorders outside of the clinical context, see, in particular, Warin 2009.

9. Prochaska and DiClemente 1994.

7. LOOSENING THE TIES THAT BIND

1. During this part of treatment, clients are expected to remain inactive (sitting or lying down) in community space observation (that is, in the common areas of the treatment center and not in bedrooms or group rooms, which are unsupervised) while awake. They are to eat or supplement 100 percent of their meal plan and complete the full fluid protocol, which may include the use of a feeding tube. If they are struggling with bulimia or have a history of self-harm or excessive exercising, they are required to be on bathroom monitoring, which means that a staff member must

be present with them in the bathroom at all times (bathrooms remain locked outside of designated restroom times and special requests). Clients are expected to attend individual sessions with members of the treatment team, attend group therapy sessions, and "accept" medication, medical tests, and procedures as discussed with their psychiatrist and physician. Depending on the client's medical status, a parent, guardian, or loved one may need to be in town in order to provide support and transportation for medical appointments outside of Cedar Grove. Privileges in the stabilization phase are limited. Patients can use the staff phone to contact family members or loved ones for fifteen-minute calls between 7:30 and 9:30 p.m. Daily supervised breaks are permitted (pending physician approval). The main goal in this initial stage of treatment is to lay the foundation for engagement in the clinic's program by creating a disposition in clients to accept such things as medications, medical tests and procedures, and treatment guidelines.

2. Delvecchio-Good 2007.

3. Winnicott 1953.

4. Anthropologist Helen Gremillion (2003) has evocatively documented the irony of such forms of measurement and accounting in eating disorders clinics and the ways they replicate many of the practices of the eating disorders themselves.

5. See Bruch 1978 for an emblematic discussion of this view. Although Bruch's book was first published forty years ago, key components of her understanding of eating disorders still hold strong sway in the treatment of these conditions today.

6. See Minuchin, Rosman, and Baker 1978 for a classic articulation of this approach. Although much work has been done since then, the authors' views still heavily inform clinicians' perspectives today. It may be worth noting that my own family did not fit this model at all; I experienced my anorexia not as helping me become childlike (a state that I wanted to flee) but as a way of maturing and acting like a "grown woman."

7. See Humphrey 1989 for a classic articulation of these views, which continue to influence clinician perspectives in practice.

8. This kind of manipulating is not unique to eating disorders—it is common in situations where people experience significant limitations on their ability to get basic needs attended to.

9. Dare et al. 1994.

10. Raikhel and Garriott 2013.

8. ME, MYSELF, AND ED

1. Motivationally, clients at this stage are expected to participate more actively in their treatment—to take the initiative to follow guidelines consistently rather than having to be reminded to do so. For example, the patient handbook notes that clients should "demonstrate the ability to consistently follow the basic program guidelines, including community space guidelines, group therapy attendance, the

electronics policy, and participation in post-meal group" and that they should arrive on time for morning weights, vitals, and breakfast (in the case of residential clients) or programming (in the case of partial hospitalization clients). To complement this increased participation in treatment, clients are provided with a personal cubby to store items and may access electronics for thirty minutes in the morning and after dinner until 9:30 p.m. They may attend daily staff-supervised breaks (usually outside) and staff-supervised outings. They are also eligible for one therapeutic pass per week to spend with family or loved ones. This stage also includes "nutrition challenge opportunities" (participating in meal passes and self-portioning meals, with treatment team approval) and "fitness privileges" (participation in yoga, dance therapy, authentic movement, and healthy movement groups, as well as daily, supervised walks).

2. Schaefer and Rutledge 2003.

3. Schwartz 1995, 57.

4. Schwartz 1995, 17.

5. Schwartz 1995, 17.

6. See Skyttner 2010 for an overview of general systems theory, and Flood 1990 for a comprehensive critique of systems thinking.

7. Parts can be male or female, regardless of the gender identification of the individual. Yet notably absent from IFS is an engagement with issues of gender and the intersections of gender and power within social networks. How the gendering of parts comes about and how it affects a person's perceived inner processes are questions of critical importance, particularly in the treatment of eating disorders, which are often thought to be linked to cultural ambivalences about gender and power. See, e.g., Bordo 2004.

8. Frankfurt 1971; Oshana 2007.

9. Oshana 2007.

10. Fischer 2005.

11. Fischer 1995, 38.

12. Schwartz 1995, 38.

13. Csikszentmihalyi 2009.

14. Schwartz 1995, 45.

15. Cedar Grove draws this characterization from Jenni Schaefer's popular book *Life Without Ed,* in which the author describes her relationship with her eating disorder as similar to an abusive marriage from which she escaped. Although I do not discuss the significance of the gendering of Ed as male in detail here, I will briefly note that Ed as male sits in contrast to feminized personifications of eating disorders commonly found on pro-anorexia and pro-bulimia websites. In these online communities, "Ana" and "Mia" are portrayed as friends, goddesses, or harsh mistresses to be appeased.

16. Hermans and Dimaggio 2016.

17. Understanding self-transformation through altering one's internal dialogue or "self-talk" is certainly nothing new in the world of psychotherapy, and it was particularly central in approaches developed during the 1970s and 1980s. What

distinguishes IFS from these other models is the degree to which it elaborates self-talk as multidirectional (rather than unidirectional) and polyvocal (as opposed to monovocal). That is, the talk does not emanate from an introject of a parent or other authority figure toward the vulnerable self but involves ongoing, multilayered dialogue among multiple endogenous internal orientations—dialogue that occurs in the *presence* of Self but does not touch Self directly. This distinction is important for understanding the utility and possible risks of IFS in the contemporary American context of managed mental healthcare, both of which center on issues of agency.

18. Boddy 1989.
19. Rawls 1972.
20. Schwartz 1995, 15.
21. Rose 2005, 7.
22. My clinical practice is a not-for-profit entity and uses a sliding fee scale. I do not accept any payments from insurance companies.
23. Rose 2005.

9. "FAT" IS NOT A FEELING

1. Mol, Moser, and Pols 2010.
2. See Lester 2014 for a full discussion.
3. Seligman 2014.
4. Schüll 2014, 227.
5. Schüll 2014, 229.
6. Schüll 2014, 230.
7. Rose 2003a, 430; 2003b, 58.
8. Keane 2002, 159.
9. Schüll 2014, 233.
10. Schüll 2014, 239.
11. Schüll 2014, 241.

SECTION 4. RECURSIONS

1. Wetherell 2012.

10. RUNNING ON EMPTY

1. Ahern 1999.
2. Winnicott 1953.
3. See Lester 2009 for a more extended discussion.

4. Dumit 2012.

5. Dumit 2012.

6. Luhrmann 2000.

7. Lakoff 2009.

8. Van der Geest and Whyte 1989; Carpenter-Song 2009.

9. Crowley-Matoka and True 2012; Anderson-Fye and Floersch 2011.

10. Jenkins 2011.

11. Jenkins 2011; Carpenter-Song 2009.

12. Anderson-Fye and Floersch 2011.

13. See, e.g., Lester 2004, 2009.

11. CAPITALIZING ON CARE

1. This is a pseudonym.

2. William Bithoney, "Behavioral Health: A Market Ripe for Growth and Consolidation," *BDO Health & Life Sciences RX* (blog), March 17, 2015, www.bdo.com /blogs/health-and-life-sciences/march-2015/behavioral-health-a-market-ripe-for-growth.

3. In 2008, Congress passed the Mental Health Parity and Addiction Equity Act (MHPAEA), which requires insurers to equalize coverage for behavioral health and medical health benefits in terms of copayments, deductibles, lifetime caps, and access to providers. Also in 2008, the Medicare Improvements for Patients and Providers Act was passed, which increases access to mental health treatments in federal programs. In 2010, the Affordable Care Act (popularly known as Obamacare) allowed adult children aged eighteen to twenty-six to remain on their parents' insurance. It also built on to the MHPAEA by requiring most insurance plans to cover certain identified mental health and substance abuse services. See Cockrell et al. 2014.

4. Allison Kodjak, "Investors See Big Opportunities in Opioid Addiction Treatment," *All Things Considered,* National Public Radio, June 10, 2016.

5. Goode 2016.

6. Goode 2016.

7. Attia et al. 2016.

8. Some therapreneurs (myself included) bypass some aspects of this process by refusing to accept insurance directly, instead having clients pay up front and obtain reimbursement on their own. Regardless, therapreneurs must contend with the realities of managed care, as this structures most clients' abilities to obtain services.

9. Wilson and Yochim 2015.

10. Ho 2009.

11. Stewart 2007.

12. Wilson and Yochim 2015; Berlant 2011, 5.

13. Butler 2010.

14. Muehlebach 2013.

15. Butler 2004, 25.

16. Tsing 2015, 2.

17. Allison 2016. For more on precarity, see Allison 2013; Butler 2004; Dave 2014; Han 2012; Millar 2014; O'Neill 2014; Stewart 2012; and Tsing 2015.

18. Muehlebach 2013, 300.

19. Ollove 2012.

20. Ollove 2012.

21. "Estimates of Funding for Various Research, Condition, and Disease Categories (RCDC)," NIH Categorical Spending, National Institutes of Health, May 18, 2018, https://report.nih.gov/categorical_spending.aspx.

22. Butler 2004; see also Butler 2010.

23. Puar 2017, 13; see also Dumit 2012.

24. Ettlinger 2007.

25. Ettlinger 2007, 319.

26. Ettlinger 2007, 320, 323.

27. Ettlinger 2007, 324.

28. Ettlinger 2007, 320.

29. Ettlinger 2007.

30. Ettlinger 2007.

31. Ettlinger 2007, 326.

32. Ettlinger 2007.

33. Berlant 2011.

34. Berlant 2011, 1.

35. Berlant 2007, 754.

36. Puar 2012, 163.

37. Puar 2011, 153.

38. Lester 2014.

39. Martin, Myers, and Viseu 2015, 627.

12. CONCLUSIONS

1. Joanna Kay, "5 Things Everyone with an Eating Disorder Should Know about Their Insurance," National Eating Disorders Association, accessed April 10, 2019, www.nationaleatingdisorders.org/blog/5-things-everyone-eating-disorder-should-know-about-their-insurance.

2. "EDC Applauds SAMHSA's Recently Announced Center of Excellence for Eating Disorders Awardee—University of North Carolina at Chapel Hill," press release, Eating Disorders Coalition, September 21, 2018, http://eatingdisorderscoalition.org.s208556.gridserver.com/couch/uploads/file/press-release_center-for-excellence-award_9-21-18.pdf.

3. www.moedc.org.

4. "Get to Know Us," Missouri Eating Disorders Association, accessed April 10, 2019, www.moeatingdisorders.org/get-to-know-us.

5. "Insurance & Legal Issues," National Eating Disorders Association, accessed April 10, 2019, www.nationaleatingdisorders.org/learn/general-information/insurance.

WORKS CITED

Adams, Vincanne, Michelle Murphy, and Adele E. Clarke. 2009. "Anticipation: Technoscience, Life, Affect, Temporality." *Subjectivity* 28, no. 1: 246–65. doi:10.1057/sub.2009.18.

Ahearn, Laura M. 1999. "Agency." *Journal of Linguistic Anthropology* 9, nos. 1–2: 12–15. doi:10.1525/jlin.1999.9.1–2.12.

Ahmed, Sara. 2014. *Willful Subjects*. Durham: Duke University Press.

Allison, Anne. 2013. *Precarious Japan*. Durham: Duke University Press.

———. 2016. "Precarity: Commentary by Anne Allison." *Cultural Anthropology*, Curated Collections, September 13. https://culanth.org/curated_collections/21-precarity/discussions/26-precarity-commentary-by-anne-allison.

American Psychiatric Association. 2013. *Diagnostic and Statistical Manual of Mental Disorders: DSM-5*. 5th ed. Arlington: American Psychiatric Publishing.

Anderson, Ben. 2009. "Affective Atmospheres." *Emotion, Space and Society* 2, no. 2: 77–81. doi:10.1016/j.emospa.2009.08.005.

———. 2016. *Encountering Affect: Capacities, Apparatuses, Conditions*. London: Routledge.

Anderson, Daniel J., John P. McGovern, and Robert L. Dupont. 1999. "The Origins of the Minnesota Model of Addiction Treatment—A First Person Account." *Journal of Addictive Diseases* 18, no. 1: 107–14. doi:10.1300/j069v18n01_10.

Anderson-Fye, Eileen P. 2004. "A 'Coca-Cola' Shape: Cultural Change, Body Image, and Eating Disorders in San Andrés, Belize." *Culture, Medicine and Psychiatry* 28, no. 4: 561–95. doi:10.1007/s11013-004-1068-4.

Anderson-Fye, Eileen P., and Jerry Floersch. 2011. "'I'm Not Your Typical "Homework Stresses Me Out" Kind of Girl': Psychological Anthropology in Research on College Student Usage of Psychiatric Medications and Mental Health Services." *Ethos* 39, no. 4: 501–21. doi:10.1111/j.1548-1352.2011.01209.x.

Angell, Marcia. 1993. "The Doctor as Double Agent." *Kennedy Institute of Ethics Journal* 3, no. 3): 279–86. doi:10.1353/ken.0.0253.

Anthony, William A. 1993. "Recovery from Mental Illness: The Guiding Vision of the Mental Health Service System in the 1990s." *Psychosocial Rehabilitation Journal* 16, no. 4: 11–23. doi:10.1037/h0095655.

Arcelus, Jon, Alex J. Mitchell, Jackie Wales, and Søren Nielsen. 2011. "Mortality Rates in Patients with Anorexia Nervosa and Other Eating Disorders." *Archives of General Psychiatry* 68, no. 7: 724. doi:10.1001/archgenpsychiatry.2011.74.

Attia, Evelyn, Kristy L. Blackwood, Angela S. Guarda, Marsha D. Marcus, and David J. Rothman. 2016. "Marketing Residential Treatment Programs for Eating Disorders: A Call for Transparency." *Psychiatric Services* 67, no. 6: 664–66. doi:10.1176/appi.ps.201500338.

Banks, Caroline Giles. 1992. "'Culture' in Culture-Bound Syndromes: The Case of Anorexia Nervosa." *Social Science and Medicine* 34, no. 8: 867–84. doi:10.1016 /0277–9536(92)90256-p.

———. 1996. "'There Is No Fat in Heaven': Religious Asceticism and the Meaning of Anorexia Nervosa." *Ethos* 24, no. 1: 107–35. doi:10.1525/eth.1996.24.1.02a00040.

Barber, Mary E. 2012. "Recovery as the New Medical Model for Psychiatry." *Psychiatric Services* 63, no. 3: 277–79. doi:10.1176/appi.ps.201100248.

Becker, Anne E. 2004. "Television, Disordered Eating, and Young Women in Fiji: Negotiating Body Image and Identity during Rapid Social Change." *Culture, Medicine and Psychiatry* 28, no. 4: 533–59. doi:10.1007/s11013–004–1067–5.

———. 2007. "Culture and Eating Disorders Classification." *International Journal of Eating Disorders* 40, no. S3. doi:10.1002/eat.20435.

Becker, Anne E., Jennifer J. Thomas, and Kathleen M. Pike. 2009. "Should Non-Fat-Phobic Anorexia Nervosa Be Included in *DSM-V*?" *International Journal of Eating Disorders* 42, no. 7: 620–35. doi:10.1002/eat.20727.

Bell, Rudolph M. 1985. *Holy Anorexia.* Chicago: University of Chicago Press.

Bellack, Alen S. 2006. "Scientific and Consumer Models of Recovery in Schizophrenia: Concordance, Contrasts, and Implications." *Schizophrenia Bulletin* 32, no. 3: 432–42. doi:10.1093/schbul/sbj044.

Benjamin, Jessica. 2017. *Beyond Doer and Done To: Recognition Theory, Intersubjectivity, and the Third.* New York: Routledge.

Berlant, Lauren Gail. 2007. "Slow Death (Sovereignty, Obesity, Lateral Agency)." *Critical Inquiry* 33, no. 4: 754–80. doi:10.1086/521568.

———. 2011. *Cruel Optimism.* Durham: Duke University Press.

Blackman, Lisa. 2012. *Immaterial Bodies.* Los Angeles: SAGE.

Boddy, Janice. 1989. *Wombs and Alien Spirits Women, Men and the Zar Cult in Northern Sudan.* Madison, WI: University of Wisconsin Press.

Bordo, Susan. 2004. *Unbearable Weight: Feminism, Western Culture, and the Body.* Berkeley: University of California Press.

Bothwell, Laura E., Jeremy A. Greene, Scott H. Podolsky, and David S. Jones. 2016. "Assessing the Gold Standard: Lessons from the History of RCTs." *New England Journal of Medicine* 374, no. 22: 2175–181. doi:10.1056/nejmms1604593.

Brodwin, Paul. 2013. *Everyday Ethics: Voices from the Frontline of Community Psychiatry.* Berkeley: University of California Press.

Bruch, Hilde. 1978. *The Golden Cage: The Enigma of Anorexia Nervosa*. New York: Vintage.

Bruch, Hilde, Danita Czyzewski, and Melanie A. Suhr. 2006. *Conversations with Anorexics: A Compassionate and Hopeful Journey through the Therapeutic Process.* Lanham, MD: J. Aronson.

Brumberg, Joan Jacobs. 2000. *Fasting Girls: The Emergence of Anorexia Nervosa as a Modern Disease.* New York: Vintage.

Bulik, Cynthia M., Nancy D. Berkman, Kimberly A. Brownley, Jan A. Sedway, and Kathleen N. Lohr. 2007. "Anorexia Nervosa Treatment: A Systematic Review of Randomized Controlled Trials." *International Journal of Eating Disorders* 40, no. 4: 310–20. doi:10.1002/eat.20367.

Butler, Judith. 2004. *Precarious Life: The Powers of Mourning and Violence.* New York: Verso.

———. 2010. *Frames of War: When Is Life Grieveable?* New York: Verso.

Carpenter-Song, Elizabeth. 2009. "Children's Sense of Self in Relation to Clinical Processes: Portraits of Pharmaceutical Transformation." *Ethos* 37, no. 3: 257–81. doi:10.1111/j.1548–1352.2009.01053.x.

Chavez, Mark, and Tom R. Insel. 2007. "Eating Disorders: National Institute of Mental Health's Perspective." *American Psychologist* 62, no. 3: 159–66.

Cockrell, Geoff C., Amber McGrall Walsh, Richard S. Grant, McGuire Woods, and Jason F. Shafer. 2014. "Bullish Behavioral Health Market Drives Investment." *Law360* (blog), July 17. www.law360.com/articles/558263/bullish-behavioral-health-market-drives-investment.

Collins, M. Elizabeth. 1991. "Body Figure Perceptions and Preferences among Pre-adolescent Children." *International Journal of Eating Disorders* 10, no. 2: 199–208. doi:10.1002/1098–108x(199103)10:23.0.co;2-d.

Corstens, Dirk, Eleanor Longden, Simon McCarthy-Jones, Rachel Waddingham, and Neil Thomas. 2014. "Emerging Perspectives from the Hearing Voices Movement: Implications for Research and Practice." Supplement, *Schizophrenia Bulletin* 40, no. S4: S285–S294.

Crowley-Matoka, Megan, and Gala True. 2012. "No One Wants to Be the Candy Man: Ambivalent Medicalization and Clinician Subjectivity in Pain Management." *Cultural Anthropology* 27, no. 4: 689–712. doi:10.1111/j.1548–1360.2012.01167.x.

Csikszentmihalyi, Mihaly. 2009. *Flow: The Psychology of Optimal Experience.* New York: Harper Row.

Dare, Christopher, Daniel Le Grange, Ivan Eisler, and Joan Rutherford. 1994. "Redefining the Psychosomatic Family: Family Process of 26 Eating Disorder Families." *International Journal of Eating Disorders* 16, no. 3: 211–26. doi:10.1002/1098–108x(199411)16:33.0.co;2-x.

Dave, Naisargi. 2014. "Witness: Humans, Animals, and the Politics of Becoming." *Cultural Anthropology* 29, no. 3: 433–56. doi:10.1215/9780822372455–006.

Dawson, Lisa, Paul Rhodes, and Stephen Touyz. 2014. "The Recovery Model and Anorexia Nervosa." *Australian and New Zealand Journal of Psychiatry* 48, no. 11: 1009–16.

Debord, Guy. 1977. *Society of the Spectacle*. Detroit, MI: Black and Red.

Delvecchio-Good, Mary-Jo. 2007. "The Medical Imaginary and the Biotechnical Embrace: Subjective Experiences of Clinical Scientists and Patients." In *Subjectivity: Ethnographic Investigations,* edited by Joao Biehl, Byron Good, and Arthur Kleinman, 362–80. Berkeley: University of California Press.

Deveaux, Monique. 1994. "Feminism and Empowerment: A Critical Reading of Foucault." *Feminist Studies* 20, no. 2: 223–47.

DiNicola, Vincenzo F. 1990. "Anorexia Multiforme: Self-Starvation in Historical and Cultural Context." *Transcultural Psychiatric Research Review* 27, no. 4: 245–86. doi:10.1177/136346159002700401.

Douglas, Mary. 1966. *Purity and Danger: An Analysis of Concepts of Pollution and Taboo*. New York: Routledge.

Dumit, Joseph. 2006. "Illnesses You Have to Fight to Get: Facts as Forces in Uncertain, Emergent Illnesses." *Social Science and Medicine* 62, no. 3: 577–90. doi:10.1016/j.socscimed.2005.06.018.

———. 2012. *Drugs for Life: How Pharmaceutical Companies Define Our Health*. Durham, NC: Duke University Press.

Eating Disorders Coalition. 2016. "Facts about Eating Disorders: What the Research Shows." http://eatingdisorderscoalition.org.s208556.gridserver.com/couch/uploads/file/fact-sheet_2016.pdf.

Eli, Karin. 2014. "Between Difference and Belonging: Configuring Self and Others in Inpatient Treatment for Eating Disorders." *PLoS ONE* 9, no. 9: e105452. doi:10.1371/journal.pone.0105452.

———. 2016. "'The Body Remembers': Narrating Embodied Reconciliations of Eating Disorder and Recovery." *Anthropology and Medicine* 23, no. 1: 71–85. doi: 10.1080/13648470.2015.1135786.

Engel, George L. 1977. "The Need for a New Medical Model: A Challenge for Biomedicine." *Science* 196, no. 4286: 129–36.

Erickson, Victoria. 2015. *Edge of Wonder*. Toronto: Enrealment Press.

Ettlinger, Nancy. 2007. "Precarity Unbound." *Alternatives: Global, Local, Political* 32, no. 3: 319–40. doi:10.1177/030437540703200303.

Fairburn, Christopher G. 2008. *Cognitive Behavior Therapy and Eating Disorders*. New York: Guilford Press

Fischer, John Martin. 2005. "Free Will and Moral Responsibility." In *The Oxford Handbook of Ethical Theory,* edited by David Copp, 321–56. New York: Oxford University Press.

Flood, Robert L. 1990. "Liberating Systems Theory." In *Liberating Systems Theory: Contemporary Systems Thinking,* 11–32. Boston: Springer. doi:10.1007/978-1-4899-2477-3_2.

Fox, Harriette B., Margaret A. McManus, and Mary B. Reichman. 2003. "Private Health Insurance for Adolescents: Is It Adequate?" *Journal of Adolescent Health* 32, no. 6: 12–24. doi:10.1016/s1054-139x(03)00070-3.

Frankfurt, Harry G. 1971. "Freedom of the Will and the Concept of a Person." *Journal of Philosophy* 68, no. 1: 5–20. doi:10.2307/2024717.

Freud, Sigmund. 1918. *From the History of an Infantile Neurosis*. London: Vintage.

Gaesser, Glenn A. 2002. *Big Fat Lies: The Truth about Your Weight and Your Health*. Carlsbad, CA: Gürze Books.

Garner, David M. 2008. "Women and Dieting." In *Encyclopedia of Obesity*, edited by Katherine Keller, 801–5. New York: SAGE.

Geppert, Cynthia M. A. 2015. "Futility in Chronic Anorexia Nervosa: A Concept Whose Time Has Not Yet Come." *American Journal of Bioethics* 15, no. 7: 34–43. doi:10.1080/15265161.2015.1039720.

Goode, Erica. 2016. "Centers to Treat Eating Disorders Are Growing, and Raising Concerns." *New York Times*, March 14. www.nytimes.com/2016/03/15/health/eating-disorders-anorexia-bulimia-treatment-centers.html.

Gooldin, Sigal. 2008. "Being Anorexic." *Medical Anthropology Quarterly* 22, no. 3: 274–96. doi:10.1111/j.1548–1387.2008.00026.x.

Gordon, Richard A. 1988. "A Sociocultural Interpretation of the Current Epidemic of Eating Disorders." In *The Eating Disorders*, edited by B. J. Blinder, B. F. Chaiting, and R. Goldstein, 151–63. Rockford, IL: PMA Publishing Group.

Gremillion, Helen. 1992. "Psychiatry as Social Ordering: Anorexia, a Paradigm." *Social Science and Medicine* 35, no. 1: 57–71.

———. 2003. *Feeding Anorexia Gender and Power at a Treatment Center*. Durham, NC: Duke University Press.

Grunwald, Martin, Christine Ettrich, Bianka Assmann, Angelika Dähne, Werner Krause, Frank Busse, and Hermann-Joseph Gertz. 2001. "Deficits in Haptic Perception and Right Parietal Theta Power Changes in Patients with Anorexia Nervosa before and after Weight Gain." *International Journal of Eating Disorders* 29, no. 4: 417–28. doi:10.1002/eat.1038.

Gull, William Whitney. 1874. "Anorexia Nervosa (Apepsia Hysterica, Anorexia Hysterica)." *Transactions of the Clinical Society of London* 7: 22–28.

Gutman, Huck, Patrick H. Hutton, and Luther H. Martin. 1988. *Technologies of the Self: A Seminar with Michel Foucault*. London: Tavistock.

Hahn, Ulrike. 2011. "The Problem of Circularity in Evidence, Argument, and Explanation." *Perspectives on Psychological Science* 6, no. 2: 172–82. doi:10.1177/1745691611400240.

Han, Clara. 2012. *Life in Debt: Times of Care and Violence in Neoliberal Chile*. Berkeley: University of California Press.

Hermans, H. J. M., and Giancarlo Dimaggio, eds. 2016. *The Dialogical Self in Psychotherapy*. London: Routledge.

Ho, Karen Zouwen. 2009. *Liquidated: An Ethnography of Wall Street*. Durham, NC: Duke University Press.

Hoek, Hans Wijbrand. 2006. "Incidence, Prevalence and Mortality of Anorexia Nervosa and Other Eating Disorders." *Current Opinion in Psychiatry* 19, no. 4: 389–94. doi:10.1097/01.yco.0000228759.95237.78.

Hoek, Hans Wijbrand, and Daphne Van Hoeken. 2003. "Review of the Prevalence and Incidence of Eating Disorders." *International Journal of Eating Disorders* 34, no. 4: 383–96. doi:10.1002/eat.10222.

Horgan, Constance M., Dominic Hodgkin, Maureen T. Stewart, Amity Quinn, Elizabeth L. Merrick, Sharon Reif, Deborah W. Garnick, and Timothy B. Creedon. 2015. "Health Plans' Early Response to Federal Parity Legislation for Mental Health and Addiction Services." *Psychiatric Services* 67, no. 2: 162–68. doi:10.1176/appi.ps.201400575.

Hudson, James I., Eva Hiripi, Harrison G. Pope Jr., and Ronald C. Kessler. 2007. "The Prevalence and Correlates of Eating Disorders in the National Comorbidity Survey Replication." *Biological Psychiatry* 61, no. 3: 348–58.

Humphrey, Laura L. 1989. "Observed Family Interactions among Subtypes of Eating Disorders Using Structural Analysis of Social Behavior." *Journal of Consulting and Clinical Psychology* 57, no. 2: 206–14. doi:10.1037//0022-006x.57.2.206.

Illouz, Eva. 2017. *Saving the Modern Soul: Therapy, Emotions, and the Culture of Self-Help.* Berkeley: University of California Press.

Innis, Harold A., and Mary Quayle Innis. 1972. *Empire and Communications.* Toronto: University of Toronto Press.

Jackson, Jean E. 2005. "Stigma, Liminality, and Chronic Pain: Mind–Body Borderlands." *American Ethnologist* 32, no. 3: 332–53. doi:10.1525/ae.2005.32.3.332.

James, Erica Caple. 2010. *Democratic Insecurities: Violence, Trauma and Intervention in Haiti.* Berkeley: University of California Press.

Jenkins, Janis Hunter, ed. 2011. *Pharmaceutical Self: The Global Shaping of Experience in an Age of Psychopharmacology.* Santa Fe, NM: SAR Press.

Jones, Nev, Casadi "Khaki" Marino, and Marie C. Hansen. 2015. "The Hearing Voices Movement in the United States: Findings from a National Survey of Group Facilitators." *Psychosis* 8, no. 2: 106–17. doi:10.1080/17522439.2015.1105282.

Joyce, James. 1916. *A Portrait of the Artist as a Young Man.* New York: B. W. Heubsch.

Kalisvaart, Jennifer L., and Albert C. Hergenroeder. 2007. "Hospitalization of Patients with Eating Disorders on Adolescent Medical Units Is Threatened by Current Reimbursement Systems." *International Journal of Adolescent Medicine and Health* 19, no. 2: 155–65. doi:10.1515/ijamh.2007.19.2.155.

Keane, Helen. 2002. *What's Wrong with Addiction?* New York: New York University Press.

Keckley, Paul. 2004. "Evidence-Based Medicine and Managed Care: Applications, Challenges, Opportunities." *Medscape General Medicine* 6, no. 2: 56.

Keel, Pamela K., and Kelly L. Klump. 2003. "Are Eating Disorders Culture-Bound Syndromes? Implications for Conceptualizing Their Etiology." *Psychological Bulletin* 129, no. 5: 747–69. doi:10.1037/0033-2909.129.5.747.

Kemps, Eva, Marika Tiggemann, Tracey Wade, David Ben-Tovim, and Rolf Breyer. 2006. "Selective Working Memory Deficits in Anorexia Nervosa." *European Eating Disorders Review* 14, no. 2: 97–103. doi:10.1002/erv.685.

Keys, Ancel. 1950. *The Biology of Human Starvation*. Minneapolis, MN: University of Minnesota Press.

Klump, K. L., K. B. Miller, P. K. Keel, M. Mcgue, and W. G. Iacono. 2001. "Genetic and Environmental Influences on Anorexia Nervosa Syndromes in a Population-Based Twin Sample." *Psychological Medicine* 31, no. 4: 737–40. doi:10.1017/s0033291701003725.

Kodjak, Alison. 2016. "Investors See Big Opportunities in Opioid Addiction Treatment." *All Things Considered,* National Public Radio, June 10. www.npr.org/sections/health-shots/2016/06/10/480663056/investors-see-big-opportunities-in-opioid-addiction-treatment.

Lakoff, Andrew. 2009. *Pharmaceutical Reason: Knowledge and Value in Global Psychiatry*. Cambridge: Cambridge University Press.

Lambert, Michael J., and John C. Okiishi. 1997. "The Effects of the Individual Psychotherapist and Implications for Future Research." *Clinical Psychology: Science and Practice* 4, no. 1: 66–75. doi:10.1111/j.1468–2850.1997.tb00100.x.

Lavis, Anna. 2016. "Food, Bodies, and the Stuff of (Not) Eating in Anoerxia." *Gastronomica: The Journal of Critical Food Studies* 16, no. 3: 56–65.

Legrand, Dorothée, and Frédéric Briend. 2015. "Anorexia and Bodily Intersubjectivity." *European Psychologist* 20, no. 1: 52–61. doi:10.1027/1016–9040/a000208.

LeGrange, Daniel, Sonja A. Swanson, Scott J. Crow, and Kathleen R. Merikangas. 2012. "Eating Disorder Not Otherwise Specified Presentation in the US Population." *International Journal of Eating Disorders* 45, no. 5: 711–18. doi:10.1002/eat.22006.

Lester, Rebecca J. 1995. "Embodied Voices: Women's Food Asceticism and the Negotiation of Identity." *Ethos* 23, no. 2: 187–222. doi:10.1525/eth.1995.23.2.02a00040.

———. 1997. "The (Dis)embodied Self in Anorexia Nervosa." *Social Science and Medicine* 44, no. 4: 479–89. doi:10.1016/s0277–9536(96)00166–9.

———. 1999. "Let Go and Let God: Religion and the Politics of Surrender in Overeaters Anonymous." In *Interpreting Weight: The Social Management of Fatness and Thinness,* edited by Jeffery Sobal and Donna Maurer, 139–64. Hawthorne, NY: Aldine de Gruyter.

Lester, Rebecca J., 1999. "Let Go and Let God: Religion and the Politics of Surrender in Overeaters Anonymous." In *Interpreting Weight: The Social Management of Fatness and Thinness,* edited by Jeffrey Sobal and Donna Maurer, 139–64. Hawthorne, NY: Aldine De Gruyter.

———. 2000. "Like a Natural Woman: Celibacy and the Embodied Self in Anorexia Nervosa." In *Celibacy, Culture, and Society: The Anthropology of Sexual Abstinence,* edited by Elisa J. Sobo and Sandra Bell, 197–213. Madison, WI: University of Wisconsin Press.

———. 2004. "Eating Disorders and the Problem of 'Culture' in Acculturation." *Culture, Medicine and Psychiatry* 28, no. 4: 607–15.

———. 2007. "Critical Therapeutics: Cultural Politics and Clinical Reality in Two Eating Disorder Treatment Centers." *Medical Anthropology Quarterly* 21, no. 4: 369–87. doi:10.1525/maq.2007.21.4.369.

———. 2009. "Brokering Authenticity." *Current Anthropology* 50, no. 3: 281–302. doi:10.1086/598782.

———. 2014. "Health as Moral Failing: Medication Restriction among Women with Eating Disorders." *Anthropology and Medicine* 21, no. 2: 241–50. doi:10.1080/13648470.2014.927824.

———. 2016. "Ground Zero: Ontology, Recognition, and the Elusiveness of Care in American Eating Disorders Treatment." *Transcultural Psychiatry* 55, no. 4: 516–33. doi:10.1177/1363461516674874.

Levinas, Emmanuel. 1979. *Totality and Infinity: An Essay on Exteriority*. Pittsburgh, PA: Duquesne University Press.

———. 1996. "Ethics as First Philosophy." In *The Continental Philosophy Reader*, edited by Richard Kearney and Mara Rainwater, 124–35. New York: Routledge. First published 1984.

Levine, Michael P., and Linda Smolak. 1996. "Media as a Context for the Development of Disordered Eating." In *The Developmental Psychopathology of Eating Disorders: Implications for Research, Prevention, and Treatment*, 235–47. Hillsdale, NJ: Lawrence Erlbaum Associates.

Livingston, Julie. 2012. *Improvising Medicine: An African Oncology Ward in an Emerging Cancer Epidemic*. Durham, NC: Duke University Press.

Lock, James, and Daniel LeGrange. 2015. *Treatment Manual for Anorexia Nervosa: A Family-Based Approach*. New York: Guilford.

Loomis, Jack M. 2016. "Presence in Virtual Reality and Everyday Life: Immersion within a World of Representation." *Presence: Teleoperators and Virtual Environments* 25, no. 2: 169–74. doi:10.1162/pres_a_00255.

Luhrmann, T. M. 2000. *Of Two Minds: The Growing Disorder in American Psychiatry*. New York: Knopf.

Macleish, Kenneth T. 2012. "Armor and Anesthesia: Exposure, Feeling, and the Soldiers Body." *Medical Anthropology Quarterly* 26, no. 1: 49–68. doi:10.1111/j.1548-1387.2011.01196.x.

———. 2015. *Making War at Fort Hood: Life and Uncertainty in a Military Community*. Princeton, NJ: Princeton University Press.

Manderson, Lenore, and Carolyn Smith-Morris. 2010. *Chronic Conditions, Fluid States: Chronicity and the Anthropology of Illness*. New Brunswick, NJ: Rutgers University Press.

Martin, Aryn, Natasha Myers, and Ana Viseu. 2015. "The Politics of Care in Technoscience." *Social Studies of Science* 45, no. 5: 625–41. doi:10.1177/0306312715602073.

Masco, Joseph. 2014. *The Theater of Operations: National Security Affect from the Cold War to the War on Terror*. Durham, NC: Duke University Press.

Massumi, Brian. 2007. *Parables for the Virtual: Movement, Affect, Sensation*. Durham, NC: Duke University Press.

———. 2016. *Politics of Affect*. Cambridge, MA: Polity.

McCormick, Laurie M., Pamela K. Keel, Michael C. Brumm, Wayne Bowers, Victor Swayze, Arnold Andersen, and Nancy Andreasen. 2008. "Implications of Starvation-Induced Change in Right Dorsal Anterior Cingulate Volume in Anorexia Nervosa." *International Journal of Eating Disorders* 41, no. 7: 602–10. doi:10.1002/eat.20549.

Medway, Meredith, and Paul Rhodes. 2016. "Young People's Experience of Family Therapy for Anorexia Nervosa: A Qualitative Meta-Synthesis." *Advances in Eating Disorders* 4, no. 2: 189–207. doi:10.1080/21662630.2016.1164609.

Mellin, L. M., C. E. Irwin Jr., and S. Scully. 1992. "Prevalence of Disordered Eating in Girls: A Survey of Middle-Class Children." *Journal of the American Association Dietetics Association* 92, no. 7 (July): 851–53.

Millar, Kathleen. 2014. "The Precarious Present: Wageless Labor and Disrupted Life in Rio de Janeiro, Brazil." *Cultural Anthropology* 29, no. 1: 32–53. doi:10.14506/ca29.1.04.

Mintz, Sidney W., and Christine M. Du Bois. 2002. "The Anthropology of Food and Eating." *Annual Review of Anthropology* 31, no. 1: 99–119. doi:10.1146/annurev.anthro.32.032702.131011.

Minuchin, Salvador, Bernice L. Rosman, and Lester Baker. 1978. *Psychosomatic Families: Anorexia Nervosa in Context*. Cambridge, MA: Harvard University Press.

Mitchell, Stephen A. 2014. *Relationality: From Attachment to Intersubjectivity*. New York: Psychology Press.

Mol, Annemarie. 2002. *The Body Multiple: Ontology in Medical Practice*. Durham, NC: Duke University Press.

———. 2011. *The Logic of Care: Health and the Problem of Patient Choice*. London: Routledge.

Mol, Annemarie, Ingunn Moser, and Jeannette Pols, eds. 2010. *Care in Practice: On Tinkering in Clinics, Homes and Farms*. Bielefeld: Transcript Verlag.

Morton, Richard. 1694. *Phthisiologia, or A Treatise of Consumptions*. London: Printed for Sam. Smith and Benj. Walford, at the Princes Arms in St. Pauls Church-Yard.

Muehlebach, Andrea. 2013. "On Precariousness and the Ethical Imagination: The Year 2012 in Sociocultural Anthropology." *American Anthropologist* 115, no. 2: 297–311. doi:10.1111/aman.12011.

Mulligan, Jessica M. 2014. *Unmanageable Care an Ethnography of Health Care Privatization in Puerto Rico*. New York: New York University Press.

Myers, Neely Laurenzo. 2015. *Recovery's Edge: An Ethnography of Mental Health Care and Moral Agency*. Nashville, TN: Vanderbilt University Press.

Nasser, Mervat. 1988. "Eating Disorders: The Cultural Dimension." *Social Psychiatry and Psychiatric Epidemiology* 23, no. 3: 184–7.

National Institutes of Health. 2018. "NIH Categorical Spending." May 18. https://report.nih.gov/categorical_spending.aspx.

Noordenbos, Greta, with Anna Oldenhave, Jennifer Muschter, and Nynke Terpstra. 2002. "Characteristics and Treatment of Patients with Chronic Eating Disorders." *Eating Disorders: The Journal of Treatment and Prevention* 10, no. 1: 15–29.

Norcross, John C., and Clara E. Hill. 2004. "Empirically Supported Therapy Relationships." *Clinical Psychologist* 57, no. 3: 19–24. doi:10.1037/e533282009–008.

Ollove, Michael. 2012. "Parity for Behavioral Health Coverage Delayed by Lack of Federal Rules." *Stateline* (blog), November 30. www.pewtrusts.org/en/research-and-analysis/blogs/stateline/2012/11/30/parity-for-behavioral-health-coverage-delayed-by-lack-of-federal-rules.

O'Neill, Bruce. 2014. "Cast Aside: Boredom, Downward Mobility, and Homelessness in Post-Communist Bucharest." *Cultural Anthropology* 29, no. 1: 8–31. doi:10.14506/ca29.1.03.

Orange, Donna M. 2010. "Recognition As: Intersubjective Vulnerability in the Psychoanalytic Dialogue." *International Journal of Psychoanalytic Self Psychology* 5, no. 3: 227–43. doi:10.1080/15551024.2010.491719.

Orbach, Susie. 2005. *Hunger Strike: The Anorectics Struggle as a Metaphor for Our Age.* London: Karnac Books.

Orr, Jackie. 2006. *Panic Diaries: A Genealogy of Panic Disorder.* Durham, NC: Duke University Press.

Oshana, Marina. 2007. "Autonomy and the Question of Authenticity." *Social Theory and Practice* 33, no. 3: 411–29. doi:10.5840/soctheorpract200733315.

Palazzoli, Mara Selvini. 1985. "Anorexia Nervosa: A Syndrome of the Affluent Society." *Journal of Strategic and Systemic Therapies* 4, no. 3: 12–16. doi:10.1521/jsst.1985.4.3.12.

Peebles, Scott A., P. Alex Mabe, Larry Davidson, Larry Fricks, Peter F. Buckley, and Gareth Fenley. 2007. "Recovery and Systems Transformation for Schizophrenia." *Psychiatric Clinics of North America* 30, no. 3: 567–83. doi:10.1016/j.psc.2007.04.009.

Pike, Kathleen M., and Amy Borovoy. 2004. "The Rise of Eating Disorders in Japan: Issues of Culture and Limitations of the Model of 'Westernization.'" *Culture, Medicine and Psychiatry* 28, no. 4: 493–531. doi:10.1007/s11013–004–1066–6.

Prince, R., and E. F. Thebaud. 1983. "Is Anorexia Nervosa a Culture-Bound Syndrome?" *Transcultural Psychiatric Research Review* 20, no. 4: 299–302. doi:10.1177/136346158302000419.

Prochaska, James O., and Carlo C. DiClemente. 1994. *The Transtheoretical Approach: Crossing Traditional Boundaries of Therapy.* Malabar, FL: Krieger.

Puar, Jasbir K. 2011. "The Cost of Getting Better: Suicide, Sensation, Switchpoints," *GLQ: A Journal of Lesbian and Gay Studies* 18, no. 1 (Fall): 149–58.

———. 2012. "Precarity Talk: A Virtual Roundtable with Judith Butler, Lauren Berlant, Bojana Cvejić, Isabell Lorey, Jasbir Puar, and Ana Vujanović." In *Theater Drama Review* 56, no. 4 (Winter): 163–77.

———. 2017. *The Right to Maim: Debility, Capacity, Disability.* Durham, NC: Duke University Press.

Raikhel, Eugene A., and William Campbell Garriott, eds. 2013. *Addiction Trajectories.* Durham, NC: Duke University Press.

Rand, Ayn. *Atlas Shrugged.* 1957. Garden City, NY: International Collectors Library.

Rawls, John. 1972. *A Theory of Justice.* Cambridge, MA: Belknap Press of Harvard University Press.

Reed, G. M., and Elena J. Eisman. 2006. "Uses and Misuses of Evidence: Managed Care, Treatment Guidelines, and Outcomes Measurement in Professional Practice." In *Evidence-Based Psychotherapy: Where Practice and Research Meet,* edited by C. D. Goodheart, A. E. Kazdin, and R. J. Sternberg, 13–35. Washington, DC: American Psychological Association.

Resnick, Sandra G., Alan Fontana, Anthony F. Lehman, and Robert A. Rosenheck. 2005. "An Empirical Conceptualization of the Recovery Orientation." *Schizophrenia Research* 75, no. 1: 119–28. doi:10.1016/j.schres.2004.05.009.

Riva, Giuseppe, Fabrizia Mantovani, Claret Samantha Capideville, Alessandra Preziosa, Francesca Morganti, Daniela Villani, Andrea Gaggioli, Cristina Botella, and Mariano Alcañiz. 2007. "Affective Interactions Using Virtual Reality: The Link between Presence and Emotions." *CyberPsychology and Behavior* 10, no. 1: 45–56. doi:10.1089/cpb.2006.9993.

Rose, Nikolas. 2003a. "The Neurochemical Self and Its Anomalies." In *Risk and Morality,* edited by R. Ericson, 407–37, Toronto: University of Toronto Press.

——— 2003b. "Neurochemical Selves." *Society* 41, no. 1: 46–59.

———. 2005. *Governing the Soul the Shaping of the Private Self.* London: Free Association Books.

Rosen, David S. 2010. "Clinical Report—Identification and Management of Eating Disorders in Children and Adolescents." *Pediatrics* 126, no. 6: 1240–253.

Sackett, David L. 2000. *Evidence Based Medicine: How to Practice and Teach EBM.* London: Churchill Livingstone.

Sanchez-Vives, Maria V., and Mel Slater. 2005. "From Presence to Consciousness through Virtual Reality." *Nature Reviews Neuroscience* 6, no. 4: 332–39. doi:10.1038/nrn1651.

Sartre, Jean Paul, ed. 1964. *Nausea.* New York: New Directions.

Schaefer, Jenni, and Thom Rutledge. 2003. *Life without Ed: How One Woman Declared Independence from Her Eating Disorder and How You Can Too.* New York: McGraw-Hill Education.

Scheel, Judy. 2014. "Duplicity, Lies, Manipulation, and Eating Disorders: Are You Ready for Treatment?" *Psychology Today* (blog), July 25. www.psychologytoday.com/us/blog/when-food-is-family/201407/duplicity-lies-manipulation-and-eating-disorders.

Schrank, Beate, and Mike Slade. 2007. "Recovery in Psychiatry." *Psychiatric Bulletin* 31, no. 9: 321–25. doi:10.1192/pb.bp.106.031425.

Schüll, Natasha Dow. 2014. *Addiction by Design: Machine Gambling in Las Vegas.* Princeton, NJ: Princeton University Press.

Schwartz, Richard C. 1995. *Internal Family Systems Therapy.* New York: Guilford Press.

Seligman, Rebecca. 2014. *Possessing Spirits and Healing Selves: Embodiment and Transformation in an Afro-Brazilian Religion.* New York: Palgrave Macmillan.

Seremetakis, C. Nadia. 1996. *The Senses Still: Perception and Memory as Material Culture in Modernity.* Chicago: University of Chicago Press.

Sharma, Sarah. 2014. *In the Meantime: Temporality and Cultural Politics.* Durham, NC: Duke University Press.

Shohet, Merav. 2007. "Narrating Anorexia: 'Full' and 'Struggling' Genres of Recovery." *Ethos* 35, no. 3: 344–82. doi:10.1525/eth.2007.35.3.344.

———. 2018. "Beyond the Clinic? Eluding a Medical Diagnosis of Anorexia through Narrative." *Transcultural Psychiatry* 55, no. 4: 495–515. doi:10.1177/1363461517722467.

Skyttner, Lars. 2010. *General Systems Theory: An Introduction.* Hackensack, NJ: World Scientific Publishing.

Steinhausen, Hans-Christoph. 2002. "The Outcome of Anorexia Nervosa in the 20th Century." *American Journal of Psychiatry* 159, no. 8: 1284–93. doi:10.1176/appi.ajp.159.8.1284.

———. 2009. "Outcome of Eating Disorders." *Child and Adolescent Psychiatric Clinics of North America* 18, no. 1 (February): 225–42. doi:10.1016/j.chc.2008.07.013.

Stevenson, Lisa. 2014. *Life Beside Itself: Imagining Care in the Canadian Arctic.* Berkeley: University of California Press.

Stewart, Kathleen. 2007. *Ordinary Affects.* Durham, NC: Duke University Press.

———. 2012. "Precarity's Forms." *Cultural Anthropology* 27, no. 3: 518–25.

Stolorow, Robert D. 2011. *World, Affectivity, Trauma: Heidegger and Post-Cartesian Psychoanalysis.* New York: Routledge.

Stolorow, Robert D., and George E. Atwood. 2014. *Contexts of Being: The Intersubjective Foundations of Psychological Life.* Hoboken, NJ: Taylor and Francis.

Strathern, Marilyn. 2000. *Audit Cultures: Anthropological Studies in Accountability, Ethics and the Academy.* New York: Routledge.

Striegel-Moore, Ruth H., Douglas Leslie, Stephen A. Petrill, Vicki Garvin, and Robert A. Rosenheck. 2000. "One-Year Use and Cost of Inpatient and Outpatient Services among Female and Male Patients with an Eating Disorder: Evidence from a National Database of Health Insurance Claims." *International Journal of Eating Disorders* 27, no. 4: 381–89. doi.org/10.1002/(SICI)1098-108X(200005)27:43.0.CO;2-U.

Sullivan, Patrick. 1995. "Mortality in Anorexia Nervosa." *American Journal of Psychiatry* 152, no. 7 (July): 1073–74.

Swanson, Sonja A., S. Crow, Daniel LeGrange, J. Swedensen, and K. R. Merikangas. 2011. "Prevalence and Correlates of Eating Disorders in Adolescents." *Archives of General Psychiatry* 68, no. 7: 714–23. doi:10.1001/archgenpsychiatry.2011.22.

Swartz, Leslie. 1985. "Anorexia Nervosa as a Culture-Bound Syndrome." *Social Science and Medicine* 20, no. 7: 725–30.

Tanenbaum, Sandra. 2003. "Evidence-Based Practice in Mental Health: Practical Weaknesses Meet Political Strengths." *Journal of Evaluation in Clinical Practice* 9, no. 2: 287–301. doi:10.1046/j.1365-2753.2003.00409.x.

Taussig, Michael. 1991. "Tactility and Distraction." *Cultural Anthropology* 6, no. 2: 147–53. doi:10.1525/can.1991.6.2.02a00020.

Thrift, Nigel. 2004. "Intensities of Feeling: Towards a Spatial Politics of Affect." *Human Geography* 86, no. 1: 57–78. doi:10.1111/j.0435-3684.2004.00154.x.

———. 2008. *Non-Representational Theory: Space, Politics, Affect*. New York: Routledge.

Tsing, Anna Lowenhaupt. 2015. *Friction: An Ethnography of Global Connection*. Princeton, NJ: Princeton University Press.

Turner, Victor. 1967. *The Forest of Symbols: Aspects of Ndembu Ritual*. New York: H. N. Abrams in association with Albright-Knox Art Gallery.

Vandereycken, Walter. 2003. "The Place of Inpatient Care in the Treatment of Anorexia Nervosa: Questions to Be Answered." *International Journal of Eating Disorders* 34, no. 4: 409–22. doi:10.1002/eat.10223.

Van der Geest, Sjaak, and Susan Reynolds Whyte. 1989. "The Charm of Medicines: Metaphors and Metonyms." *Medical Anthropology Quarterly* 3, no. 4: 345–67. doi:10.1525/maq.1989.3.4.02a00030.

Van Gennep, Arnold. 1960. *The Rites of Passage*. Chicago: University of Chicago Press.

Vitousek, Kelly, Susan Watson, and G. Terence Wilson. 1998. "Enhancing Motivation for Change in Treatment-Resistant Eating Disorders." *Clinical Psychology Review* 18, no. 4: 391–420. doi:10.1016/s0272-7358(98)00012-9.

Wang, Philip S., Michael Lane, Mark Olfson, Harold A. Pincus, Kenneth B. Wells, and Ronald C. Kessler. 2005. "Twelve-Month Use of Mental Health Services in the United States." *Archives of General Psychiatry* 62, no. 6: 629–40. doi:10.1001/archpsyc.62.6.629.

Warin, Megan. 2003. "Miasmatic Calories and Saturating Fats: Fear of Contamination in Anorexia." *Culture, Medicine, and Psychiatry* 27, no. 1: 77–93.

———. 2009. *Abject Relations: Everyday Worlds of Anorexia*. New Brunswick, NJ: Rutgers University Press.

Warren, Cortney S., Kerri J. Schafer, Mary Ellen Crowley, and Roberto Olivardia. 2012. "A Qualitative Analysis of Job Burnout in Eating Disorder Treatment Providers." *Eating Disorders* 20, no. 3: 175–95. doi:10.1080/10640266.2012.668476.

———. 2013. "Demographic and Work-Related Correlates of Job Burnout in Professional Eating Disorder Treatment Providers." *Psychotherapy* 50, no. 4: 553–64. doi:10.1037/a0028783.

Wetherell, Margaret. 2012. *Affect and Emotion: A New Social Science Understanding*. Los Angeles: SAGE.

White, William L. 1998. *Slaying the Dragon: The History of Addiction Treatment and Recovery in America*. Bloomington, IL: Chestnut Health Systems.

Williams, Bernard. 1981. *Moral Luck: Philosophical Papers*. Cambridge: Cambridge University Press.

Williams, Raymond. 1977. *Marxism and Literature*. New York: Oxford University Press.

Wilson, Julie Ann, and Emily Chivers Yochim. 2015. "Mothering through Precarity." *Cultural Studies* 29, nos. 5–6: 669–86. doi:10.1080/09502386.2015.1017139.

Winnicott, D. W. 1953. "Transitional Objects and Transitional Phenomena." *International Journal of Psychoanalysis* 34: 89–97.

Woolgar, Steve, and Dorothy Pawluch. 1985. "Ontological Gerrymandering: The Anatomy of Social Problems Explanations." *Social Problems* 32, no. 3: 214–27. doi:10.2307/800680.

Zahavi, Dan. 2001. "Beyond Empathy: Phenomenological Approaches to Subjectivity." *Journal of Consciousness Studies* 8, nos. 5–7: 151–67.

INDEX

126–28; medical staff at, 114–16; milieu therapy of, 139–40; overview, xv, xix; programming at, 124–25; restructuring by MediCorp of, 305–6; stabilization phase at, 126–28, 184–87; staff roles at, 113–14; therapeutic program of, 134–39, 193; therapeutic staff at, 118–21; view of eating disorders, 121–23

Center of Excellence for Eating Disorders, 326–27

change model, 180–81

Charcot, Jean-Martin, 38–39

Chivers Yochim, Emily, 310

choice, 255–56

chronicity of illness, 143–46, 170, 173–74

chronographies models, 169–71

circularity, problem of, 107–8

Clarke, Adele, 147, 148

class. See economics and access to care

classification, 313

clinical research methods, xix–xxii

clinicians. See health professionals

coagulated temporality, 144

cognitive behavioral therapy (CBT), 45–46, 49, 54

Colleen, 220

colonialism, 342n3

combat soldiers, and vulnerability *vs.* invincibility, 74

compulsive exercise, 10, 122, 128, 136, 140, 225, 283

consent, 339n3

containment, 128–34. *See also* surveillance

contested illnesses and biomedical framework, 11–12

control, dynamics of, 50–52, 54, 196–99, 212, 237–38, 267–69

cost of treatment, 90. *See also* health insurance

countertransference, xx, 281–83, 384

"cruel optimism," 315, 318–20

Csikszentmihalyi, Mihaly, 223

culture-bound syndrome, eating disorders as, 63–65, 343n4, 344n7

cutting, 97, 155, 157, 219, 245, 260, 263, 296

dance, 121, 124, 139, 245, 352n1

Danielle, 280

Dannilyn, 90

Darcy, 136, 270

data collection in clinic, 126–28

debility, 312, 318

Debord, Guy, 144

demographics of eating disorders, xxviii, 324

denial, 207

depletion, 55–58

depression, 16, 17, 269; treatment for, 17; link with eating, 45

deprivation, 277–78, 299–301

Descartes, René, 32

desire and want, 314–15

(de)stabilization, 126–28, 184–87

determination of care process, 92–99

diagnosis process, 92–99

Diagnostic and Statistical Manual of Mental Disorders (DSM), 5–6, 8, 12, 92–93, 151, 340n2

dialectical behavior therapy, 262, 308, 347n17, 348n6

dialogical self theory, 231–32

Dickinson, Emily, 36

DiClemente, Carlo C., 181

dieticians, 117

Dimaggio, Giancarlo, 231

direct care staff, 118–19, 348n3

discharge plans, 148, 208, 290–91

distress tolerance, 128–34, 190, 272

Douglas, Mary, 83, 178–79

Dumit, Joe, 11, 12

"Duplicity, Lies, Manipulation and Eating Disorders" *(Psychology Today),* 33

dysregulation and hyper-regulation, 50–55, 248–50. *See also* regulation of the body

eating disorder not otherwise specified (EDNOS), 7

eating disorders, summary of conditions, xxvi–xxvii, 5–10, 323–26, 340n2. *See also* research; treatment; *specific condition names*

Eating Disorders Coalition, 324, 341n43

economics and access to care, 15–16, 103, 106, 324–25, 325–26. *See also* health insurance

psychological analyses *(continued)*
39–40, 41; infantilism, 40–41; Internal Family Systems Therapy (IFS), 216–19, 222–26, 232–37, 308, 348n6, 352n7, 352n17; interpersonal model, 48; phenomenological model, 48; psychodynamic approaches, 41–42; psychosomatic family theory, 42–44. *See also* research
Psychosomatic Families (Minuchin et al.), 42–43
Puar, Jasbir, 312, 318
public awareness and education on eating disorders, 323–24, 326, 329
"puckers," 160–61

race and ethnicity, xxviii, 57, 116, 324–25
randomized controlled trials (RCTs), 105–6
recognition, 22–24, 57
recovery: ambivalence to, 250–52; caregiver connections for, 269–71; choice and, 255–56; discharge plans, 148, 208, 290–91; ideal treatment scenarios for, 271–72; lapses and relapses, 257–60; "outside" motivations for, 254–57; psychic life of biopolitics, xxiii; recovery model of mental illness, 152–54, 162, 165, 166 table, 212; reintegration phase, 178; will and, 37, 154, 170–74, 350n44. *See also* treatment
Reed, Geoffrey, 105, 106
refeeding, 58–59, 168, 270, 350n42
regimes of anticipation, 147–50
regulation of the body, 50–55, 248–50
Rehab (TV show), 32
reintegration, as phase in transformation, 178
relapse, 123, 154, 173, 240, 257–60
relatedness, 34–35, 343n7. *See also* interpersonal relationships
relational practice, 293–94
release and flow, dynamics of, 134–39
religion, 31, 34, 36–37, 66, 342n3
Renaissance period, 37
research: evidence-based practice (EBP), 105–8, 314; funding on eating disorders, 311; future recommendations for,

324–25; methods used in this book, xix–xxii, xxvii, 339n3; psychological studies and theories, 37–50
resentment, 237
residential program, 13–14; intake assessment and, 90. *See also* Cedar Grove eating disorders clinic
resistance, 58–61, 250
responsibility–agency entanglement, 201–5
rites of passage, 178
Riva, Giuseppe, 67
Rose, Nicolas, 267
Rosman, Bernice L., 42–43
rumination disorder, 340n2

Sackett, David, 105
Scheel, Judy, 33
schizophrenia, 7, 16, 18; research on, 19, 311; treatment for, 17, 144, 153, 171
Schüll, Natasha Dow, 266–68
Schwartz, Richard, 217–18, 223–24, 233
sculpting, 226–29
Seal, Annie, 327–28
second-order desires, 219–22
selective eating disorder, 340n2
self-harm. *See* cutting; starvation
self-realization, 56–58
self-starvation, acute. *See* anorexia nervosa
self-surveillance, 191. *See also* surveillance
self-system, development of, 233–35
Self *vs.* a self, 222–30, 352n17
sensorimotor psychotherapy, 307, 308
separation, as phase in transformation, 178, 179, 196
separation anxiety, 183
sexual conflicts, 31, 38–42, 130, 295, 345n32
sexual identity, xxviii, 32, 66, 68, 348n3
shame: for accepting treatment, 298–301, 301; for existing or needing care, xxiii, xxv, 75, 134, 192, 251–52, 298–99, 200; for having a body, 244, 331; for having an eating disorder, 7, 18, 95, 252, 259; in IFS model, 218–19. *See also* erasure
Sharma, Sarah, 147
Sheila, 201–3; attending Allison's funeral, xvi–xvii; on fragility of her body, 59;

treatment and recovery of, xxv–xxvi, 150, 154–61

Shelly, 19–20, 138, 243, 245, 246

Shohet, Merav, 343n5

slow death, as concept, 318–20

Smith-Morris, Carolyn, 146

social justice and eating disorder treatment, 323

soma-psyche entanglement, 38–40, 48–50

speaking *vs.* silent experience, 25. *See also* agency; erasure

spirit. *See* will and recovery

stabilization, 125–28, 184–87, 193–94, 257, 350n1, 350n1 (ch. 7)

standardized treatment manuals, 106

starvation, 6, 36–37, 38, 40–41, 342n3. *See also* anorexia nervosa

Stevenson, Lisa, xxiii

Stewart, Kathleen, 309–10

stigma, xxvii, 33, 47, 152, 307, 322, 323–24

Substance Abuse and Mental Health Service Administration, 326

suffering, 11–12

suicidality, 13, 18, 161, 201, 260, 274, 299

supplements, nutritional, 4, 58, 131, 293, 295, 299, 300

surveillance, 126, 134, 191–92. *See also* containment

Susan, 93–94, 114, 194, 203–4, 316

Suzanna, 260–66

Tanenbaum, Sandra J., 105

Taussig, Michael, 74

technologies of presence, 65–69

technology, as term, 66

telemedicine, 325

Teresa of Ávila, 36

therapeutic program of Cedar Grove, 134–39, 193. *See also* treatment

therapists. *See* health professionals

therapreneurism, 308–9, 354n8

Theresa, 131, 269

Thin (film), 32

third-order desires, 222–24

360 Program, 329

Thrift, Nigel, 70

"Timeline" exercise, 136–37

To the Bone (film), 32

Transactional Analysis for Kids (Freed), 334

transference dynamics. *See* countertransference

treatment: ambivalence toward, 250–52, 293; as anticipatory project, 146–50; art therapy, 121, 134, 187, 307; behavioral program of Cedar Grove, 128–34, 193; chronicity of illness and, 143–46, 170, 173–74; chronography models, 169–71; clients on ideal, 271–72, 326; containment in, 128–34; cruel optimism of, 315–16; cultivating the idealized subject, 140–41, 248–49, 251–52, 287–88; dance, 121, 124, 139, 245, 352n1; diagnosis and determination of, 93–99; dialectical behavior therapy, 262, 308, 347n17, 348n6; distress tolerance, 128–34, 190, 272; economic considerations and access to, 15–16, 103, 106, 324–25, 325–26; evidence-based practice, 105–8, 314, 325, 347n17; future recommendations for, 325–26, 334–35; group therapy, 134–35, 226–301; health insurance and, xix, 15–18, 20–21, 90, 312–20; IFS model, 216–19, 222–26, 232–37, 308, 348n6, 352n7, 352n17; intake process for, 90–92; as investment opportunity, 305–6; liminality in, 178–80; managed care and healthcare industry of, 13–20; medical model, 150–52, 154, 165, 166 table, 212; medical necessity for, 99–100, 103; medical program of Cedar Grove, 126–28, 193; medications, 16, 114, 115, 259, 260, 268, 293–301; milieu therapy, 139–40; mindfulness practices, 121, 134, 190, 272, 348n6; recovery model, 152–54, 162, 165, 166 table, 212; refeeding, 58–59, 168, 270, 350n42; sculpting, 226–29; stabilization, 125–28, 184–87, 193–94, 257, 350n1 (chap. 7); summary of inadequacies of, xvii–xviii, xxiii, xxvi–xxvii; therapeutic homework in, 135–38; therapeutic program of Cedar Grove, 134–39, 193; unblending, 229–30; using Ed as personification of eating disorder, 183, 224–34, 236–38,

Founded in 1893,
UNIVERSITY OF CALIFORNIA PRESS
publishes bold, progressive books and journals
on topics in the arts, humanities, social sciences,
and natural sciences—with a focus on social
justice issues—that inspire thought and action
among readers worldwide.

The UC PRESS FOUNDATION
raises funds to uphold the press's vital role
as an independent, nonprofit publisher, and
receives philanthropic support from a wide
range of individuals and institutions—and from
committed readers like you. To learn more, visit
ucpress.edu/supportus.